Ayurvedic Curative Cuisines for Everyone
DR. LIGHT MILLER

MOONLIGHT BOOKS

Ayurvedic Curative Cuisine for Everyone

FIRST INDIAN EDITION: **2017**
ISBN : 978-81-932643-2-4

Published by
MOONLIGHT BOOKS
20 Ekjot Apartment, Pitampura, New Delhi-110034, India
Email : moonlightbooks2016@gmail.com
Website : www.moonlightbooks.in

Copyright © 2011 Dr. Light Miller
Published by
Lotus Press, P.O. Box 325, Twin Lakes, WI 53181 USA
Web: www.lotuspress.com Email: lotuspress@lotuspress.com

For Sale in Asia

ALL RIGHTS RESERVED. No part of this book may be reproduced in any form or by any electronic or mechanical means including information storage and retrieval systems without permission in writing from the publisher, except by a reviewer who may quote brief passages in a review.

This book is not intended to treat, diagnose or prescribe. The information contained herein is in no way to be considered as a substitute for a consultation with a duly licensed health care professional.

Library of Congress Cataloging-in-Publication Data
Name: Dr. Light Miller author
Title: Ayurvedic Curative Cuisine for Everyone
Description: First edition
Subjects: Ayurveda | Food |
Classification:2010926699 (print)

Printed by Replika Press Pvt. Ltd., India

Table of Contents

Dedication 4
Author Introduction 5
Introduction to Ayurvedic 7
Questionnaire 17
Introduction to Foods 20
Fruits 28
Vegetables 118
Seaweeds 228
Beans 248
Grains 283
Poultry 312
Meat 317
Fish 329
Condiments 336
Herbs & Spices 351
Nuts & Seeds 401
Dairy Products 426
Sweeteners 450
Oils 461
Immunity 470
Resource List 474
About the Authors 476
Raw Food Recipes 478
Measurement Chart 478
Index 479

Dedication

This book honors all teachers of ayurveda, I also send heartfelt acknowledgements To my son Bodhie, who has taught me a tremendous amount about cooking, food storage, and preparation.

To my younger son Cedar, who has loved broccoli since he was 2 years old and still loves his mama's cooking.

To my grandchildren – Noah, who eats all my mangos and apples, and Nina, who always wants blueberries and cookies yet eats whatever grandma gives her.

To Allan and Jess Miller, for letting me test the recipes on them.

To Rene Gates, a great chef herself, for her input and ideas, and for coming up with the book's title.

To Emma Bustamante, who is always ready to support me in whatever I do.

To Elizabeth Catenacci, for keeping track of my recipes for 15 years.

To Linda Ranweiler, who took the project on not knowing what she was getting into, beginning on her last day of Pancha Karma and working over 100 hours on editing. There are no words I can use to express my gratitude – without her help (and her gift as a writer) this project still might not be finished.

To Oleana Greek, for all the photographs, and the special touches of her assistant, Irena Grissom.

To my Pancha Karma clients who asked for this cookbook to be written, and to all my students who have helped in the kitchen.

To my earthly spiritual father Yahova, who was my first teacher on nutrition.

To my friend Brigitte Mars, who is my inspiration for writing.

To my god-daughter Rainbeau Mars, who always inspires me to keep a raw food awareness.

And to Kathy Biehl for proof-reading and helping with the completion of the book.

My gratitude to Mindy Reser at Villa Ananda who provided beautiful space for me to write parts of this book.

Cover Photo: To Christian Saretzki for his gifted photographic skill in creating this beautiful book cover.

Introduction

Writing and teaching about health and well-being is one of my greatest passions. I am convinced that dietary changes – particularly eating more fruits and vegetables – is one of the ways for one to regain one's health. In my many years of practice, I discovered that making small changes in people's diets can prevent many diseases, and promote health and vitality.

We have all heard the statement "one man's food is another man's poison." This does not mean that food is poison, what it means is that one can choose the energy that is most beneficial.

Ayurveda teaches that eating for your body type promotes longevity and wellbeing. Each person's nutritional needs are unique. In evaluating nutritional needs, the Ayurvedic practitioner recognizes and identifies the immune system as a fragment of the Divine Mother. This gift from her sustains us, nourishes us, and protects us from outside invasions. As long as the immune system is strong, we suffer no disease. By choosing the appropriate foods we enhance our immunity.

Cooking is one of my greatest joys in life. I am happiest when feeding lots of people healthy foods. In this book, I share many wonderful moments of serving good food to my loved ones. I just go to the refrigerator and create from whatever I have available at the time. Trust your instincts when preparing food for the people you love. Let your intuition be your guide in the kitchen.

It is evident that our nation is having a health crisis – all we have to do is look at the children's school lunches and the diseases of today: diabetes, high blood pressure and many auto-immune diseases. The proliferation of fast food places and packaged food continues. My friend Tom Pfeiffer always says we vote with our dollars – whatever we buy, we will have more of. So buy in bulk, and support organic growers. When we buy packaged vs. bulk food, the price doubles – compare the prices in your own stores. A great number of health experts today are encouraging people to eat fresh food and follow a cleaner diet. According to the L.A. Times, 40–50% of Americans eat most of their meals out or buy deli food or food that has been refrigerated for a long time. Freshly prepared food – prepared by your own hand – is always preferable. You never know how long it has been since commercially prepared food was made, or how long it sat in a truck waiting to be delivered. Ayurveda teaches that freshly made foods are more easily digested, particularly when well-spiced.

My son, an award-winning chef who has worked at many 5-star restaurants, is horrified by the way food is stored in most restaurants – meat often stored on top of vegetables, for instance. In many restaurant kitchens the employees are rushed for time, people are cursing, the kitchens are crowded, the pressure to produce is high, and the morale is low. The quality of food that goes into the prepared dishes is often poor. There is no time to send blessings to the food, or to put love into its preparation. The restaurant industry has one of the highest

Ayurvedic Curative Cuisine for Everyone

rates of alcoholism and drug addiction in our country. As customers, we only get to see what goes on outside the kitchen. My preference is always to eat at home. Even when I travel, I take my crock-pot, a skillet, my hand grinder, and my vata, pitta, and kapha churnas (spices for each body type). I do not want to generalize about the restaurant business; every city has conscious and good places at which to eat – you just have to find them and ask questions.

When you learn how easy is to make your own food, it becomes joyful to prepare your lunches for work. I share with you simple, quick, well-spiced recipes, some history or story about the food, therapeutic healing properties of each food, which foods work best for each body type, and taste the energy of each food, which is very important in Ayurveda. This book encourages you to try new foods and spices, and to eat more vegetables. There are recipes for everyone's dietary needs. To fit healthy cooking into our busy life styles, most of the recipes can be made in less than an hour – some in as little as 10 or 15 minutes.

Mother Divine has given us many herbs and foods for healing ourselves. It is fun to explore the many choices of foods available to us. The more variety in your diet, the better nourished you are. Health experts have found that eating the same foods over and over can create food allergies. Rotating your diet is very important, particularly with grains and dairy, foods that are the most common allergens.

This book encourages you to try new foods and spices and eat more fruits and vegetables. Cooking can be a fun family activity; get the children involved in chopping, cutting, and peeling. Some of the finest memories I have include preparing food with my children. Today my son continues the family legacy with his own children. Encourage kids to eat vegetables by disguising them in sauces and nut dressings. Make cooking fun and exciting. When preparing food, give thanks and bless all those who participated in getting it to us – the farmer, the truck driver, the people at the grocery store.

Thanks be to Mother Divine for the cornucopia of foods… OM SHANTI.
NAMASTE
LIGHT (jyoti)

Ayurveda

"The Science of Life"

Ayurveda is the world's oldest recorded healing system. Used for 5,000 years by many thousands of doctors on millions of patients, it is a proven system of prevention and healing. Ayurveda is the current rage in alternative medicine, with people paying to hear lectures by best selling author Dr. Deepak Chopra, MD, and spending large sums for consultations and treatments at "swank" Ayurvedic clinics around the country. Fortunely Ayurveda has several levels of treatment. At its most basic level, patients are able to treat themselves with simple diet and lifestyle changes, assisted by under standing of the metabolic type and any inherent strengths and weaknesses.

History

Ayurveda was discovered and developed by ancient Indian holy men known as "Rishi." Due to their relationship (connectedness) to both the spiritual and physical worlds, they were able to discern a basic nature of the universe, and man's place in it. They developed an oral tradition of knowledge that was fluid and allowed for growth. Ayurveda was built upon as new therapies and herbs were discovered, and trade brought on new information from other cultures.

These practitioners were scientists who made huge advances in the fields of surgery, herbal medicine, the medicinal effects of minerals and metals, exercise, physiology, human anatomy and psychology. Over a very long period of time, this information was recorded; as written language developed, the first came Rig Veda(4500 years old) followed by the Atharva Veda (3200 years old) and others.

As Ayurveda spread into other civilizations, its versatile adaptability was recognized and it was often integrated into local forms of medicine. Ayurveda had a profound effect on the medicine of Tibet, China, Persia, Egypt, Greece, Rome and Indonesia. Ayurvedic medicine was suppressed in India during British Colony rule. In 1833, the East India Company closed and banned all Ayurvedic colleges. For almost 100 years Ayurveda was known as "the poor man's medicine," practiced only in rural areas where "western medicine" was too expensive or unavailable."

With the independence of India, Ayurveda has reemerged to gain equal footing with western medicine. Currently 70% of India's population is treated ayurvedically. In 1978, at a conference on "Third World Medicine" sponsored by the World Health Organization (WHO) of the United Nations, it was concluded that Ayurveda would be the best system for undeveloped countries. Its low cost, use of herbs and remedies, adaptability to any climate, and reduced dependence on pharmaceutical products were in favorable aspects for the world's population. There is hope that a global medicine will base created with

Ayurveda as its base, and western, Chinese and traditional native medicines appropriately-blended in each locale.

Philosophy

Ayurvedic theory states that health initially results from harmony within one's self. To be healthy, harmony must exist between your purpose for being, your thoughts, your feelings and your physical actions. If your purpose is peaceful, yet your thoughts are selfish and your emotions negative, your physical body will manifest some disease symptom as a "wake up call to change." In Ayurveda the manifestation of disease is actually considered to be a good sign, because it reveals a previously hidden aspect of oneself- an aspect to be healed. This inner harmony also becomes manifest as harmony with family, friends, co-workers, society and nature.

Often the first questions an Ayurvedic physician may ask are: " What is your purpose in life? And what is the appropriate form (work, job, activity, etc.)? How are your relationships?" When harmony exists in these areas, physical healing is so much easier. The ultimate goal of Ayurvedic medicine is uninterrupted physical, mental and spiritual happiness. According to Ayurvedic philosophy, enjoyment is one of life's purposes. However, we can lose our ability to enjoy if we overindulge, and disease is one of nature's ways of saying we've overindulged. This idea is supported by a fact that we all intuitively know: either you limit yourself, or Mother Nature will limit you. Indulgence is part of enjoyment, but in Ayurvedic philosophy, indulgence is only one of the four legitimate life goals. These include:

The fulfillment of your duties to society.

The accumulation of possessions while fulfilling duties.

Satisfying legitimate desires with the assistance of one's possessions.

The realization that there is more to life than duties, possessions and desires.

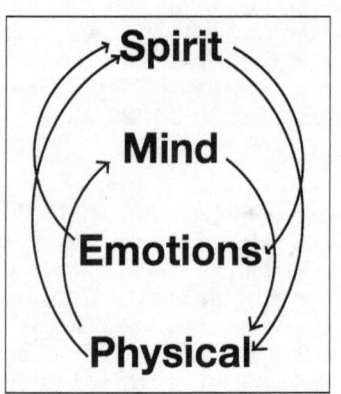

```
   Spirit
     ↕
    Mind
     ↕
  Emotions
     ↕
  Physical
```

Ayurvedic philosophy states that only a person with strong immune system can be healthy. The practitioners identify the immune system as a fragment of nature (the Divine Mother). This gift from her creates us, sustains us, nourishes us, and protects us from outside invasion. As long as our immunity is strong, we suffer no disease. "The ancient "vedic" word for immunity means forgiveness of disease," which comes from the concept that negative thoughts and lifestyles cause disease. Disease, therefore, is a message about a need for change-if only we can understand this. In this sense, strength comes from transforming our projections about our symptoms. Healing comes from seeing adversity as a challenge, by taking back our negative thoughts about people and events. We can transform disease into a "perfect opportunity." Spiritual health, then, is a dynamic balance between a strongly integrated individual personality and nature (a nature that's understood to encompass all aspects of existence.) This is only possible when people remember their debt to nature.

In summary: Ayurvedic philosophy states that health results from the relationship (the connectedness) between self, personality, and all the rest that goes into our mental, emotional, psychic and spiritual being, It believes that health also results from good relations with others; from an acknowledged indebtedness to mother nature; from the realization of ones' purpose; and from the pursuit of legitimate goals in life. Ayurvedic philosophy maintains the importance of a strong immune system, that immortality is possible, and that forgiveness is strengthening.

While it is true that food, herbs, oils, and lifestyles are important healing modalities to be embraced, we should acknowledge that our thoughts and feelings regarding our level of connectedness to all things, may be the most important factor in our wellbeing.

The act of forgiveness is profoundly healing. Ancestral healing releases constraining thoughts and feelings that we hold about ourselves and our relationships and frees us from negative behaviors. A place of peace is established within our being and we are empowered to become active co-creators of our life.

We in the West often consider the Eastern belief of ancestor worship/healing to be very primitive. However, it has long been a practice in the Catholic Church on All Soul's Day, for family members to go to cemeteries and sit by the graves of ancestors, bring them plates of food, and have conversations with them. This is also a practice within the Hawaiian community and certain Native American tribes.

The Five Element Theory

According to the Five Element Theory, the human being is a small model of the universe. What happens in the human body exists in altered form in the universal body. Ayurveda believes that everything is made up of 5 elements, or

Ayurvedic Curative Cuisine for Everyone

building blocks; earth, water, fire, air and ether. Their properties are important in understanding balances and imbalances in the human body.

Earth-representative of the solid state of matter (material), it manifests stability, fixity, and rigidity. We see around us rocks and soil standing against the wearing forces of water and wind. Our body also manifests this earth/solid-state structure: bones, cells, and tissue are physical structures through which our blood courses and oxygen is transported. Earth is considered a stable substance.

Water- liquid matter (material) characterized by change. In the outer world we see water moving through its cycles of evaporation/clouds/condensation/rain, we see it moving around solid matter such as rocks and mountains, we see it eventually wearing away solid, immovable matter as it flows from the mountain to the sea. We see rivers carrying dissolved soil and nutrients, carrying economic trade and exchange of information and culture-we see the earth's bodies of water nurture life everywhere. Our blood, lymph and other fluids move between our cells and through vessels, bringing energy, carrying away wastes, regulating temperature, bringing disease fighters and carrying hormonal information from one area to another. Water is considered a substance without stability.

Fire- the power (immaterial) to transform solids to liquids, to gas, and back again. The heat of the sun melts ice into water that becomes vapor under its influence. Fire runs the cycles of water, and it runs the cycle of weather. The sun's energy is the initiator of all energy cycles on earth- including all food chains and food webs. Within bodies it's fire-energy that binds the atoms of our molecules together; that converts food to fat (stored energy) and muscle; that turns (burns) food into work; and that creates the impulses of nervous reactions, of our feelings and even our thought processes. Fire is considered form without substance.

Air- the gaseous form of matter (material), which is mobile and dynamic. We do not see the air that blows through the tree leaves, but we do feel it. We know how material it can be- how it can respond to energy, absorb, it, and give it off-when we experience or watch a hurricane, typhoon or storm. We feel air as it courses down our throats and into our lungs. Cut that feeling off for more than a few minutes and we know with our whole being how fundamental air is to life. Within the body, air (oxygen) is the basis for all energy transfer reactions – oxidation. Clean and pure, it is a key element required for fire to burn. Air is existence without form.

```
Ether   Air   Fire   Water   Earth
    \  /       \   /     \   /
    Vata       Pitta    Kapha
```

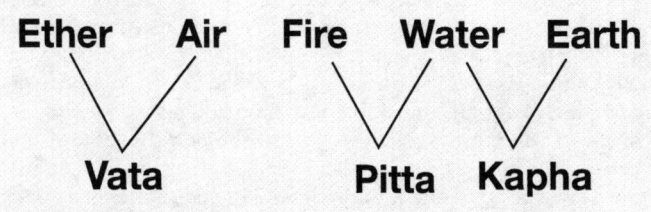

Ether- the space in which everything happens. Like outer space with millions of miles between celestial bodies, or the inner space of our bodies where our very atoms are only .00001 particles and .99999 emptiness. Space, the distance between things that which helps to define one thing from another. It may be as thin or thick as an idea, and how do we measure an idea? Subatomic concepts are posed in dimensional terminology that cannot be measured, but only thought about in relative terms. Cosmic concepts are posed in terms of infinity. One smaller than thought, the other bigger than thought. Ether is only the distance which separate matter thinner than a thought and bigger than a thought.

The Three Doshas

In Ayurvedic philosophy, the five elements combine in pairs, to form three dynamic forces (interactions) called Doshas. Dosha means, "that which changes," because they are constantly moving in dynamic balance, one with the others. Doshas are primary life forces or biological humors. They are only found in life forms (similar to the concepts of organic chemistry) and their dynamism is what makes life happen.

The five elements are Ether, Air, Fire Water and Earth. These five elements combine to create the following three Doshas – or forces: Vata, Pitta and Kapha.

Vata (va-ta) is a force conceptually made up of the elements ether and air. The proportions of ether and air determine how active Vita is. When the movement of air is unrestricted by space (as in the open ocean), it can gain momentum to become hurricane winds moving over 150 mph. When air is restrained in a box, it cannot move and becomes stale. So you can see how the amount of ether (space) affects the ability of air to gain momentum as expressed in Vata.

In the body, Vata is ***movement*** (a dynamism of the combination between ether and air), and manifests itself in living things as the movement of nerve impulses, air, blood, food, waste, and thoughts. The characteristics of Vata are: cold, light, irregular, mobile, rarefield and rough. These qualities characterize their effect on the body. Too much Vata force can cause nerve irritation high blood pressure, gas and confusion. Too little Vata can mean nerve loss, congestion, constipation and thoughtlessness.

Pitta (pit-ta) is a force conceptually created by the dynamic interplay of water and fire. These two seemingly opposed forces represent transformation. They cannot change into each other, but they modulate each other but they modulate each other and are vitally necessary to each other in the life processes. When you boil water on a fire, if the fire is too hot, all the water boils away, the pot burns. If you put too much water into the pot, it overflows and puts out the fire. In our bodies, Pitta is manifested by the quality of transformation. It is the enzymes that digest our food and the hormones, which regulate our metabolism. In our mind the Pitta force is the transformation of chemical/electrical impulses into understood thoughts.

Too much Pitta can cause ulcers, hormonal imbalance, irritated skin (acne) and consuming emotions (anger). Too little Pitta can result in indigestion, inability to understand and sluggish metabolism. The Pitta force is described according to 8 characteristics: hot, light, fluid, subtle, sharp, malodorous, soft, and clear, each of which affect the body.

Kapha (Ka-fa) is the conceptual equilibrium of water and earth. When a handful of sand is thrown into a container of water, the two will separate as the sand settles to the bottom. Only by continuous stirring will the mixture remain in balance. The force of Kapha is like stirring- it maintains balance. Kapha is structure and lubrication; it draws on the conceptual characteristics of the elements of earth and water. At one level, it's the cells, which make up our organs and the fluids, which nourish and protect them.

In the Ayurvedic organization of cause and effect, too much Kapha- force causes mucous buildup in the sinus, nasal and lung. In the colon it also causes excess mucous buildup. In the mind it creates rigidity, a fixation of thought and inflexibility. Not enough Kapha force causes the body to experience a dry respiratory track, burning stomach (due to lack of mucous, which gives protection from excess stomach acids), and inability to concentrate. Kapha force is expressed according to the following qualities: oily. Cold, heavy, stable, dense and smooth.

The Changing Forces

These three dynamic forces are constantly changing and balancing each other in all living things. They make life happen. In plant Vata is concentrated in the flowers (which reach farthest out in space and air), Kapha is concentrated in the roots (where water is stored in the embrace of earth,) and Pitta is found in the plants essential oils, resins and sap (especially in spices which stimulate digestion). Different plants have different concentrations of V-P-K. Eating root vegetables, milk products, or sedating herbs like valerian increases our Kapha. Drinking herbal flowers like lavender, or eating dry grains increases our Vata forces. Eating hot, spicy foods like cayenne or concentrated protein like bee pollen increases our Pitta tendencies.

Climactic Influences

The climates we live in and the change of seasons also add or subtract from our V-P-K balance. Hot summers or hot climates increase our pitta. Dry climates or cold autumn winds increase Vata. Wet winters or damp climates add to Kapha.

Life Stages

The stage of life we are in also affects V-P-K balance. The increase in the substance of the body, which occurs during childhood growth, means that Kapha forces are dominant during this cycle of life. The hormone changes that transform us into adults indicate that our early and middle years are under Pitta influences. As we age we can shrink and dry out, indicating an increase in Vata forces.

Individual Balance

Each of us is born with a unique balance of V-PK that makes us who we are and determines our strengths and weaknesses. No two people are the same, but there are said to be three pure types and seven mixed types this typing is used for evaluation and treatment. Compare this Ayurvedic view of the individual patient to our medical system were everyone is treated the same. For example, a person born with a particular proportion of V-P-K would be said to be a Pitta dominant individual. Due to climate, season, life stage, diet or lifestyle changes over time they may get out of balance. If they gained 30 pounds their V-P-K would change. There would be an unnatural balance of V-P-K and their health would suffer (and they wouldn't feel "themselves") until they return to the V-P-K combination they were born with. Ayurveda can help individuals discover their *original* balance.

Vata Dominant Type

An individual with primarily Vata influences will exhibit many of the following characteristics: They will have a thin-framed body whether they are tall or short. There joints crack easily and irregularity is the rule, including possible protruding joints, bow legs, disproportionate bodies with long legs, short waist, scoliosis uneven facial structure, deviated septum and crooked nose etc. If they do gain weight it will be around the middle. Their skin will have a tendency to be dry, rough and cool to the touch. Their skin will be darker than the rest of their family. Their hair may be dark, dry and kinky. Teeth often crooked, protruded with spaces and tendency toward receded gums. Their eyes can be small, dry, active, brown or black. Appetite is often variable or low, although often they will skip meals due to distractions and become ravenous, loading up their plate with more than they could possibly eat. Their fingers and toes are long and thin with nails which are brittle and crack easily. If they become sick, pain and nervousness disorders are likely. Their thirst is variable and their bowel movements are gassy, dry, hard and constipated. They are physically active, but expend their energy easily and may rely on caffeine, sugar and stimulants

Ayurvedic Curative Cuisine for Everyone

to continue, their mind is restless, curious, active and creative. Under stress they can become fearful, insecure and anxious. They change their mind easily, have a good short-term memory but often forget easily. They often dream about running, flying, jumping and fear. Their sleep is difficult interrupted and they can experience insomnia. Their speech is fast, chaotic and impulsive, and they often talk with their hands. Money goes through their hands quickly as they spend impulsively. Their pulse thready, feeble and erratic. Vata predominant types will vary greatly from one to another, but will share many of the above characteristics.

Pitta Dominant

An individual who is primarily Pitta will have a moderate frame that demonstrates good proportions. They can gain or lose weight relatively easy. Their skin is often delicate, oily, burns easily, has a coppery or yellowish tone, and is warm to touch. Freckles and moles are common with a tendency to acne. They perspire readily. Their hair is soft, blonde or red, grays early with a tendency to early thinning or balding, Fingers are well formed and proportionate. Fingernail beds have a pink appearance. Eyes are sharp, penetrating gray, green, with a yellowish tint to the sclera(white). If they become ill they will experience fever, inflammation and infection. They are often thirsty. Their bowel movements are soft, oily and loose, 3 times a day or more. They enjoy moderate activity and love competition due to their aggressive nature; they are intelligent and determined with a sharp memory. Under stress they can be irritable, driving, angry and jealous. Dreams are fiery, passionate and colorful. Their sleep is moderate and sound. Speech is sharp, clear, fluid and can be cutting and sarcastic. Pittas spend moderately and methodically. Their pulse is strong and regular. You can often tell a Pitta by their passion, high-directed energy and their commitment.

Kapha Dominant

The pure Kapha is easy to recognize- large bodies on large frames. The Hawaiians are Kapha people. Their skin is thick, oily, cool to touch pale and white. Sweat is moderate. They gain weight easily and must exercise to lose it. Their hair is thick, oily, and wavy with thick eyebrows and lashes. Teeth are strong, white large and well formed. Eyes are big and attractive. Appetite is slow and steady, although they can easily skip meals without effect. If Kaphas become ill, congestion, excess mucous and water retention are common. They rarely experience thirst. Bowel movements are thick oily and regular. Peaceful and content, they move slowly and waste no energy. Endurance is good. Negative emotions may be self-centeredness, greed, over sensitivity. They are steady and loyal friends and employees. Slow to learn new things they seldom forget anything. Dreams are often romantic involving water. Their speech is slow and monotonous or melodious; they spend slowly, save easily and always have full cupboards. Their pulse is slow and steady.

Spirit Of All That Is

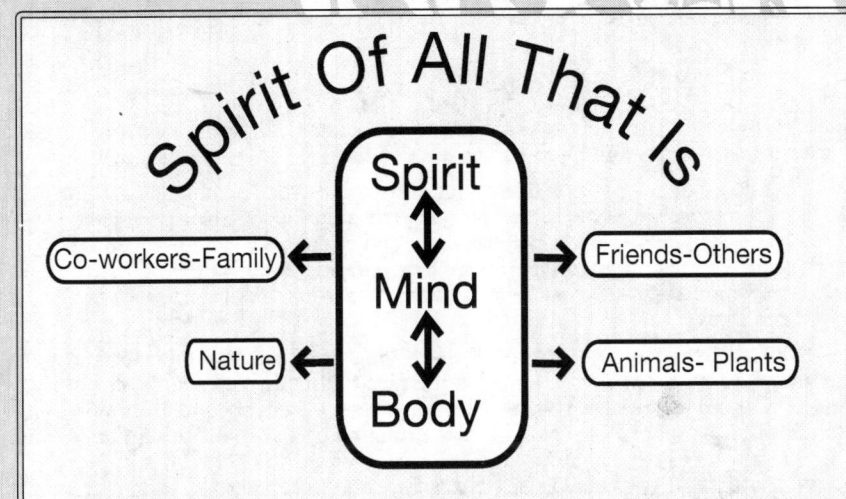

```
        Spirit
          ↕
Co-workers-Family ←→ Mind →→ Friends-Others
          ↕
Nature ←              →  Animals- Plants
          Body
```

Mixed Types

(V-P, V-K, P-V, K-V, P-K, K-P and V-P-K) In India where people largely marry into their own tribe or group, single Dosha types are predominating. In the west, we are a mixing pot; for the most part everyone is able to marry as they wish, and so mixed types predominate. Usually in a mixed type the Dosha will be dominant, with a second Dosha being very prominent. For example a Vata Pitta person will have more and stronger Vata tendencies than Pitta. A Pitta-Vata person will be similar to a Vata-Pitta person, but will have more Pitta qualities. And finally there is a type called balanced tri dosha where no one type is predominate.

Vata-Pittas are thin like a pure Vata type quick moving, friendly, talkative, but more enterprising and sharper of intellect. They don't have the extremes of Vata, and are not as high-strung or irregular. They have a stronger digestion and greater tolerance to cold. They are more tolerant of noise and physical discomforts. They have the strong drive of a Pitta with the imagination of a Vata type. They can easily fall into patterns of addictions and they need stability.

Pitta-Vatas are more of medium build with more musculature than V-P's. They're also quick in movement, good stamina, often assertive, with obvious intensity, but with Vata- type's lightness. They have strong digestion and more regular elimination than V-P or V. If they are under stress, they can react with fear or anger, which can make them insecure, tense, and hard driven. They love to eat, have a good memory and are fluid speakers.

Vata-Kaphas are often hard types to identify with a questionnaire due to the presence of opposites in many characteristics, and Vata's indecisiveness. They often have a thin Vata frame with a Kapha like relaxed, easygoing manner. They will be even tempered unless stressed. Often quick and efficient they are aware of their Kapha tendency to procrastinate. They desire to store up and save, and strongly dislike the cold. They can have slow or its irregular

Ayurvedic Curative Cuisine for Everyone

digestion.

Kapha Vatas are similar to a V-K but are more solidly built and slower moving. They are even tempered and even more relaxed than V-K's, but with less enthusiasm. They tend to be athletic, with greater stamina. They may also have digestive irregularities and complain of cold.

Pitta-Kaphas are types with Pitta intensity in a strong Kapha body. They are more muscular than a K-type and may be quite bulky. Their personality exhibits a K- type stability with Pitta force and a tendency toward anger and criticism. They are a good type for athletics, having energy and endurance. They never miss a meal. They have Pitta type digestion and Kapha type resistance to disease.

Kapha-Pittas are people who have a Kapha type structure but more fat than a P-K type. They are rounder in the face and body, move more slowly, and are more relaxed than P-K's. They have a steady energy and even more endurance than P or P-K type. They like exercise but are less motivated to do it than a P-K.

Vata-Pitta Kaphas are the hardest to describe, because they have equal amounts of each Dosha. They are the most balanced with a tendency to long life, good health and immunity. Ayurvedic physicians say that these types are the most difficult to treat when they do get out of balance. There are very few true V-P-K types. Many people who think they are V-P-K are usually two Dosha mixed type.

In studying the 10 preceding body types and looking at yourself, remember that you are unique and that this is an opportunity to learn about yourself.

Ayurvedic Questionaire

The following questionaire will allow you to find your type.
On each line circle the one that best describes you.
Occasionaly no statement or more than one will best describe you.

	Vata	Pitta	Kapha
Frame	Small & thin tall & thin underdevloped developed	Medium build, moderate physique good muscle tone	Thick, tall or short
Eyebrows & Lashes	Thin and small	Medium	Thick & bushy
Nose	Crooked, thin, small thick	Medium, reddish	Large, wide
Lips	Thin, small, irregular, full	Medium, red, pink, pointed	Large, very full
Teeth	Irregular, crooked, large had braces	Even medium	Gleaming
Shoulders	Narrow & thin	Medium, balanced	Thick, broad, firm
Chest	Narrow, twisted, pigeon or concave	Medium balanced	Large broad
Hips	Narrow	Medium	Large
Hands & Feet	Small & thin or long & thin	Medium, well proportion	Large fingers squatish/ thick toes
Skin Thickness	Thin, less than 1/4" on forearm	Medium 1/4-1/2" on forearm	Thick 1/2" or more on forearm

Ayurvedic Curative Cuisine for Everyone

	Vata	Pitta	Kapha
Childhood	Thin as a child	Medium build periods of losing and gaining weight	Gained weight easily
Weight Issues	Difficulty gaining weight even if they try to gain	Can gain or lose weight if they put their mind to it	Gains weight easily, hard time losing it unless excercises regularly
Skin Temp.	Cold hands & feet	Skin warm to the touch	skin cool but not cold
Skin type	Dry skin chaps easily	Oily skin, prone to pimples and rashes	Thick skin well lubricated
Weather	Dislikes dryness, cold & wind, (craves warmth)	Dislikes heat and sun (craves cool)	Dislikes humidity (craves dryness)
Bowels	Dry and irregular	Loose- more than twice a day diarrhea	Large, full, regular, once a day
Craving Preferences	Either indulge in rich foods or don't eat at all	Love proteins, caffeines and hot, spicy and salty foods	Loves sweets, pastries and rich foods
Endurance	Poor, tires easily	Medium, ready to go	Strong and stable
Resistance	Poor, tendency can get sick easily prone to allergies	Medium, prone to infections	Strong, prone to mucus and sinus congestion
Memory	Short term, forgets quickly	Good short & long term memory	Takes time to learn things once learned never forgets
Routine	Dislike routine-hard to structure	Enjoys planning & organizing	Works well with routine follows orders well

	Vata	Pitta	Kapha
Desision making	Difficulty making decisions, changes decisions and mind easily	Rapid decision making sees things clearly	Takes time making decisions and sticks with them
Types of thinking	Creative thinker	Organized thinker	Prefers to follow a plan or idea
chaos vs order	Likes to do many projects at once	Constantly organizing likes to proceed orderly	Resists change, likes simplicity
Emotions 1	Anxious	Irritable	Attached
Emotions 2	Nervous	Angry	Loves possesions
Emotions 3	Communicative	Caring	Devoted, loyal
Opinions and emotions	Feelings and emotions change easily	Aggresive about opinions & feelings gives opinions even if they are not asked	Avoids giving opinions in difficult situations. Does not like confrontation
	Vata Total	**Pitta Total**	**Kapha Total**

We live in a Vata Society most people will find themselves in a vata imbalance.

Food Introduction

We are what we eat. More than herbs, vitamins, enzymes, or mineral supplements, food is the major factor that most affects our metabolism. Supplements or herbs can never make up for an imbalanced diet. It is seriously delusional to think popping a handful of supplements will make up for a poor diet of soda and TV dinners. For good health and wellbeing, a heavy emphasis is placed upon quality food.

To follow an Ayurvedic diet, it is necessary to know your doshic condition so that you may follow the appropriate recommendations for your body type. A questionnaire has been provided in this cookbook to assist you in determining your constitution.

In this book, we have listed the genus and species of foods to avoid confusion. Methods of gathering or preparation specific to certain foods have also been presented herein. Historical notes were added for reasons of interest and genetics. A family's country of origin will often be a region where particular foods are grown or originated from, and are especially suited to the metabolism of individuals; e.g., olives for Mediterranean people, whale blubber for Eskimos, and corn for Mexicans, etc. Sometimes, those who stray from their "native" foods often suffer vague, disquieting symptoms, which could be related to specific nutritional factors which they are now missing.

Energy: Will be either Cooling (good for Pitta and for summer diets) or Heating (good for Vata, or Kapha and cool weather).

Taste: Defines each food elemental background (Earth, Fire, Air, Water) and allows each specific doshic type to know whether the food should be avoided, eaten occasionally, or a major part of their diet.

Post Digestive: This refers to the remaining taste energetic after digestion. Sweet builds tissue; pungent burns up tissue; and sour promotes secretions. This is more important in continued long term use than occasional use.

Indications: Various conditions for which the food would be medicine; e.g., pomegranate is good for kidney and bladder infection. "Let food be your medicine and medicine be your food."

Systems: The systems of the body most helped; Digestive System, Circulatory, Endocrine, Lymphatic, Muscular, Skeletal, Excretory, Immune, Urinary, and Epithelial.

Dosha Affect: This provides guidance for doshic types; e.g., Bean Sprouts -

   Vata: Avoid; **Pitta**: Good; **Kapha**: Excellent.

Note: Any dosha in balance can handle any food occasionally.

Strictness is more important when you are significantly out of balance.

Mixes Well With: Provides food combining tips; e.g., walnuts mix well with green, leafy vegetables, etc.

I encourage you to be kind to yourself on this new diet. If you follow the diet for five days out of seven, you will begin to experience changes as you progress. Certain foods can aggravate a specific dosha type, therefore, particular foods are to either be avoided or included in your diet. In the beginning, do not become too strict because it might seem like a hardship and you may then let it go altogether. It is what you do most of the time that counts. If you experience laziness and break the diet once in a while, it is not so bad. You can then look forward to returning to your diet. You can make it easier on yourself by taking small steps and then gradually incorporate the bigger changes. On the days that you follow your diet, you are working towards a great shift in your physical and emotional wellbeing. Always keep your goal in mind and do your best. Having your kitchen well stocked with foods that are appropriate for your diet makes meal preparation relatively easy and provides an added incentive towards success.

Some of the sickest people are those people who are so "stuck" on their diet that they have become neurotic. They are very uptight and hard on themselves; their attitude has made them very ill. These people are hard to be with and hard to treat.

Food is a major part of our social interactions. When dining at a friend's home, it is best to eat what they have prepared. Otherwise, it is easy to feel deprived and restricted by your diet. If the hostess is a friend, you may wish to inform her of your eating patterns ahead of time and that you require certain foods. If this is not possible, then eat what has been prepared and enjoy the meal and the company, returning to your diet when at home.

It takes a while to adjust to a new way of eating. For someone who is used to eating foods that are aggravating, it is hard to break the pattern; e.g., Pitta's are often very fond of hot, spicy foods. "One man's food is another man's poison." We need to let go of our preconceptions about what are "good" or "bad" foods. People are always talking about how "good" salads are for us. Yet for Vata types, eating too much salad and raw foods can make them ill. You often hear how cooking destroys food, but cooking is what makes starches available for digestion. Human digestion cannot break down cellulose, but heat can.

Those who change from eating a high protein diet (especially beef), to a diet of only fruits and vegetables, may cleanse too quickly and experience gas or diarrhea. If you experience poor digestion or malabsorption, it is necessary to attend to those issues first. Always transition gradually into the new way of eating. If you eat fried foods, transition to foods that are baked, broiled and steamed. Your meat consumption could be cut from seven days a week to 4-5 days per week. Remember, do not drink much with your meals because liquids dilute your digestive power. As you experience observable benefits in your wellbeing, it is easier to feel inspired to cut inappropriate foods from your diet. A difference can be felt within one month after being consistent on your new diet.

Ayurvedic Curative Cuisine for Everyone

Food should be eaten as fresh as possible or freshly cooked or juiced. Always buy organic when available. It is best to stay away from foods grown with pesticides or inorganic fertilizers. Eat as much fresh fruit and vegetables as possible.

Food combining is important. Improper food combining causes poor digestion and malabsorption of nutrients because different types of foods require different kinds of digestive enzymes. Digestion is easier if the foods within the stomach at any particular time require the same enzymes. Also, do not become focused on limited choices. Be sure that you do not eat too much of a few foods and not enough of others. Remember, variety is the spice of life. Getting too much of one food, combined with poor digestion, may cause allergies. If you are allergic, a diet diary is recommended. This is often useful so that you can see for yourself what your symptoms are and how often you are eating the same foods over and over again.

The stomach is a muscular, hollow organ, the size of our hands put together as follows: With palms facing each other, place the heels of your wrists together and then put all fingertips together. Then arch the palms outward creating a ball. This demonstrates the natural size of your stomach before any food expansion. When you fill your stomach more than its natural size, the muscular activity is not as efficient and digestions will take longer. Any excess turns into Ama, which is toxic waste matter that is inadequately digested, and then deposited within the body. In most cases, when overeating occurs, it means that the body is not getting enough nutrition and continually wants more. Proper chewing is also important because digestion begins in the mouth. Chewing is the first stage of digestion. Small particle size ensures that the enzymes can do their work. Chewing each bite 30+ times is necessary to liquefy the food for easier digestion. This will ensure complete assimilation of all the nutrients. You won't need to eat so much.

It is important to remember that eating should be a time of quiet, not for handling business, or discussing the challenges of life. Eating on the run or in stressful situations is extremely harmful. If at all possible, sit down and have a peaceful meal. This is imperative to the achievement of perfect health. Always remember to bless your food and remember the Mother Earth who provides for us all.

Preparing Foods

When cooking food, it is often best to slow cook and keep it well covered in order to maintain the nutritional value and to make it easier to digest. Do not use large amounts of oil in cooking. While raw foods do have more enzymes and more life force, the average person does not have adequate digestive power to break down the food. When food is cooked, it is easier on the digestive fire. Raw foods are best used in reducing and cleansing diets due to their lightness. It is usually recommended that fruit be eaten raw. However, when someone is in a high Vata condition, it is recommended that they even cook their fruits. Most grains are best when cooked, although when sprouted, they are easily digested. At this stage, they become a vegetable and are no longer so starchy. When building tissue within the body, starch is important.

Cooking is an art! A personal experience of enjoyment and creativity! A gift to people you love! Always enter the kitchen free of negative thoughts, with clean hands, a clean apron, and a tidy work area. Never fight, be in a bad mood, or have negative thoughts while preparing food. We are energetic beings, and our energy can enhance or deplete the food that we are preparing. Chanting, positive affirmations, and singing are positive energies that you can bring to the preparation of food. Listen to the vibrations of the vegetable. When you listen, they will be guiding you as to how they want to be prepared. The way the food is presented provides an important vibration that is taken into our body-mind-spirit. The way we eat is a reflection of the conditions in which we live our life.

Equipment to have in the kitchen:
- A good wok
- Wood lids for pots
- Steam basket
- A pressure cooker
- Good cast iron skillet
- Stainless steel pans - Never use aluminum or Teflon.
- Glass pans
- Good quality stainless steel knives
- Plastic cutting board for meat (to prevent bacterial contamination) and a separate one for cutting vegetables and breads
- VitaMix or a good food processor and blender
- Whenever you can, use spring or good purified water or boil your water before cooking to remove the chlorine.

Always keep your equipment handy in a clean and well organized kitchen as this provides easy access to an enjoyable working environment.

We are a multi-cultural society. The average American is afraid of Indian food because it is foreign to them and most seem to think of this type of food as "hot." Not everyone is ready for Indian foods all the time, especially when beginning a new diet. Include a variety of other forms of food preparation, such as Thai, Chinese, and Macrobiotic, yet keep the Ayurvedic principals. Once the Ayurvedic energies of food are understood, they can be adapted to many recipes. Slowly, you can transition into a full Ayurvedic Indian cooking lifestyle. For those times when you have a busy schedule, it is good to create a menu for each week. Use a shopping list to avoid numerous runs to the store and always buy certain foods in bulk, such as grains and nuts. If possible, al-

Ayurvedic Curative Cuisine for Everyone

ways use foods that are in season. In the tropics, sometimes foods will need to be stored in the refrigerator, even grains, nuts, etc.

As you go through this cookbook, you will see that each food has its own balancing and energizing qualities. Many forms of energy can be experienced as we incorporate these foods into our diet. We need warm foods to keep our digestive fire burning. Too much cold food or liquid depletes this digestive fire and when we continually lack digestive fire, we become ill and weak. It is important to experience all tastes and energies in order to nutritionally satisfy the body and support wellbeing. It is important to keep in mind your doshic condition so that you may follow the appropriate recommendations for your body type.

Springtime - This is a good time to add the many greens and fresh herbs that are now peaking, unfolding, and available. The dandelions and the young mustards can be added to soups or quickly sautéed. Work to reduce salt intake and stay away from fermented foods or pickles. During the summer months you may want to add a bit of raw food to your diet.

Summer - Many fruits and vegetables are now available at their peak of growth. The foods that grow during this season have more active, expansive energy; more Vata. Salads can be served more frequently for the appropriate body type. Vatas must still maintain their oil intake during the summer months. Begin to cook simple meals and prepare foods that are tasty. Summer is a good time for outdoor parties and barbecues, and you may even want to have dinners in the park with friends and families. Fruit gelatin with melon would be a great addition to the menu.

Autumn - The tubers and root vegetables are ready for harvest. We begin to slow down, and our energies turn more inward. We start feeling the seasonal changes with the onset of cold, dry winds. Start preparing yourself for winter by building up the immune system with foods that provide good physical nourishment; squashes, apples, oranges, onions, cabbage, and turnips. Many of these harvested crops will last through the winter by drying, canning, pickling, freezing, or storing in a food cellar.

Winter - During the winter season, strong winds start moving in and snow covers parts of the northern hemisphere. As this inward movement deepens, eating cooked foods prepared with a variety of spices is recommended. This is a time for warm, nourishing, bountiful, homemade soups, stews, and casseroles to invigorate the body. More oil may be added for all doshas to keep the body warm. Other helpful additions to a winter diet are salt, fermented foods, more grains, wheat breads, jams, roasted nuts, and nut butters. It is the time to clean and burn off any excess nutrition built up during the summer months.

When preparing foods, keep the visual presentation in mind. Color is a form of energy, therefore, decorating your plate with the various food colors will nurture the body-mind-Spirit.

Lemon and Lime - A slice of citrus can add a sour touch to the palate, which helps to break down foods, increase digestion, and stimulate the liver and gastric juices. Especially good to serve with fish.

Green Foods - Like chard, cabbage, spinach, broccoli, green onions, and scallions. They are calming and help with detoxifying effects.

Yellow Foods - Like millet and squashes. Good for the stomach and spleen.

Red Foods - Like beets and berries. Stimulate the heart and blood circulation.

Orange Foods - Like carrots, sweet potatoes, and yams. Helps build the immune system.

White Foods - Like potatoes, rice, and barley. Helps the lungs and intestines.

Currently, most Americans eat at least 50-60% of all meals in restaurants or fast food places. Restaurant eating should be left for special occasions and fast food should be avoided. Microwaves devitalize foods, altering their molecular vibrations. Gas stoves are better than electric stoves for cooking.

I always recommend a crockpot because it is easy; slow cooking is healthy and makes food available throughout the day. You can prepare it before you go to sleep or before going to work. It is one of our western conveniences. It does not take a lot of attention and space and all kinds of food can be cooked in it. When the food is prepared overnight in slow cookers, it is ready for the next day and also allows for the possibility of taking some to work.

Food Combining

Food combining is very important for good digestion, weight reduction, and for the prevention of cellulite. Avoid eating protein and starches together; e.g., meats with potatoes. Proteins, such as meat and dairy products, should be eaten with non-starchy vegetables. No fruit with proteins. Fruits and starchy veggies are best not mixed together. Grains mix well with all vegetables. Nuts mix with green vegetables, citrus fruits, or sour fruits. Starchy vegetables, like squashes and potatoes, mix best with green vegetables.

It takes different enzymes to digest different types of foods. Proteins call for hydrochloric acid and pepsin to be released onto the stomach contents for acid protein digestion (breaking down proteins into amino acids). Starch digestion begins in the mouth (with ptyalin from the saliva) and will continue in the stomach if no acid is released. This is why proteins and starches are more efficiently digested separately. This is important for the sick, weak, or persons with poor digestive fire. Healthy people need not pay as much attention to "food separation." Beans and grains are a natural combination of starches and proteins. For healthy people, restricting fluid intake with meals and eating fruits separately is recommended.

Ayurvedic Curative Cuisine for Everyone

For more efficient digestion, it is best to follow this rule: Never drink with your meals with the exception of milk unless an herbal therapy drink has been recommended. When too much liquid is taken at mealtime, this dilutes digestive enzymes; liquids weaken digestion and create fermentation (gas). Example: You set your washing machine for a small load with enough detergent and a low water level. Then if someone comes and raises the water level too high, your clothes will not come out clean. You also don't mix white and colored clothes when you wash. It can be the same with starches and proteins.

Only eat when you are hungry. Check and see if you actually are hungry... or are you feeling empty or anxious, and covering up those feelings with food.

Vata: Needs to eat more often. Their blood sugar drops easily, making it challenging for them to go long periods without food. Snacking between meals is important to their wellbeing.

Pitta: Needs to have regular solid food. It is important that they have a large meal in the middle of the day; they should eat at least three full meals per day.

Kapha: Can get by with one or two meals per day. Eat the largest meal in the middle of the day and a light meal at night. Snacking is not good for them. Never exercise after a heavy meal unless it is a mild walk. For other forms of exercise, it is best to wait a couple of hours after mealtime. Sex should be avoided immediately before or after a meal....Never watch television while eating as it increases Vata.... Smoking disturbs the digestion.... Do not go to sleep immediately after a large meal.... A small amount of wine (4 oz.) is best before mealtime to stimulate appetite, which is especially good for Vata. Desserts are usually best as a snack apart from a regular meal because it adds to the amount of food that requires digestion. Also, the sweetness interferes with protein digestion (causing putrification).

Restaurant Eating

Due to busy schedules and fast lifestyles many people purchase prepared foods. Restaurant eating is a convenience and is part of day-to-day survival for some people. The quality of food in a restaurant could never replace that of home cooking. The person who is preparing the food is not able to connect with the people who eat in his restaurant. However, that is not to say that there are no conscious chefs. Generally, restaurants buy large quantities of food, and quality is not a priority, unless you go to a small gourmet food restaurant and pay the price. The $50-$100 that you pay for a truly fine meal can go a long way towards shopping in a health food store.

Fine ethnic foods are often better than just plain American cooking. Chinese, Indian, Korean, Thai, Japanese, Vietnamese, Greek, Italian, and Mexican foods use plenty of fresh vegetables, spices, herbs, beans, rice, guacamole, fresh cilantro, and freshly made sauces. More and more restaurant owners and chefs are assisting the transformation that is taking place concerning food consciousness of the people, especially in this part of the world. A restaurant that is dedicated to providing good service will make substitutions for specific foods that a patron is unable to eat and will accommodate "off the menu" requests (e.g., no MSG, or please add extra basil).

Always stay away from restaurants that prepare foods with microwaves, use lard or MSG (especially found in Chinese cooking). Visit and support health food restaurants; they adhere to healthy food principles and use as much organic food as possible. Fast food restaurants are not recommended; yet in today's busy world, sometimes we must use them. Wendy's has a Pita sandwich with shredded veggies and romaine lettuce. Subway offers a veggie burger, and The Harvest carries sweet potatoes and many vegetarian dishes. Even in McDonald's you can choose a fish burger or charbroiled chicken sandwich over a Big Mac. Remember, we vote with our money. Whatever you buy, you are asking for more of. Money talks.

Always stay away from busy, crowded restaurants. The idea of dining out is to have time for yourself, free from preparation and clean up.

Questions to ask at the restaurant:

- Do you have filtered water?
- Are the vegetables fresh?
- Do you have romaine lettuce?
- Do you fry, boil or bake?
- Do you use lard or vegetable oil?
- Do you use whole grains?
- Do you carry herbal teas?
- Are there preservatives in the salad bar?
- Do you have honey?
- Do you have vegetarian food on the menu?

Vata does well with any place that has warm soups and vegetables.

Pitta does well with Thai and Chinese foods.

Kapha does well with salads and all vegetable dishes.

Ayurvedic Curative Cuisine for Everyone

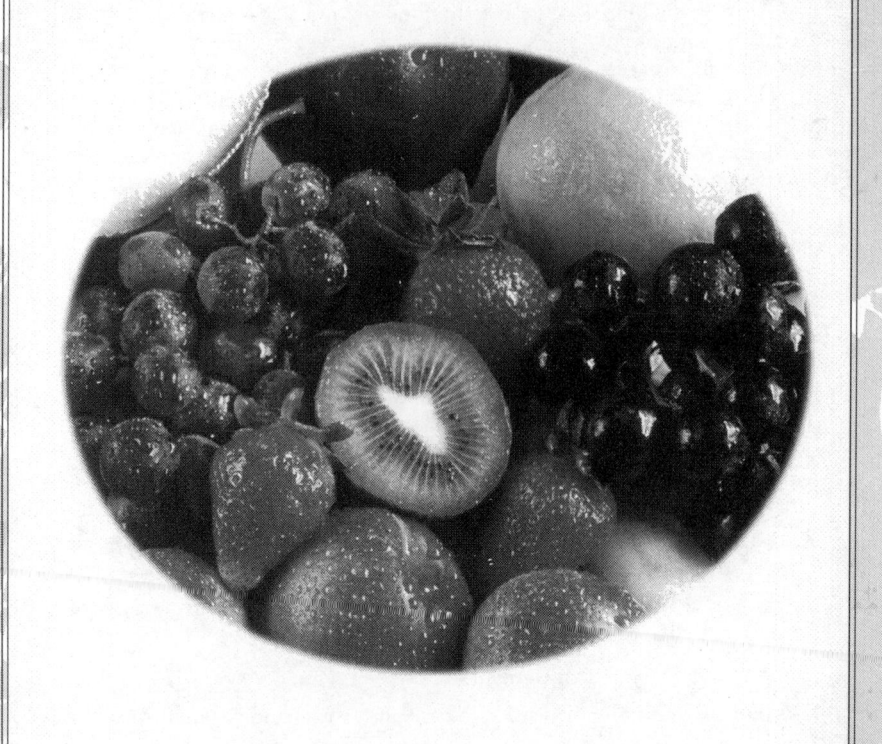

Fruits

Fruits

General Considerations

Most fruits have a high water content – between 80 and 95% – and are, therefore, thirst quenching. An average fruit is 13 to 23 grams of carbohydrate sugar and is low in fats and proteins.

Fruits are rich in vitamins A, B-6, and C, and contain generous amounts of minerals such as potassium, calcium, iron, and manganese. Fruits stimulate the secretion of gastric juices, are rich in soluble fiber, and aid in maintaining a healthy balance of intestinal flora. Organic fruit is best, because commercially grown fruit comes in contact with fertilizers, dyes, insecticides, or herbicides. Always wash fruit well before eating.

Fruits emit a large amount of ethylene gas produced by the fruit during the ripening process. If fruit is purchased unripe, place it in a paper bag to ripen. Do not use a plastic bag, because plastic holds the moisture in and will cause the fruit to rot. Overripe fruit becomes fermented, and the sugar turns into alcohol. Acetic acid is created, which causes gas and intestinal problems. Fruits that are unripe are high in starch with a bitter or astringent taste, because as fruits ripen, the starch turns to sugar. Some fruits are best to eat tree-ripened, while some ripen fine after picking.

Eat fruit fresh, either alone or with other fruits. Fruit makes an excellent snack or a good quick meal that is palatable, delicious, and energy-producing. Very sweet fruit is best eaten in the afternoon when it is Pitta time. Most fruits are sweet, acid or sub-acid, yet all fruits have a sweet flavor when ripe but become alkaline after the process of digestion. It is best not to combine too many fruits together, especially acid and sweet fruits. Sweet fruits may be combined with grains, (i.e., raisins in oatmeal), and acid fruits do well with green vegetables, (i.e., oranges with Romaine lettuce). Some starchy fruits can be baked, boiled, or fried while still hard and green and are then treated like a starch (e.g., breadfruit and plantain).

It is recommended to serve only one to three kinds of fruits per meal, and eat at room temperature. A great way to assist digestion, especially in the winter, is to season fruit with spices such as ginger, cardamom, cinnamon, fennel, anise, cloves, nutmeg, and/or allspice. Canned fruits are not recommended as they have added sugar. Fresh fruits are always the first choice.

Most fruits are sweet, creating contentment and satisfaction. During a spiritual retreat, fruits are a good diet, because most are Sattvic in nature. Fruit does not, however, increase intelligence or strength for physical work.

When drinking fruit juices, sip slowly instead of drinking in one gulp. Bottled juices can contain a larger amount of sugar due to the boiling process; it is best to dilute with good drinking water or herbal teas. Bottled juices, with a higher concentration of sugars, can also be decaying to the teeth. Many

Ayurvedic Curative Cuisine for Everyone

parents give their children too much fruit juice to the detriment of their teeth. There is much evidence that primitive man ate great quantities of fruit, which was a main source of nutrition.

Some of the fruits discussed in this course are rare fruits. Yet, for those who travel to other parts of the world, it can be interesting to learn about them. Having an understanding of these foods will be of assistance in staying balanced. Many of the metropolitan cities have international markets where these foods may be available. We invite you to try new foods to increase nutritional variety and appreciate other cultures.

Dried Fruits

Fruits are best eaten fresh during the winter season, unless the nutrients are necessary for a specific problem. Dried fruit is best for Kapha and, if they are sun-dried, it brings the sun's Pitta force. When Vata or Pitta use dried fruit for medicinal reasons, they are to be soaked overnight and blended. One must be careful when purchasing any dried fruit as they are often dried with preservatives such as sulfates and sulphur dioxide to keep them attractive. These agents are quite toxic to the kidneys.

Apple

Botanical Name: Malus sylvestris domestica

Apples have been respected as a source of nutrition by many cultures. There are approximately 2,000 varieties of apples. It is one of the easiest fruits to ship and store. There is no question that the apple is, and should be, at the head of the list of fruits. It is delightful to the eye and is excellent for nutritional value, as well as very practical to travel with. It is known for its high alkalinity. Apples contain a small amount of malic acid and are easily oxidized in the process of digestion. Malic acid helps the body utilize energy more effectively. The pectin binds with cholesterol. Good for arthritic conditions.

Energy: Cooling

Taste: Sweet, Sour, Astringent

Post Digestive: Sweet

Indications: Excellent for intestinal problems, bleeding ulceration, pectin helps bind stool, assists digestion and promotes healing of colon, arthritis, backache, cancer sores, and allergic reactions, and helps to reduce heavy metals. Used for detoxifying and adds flavor to other juices.

Systems: Digestive, Excretory, Circulatory, Endocrine, Respiratory

Dosha Affected:

Vata: When sour can be eaten. Best cooked into an applesauce spiced with ginger, cinnamon, and cardamom

Pitta: Sweet apples are excellent; best to avoid sour

Kapha: Good because of astringency

Mixes Well With: Sub-acid fruits and sweet fruit

Season: Fall & Winter

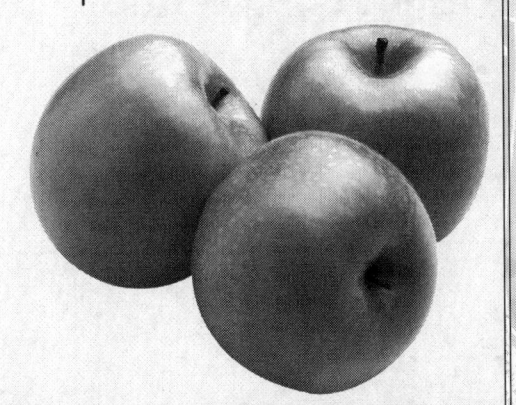

Stuffed Apples

Serves 2

- 4 apples
- 8 Medjool dates, pitted
- ¼ cup raisins
- 2 cups water (divided)
- ¼ cups fresh ginger, grated fine
- 1 teaspoon coriander, ground
- 1 teaspoon cinnamon
- 1 teaspoon fennel, ground
- 1 teaspoon nutmeg
- 1½ teaspoons sucanat or jaggary

Soak dates and raisins overnight in approximately one cup of water. The next day, cut apples in half (vertically); remove core of apple and about ½ inch of apple around the core (creating hole in which to place stuffing).

Drain half of the water from dates and raisins; set this "soaking water" aside. In blender, put date/raisin/water mixture, ginger, and spices; blend until it looks like fruit butter; set aside.

In saucepan, put remaining cup of water plus the soaking water, and add sweetener. Reduce liquid at a very low heat until it becomes a smooth syrup. Place apples in baking dish, stuff centers with date/raisin mixture, and pour the syrup over the apples. Bake for 15 minutes at 350°.

Apple Ginger Juice

Serves 2

- 3 Macintosh apples
- ¼ thumb of fresh ginger

Place ingredients in juicer. Add fresh mint or fennel if desired.

Applesauce

Serves 2

4 apples, chopped

1 teaspoon jaggary, maple syrup, or honey

2 cups water

¼ teaspoon cinnamon

¼ teaspoon cardamom

Steam apples for 10 to 15 minutes, until soft. Place in blender or food processor, add other ingredients, and blend until smooth. Serve over fruit or toast.

Apple Fritters

Serves 2

4 apples

½ cup pastry flour

½ cup oat bran

1 teaspoon baking powder

1 teaspoon cinnamon

1 teaspoon cardamom

1 teaspoon coriander

¼ cup sucanat or jaggary

2 eggs (or egg substitute)

½ cup warm water (approximately)

¼ cup ghee

Peel, core and cut apples in half. Slice thin. In bowl, mix flour, oat bran, and baking powder together. Add seasonings and sugar.

In separate bowl, beat the eggs. Put apple slices into eggs to soak for half an hour. (If eggs do not cover apples, add a little water.) Then dip each apple slice in the flour mixture, coating completely. Heat pan with ghee and lightly sauté apple slices until golden brown.

Serve with any fruit or chutney.

(This is a treat – not the best food combining!)

Apricot

Botanical Name: Prunus armeniaca vulgaris

The apricot's native countries are Arabia, Armenia, and the higher regions of Central Asia. Today they are grown all over the world. The fruit ripens in the middle of the summer after cherries and plums. There are about 45 different varieties and many different sizes, from 2½ to 3 inches. Most apricots in the market are prematurely harvested. Dried apricots are good provided they are sun-dried. They are a good source of fiber. The yellow color makes them high in beta-carotene and iron. They contain Vitamin B-5, which supports the adrenals. High in vitamin C.

Energy: Cooling

Taste: Sweet, Sour

Post Digestive: Sweet

Indications: Good for coughs, colds, fevers and inflammation. The seeds help destroy tumors due to a high level of laetrile, but one must be careful because they are toxic.
Best used under supervision.

Systems: Respiratory, Excretory, Epithelial

Dosha Affected:

Vata and **Pitta**: Good

Kapha: Moderation (if not out of balance)

Mixes Well With: Other sub-acid fruits and sweet fruits

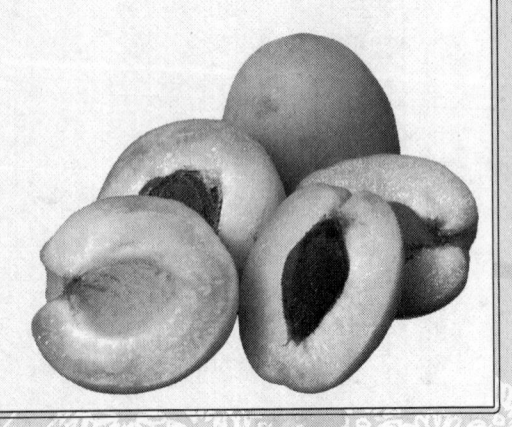

Apricot Delight

½ pound dried apricots
2 cups fresh orange juice
2 tablespoons ghee
1 tablespoon agar-agar

Soak apricots in orange juice overnight. The next morning, blend apricots and juice in blender. Melt ghee in saucepan, add apricot mixture, and bring to a boil. Stir in agar-agar to gel the mixture; remove from heat and let set until cool, then refrigerate.

Serve as topping on fruit salad.

Apricot Crisp

Serves 4

8 apricots
½ cup almond milk
2 tablespoons arrowroot powder
2 tablespoons almond flour
2 tablespoons amaranth flour
2 tablespoons ghee
½ teaspoon cardamom
¼ teaspoon nutmeg
¼ teaspoon ginger
¼ teaspoon cinnamon
2 tablespoons ground jaggary

In a medium sized baking pan, use some of the ghee to oil the pan. In a bowl mix all ingredients together. Mix well.

Put in pan. Bake at 325 for 30 minutes.

Avocado

Botanical Name: Persea gratissima, Persea drymifolia Persea americana

The avocado is also known as "alligator pear" because of its shape, color, and rough skin. Avocado trees are large evergreens. An acre of avocado trees can produce a large amount of fruit, more than any other fruit crop in the world. They are not native to the United States but are highly cultivated, and it is one of our largest industries. For many people in Mexico and Central America, an avocado is like a potato is to an American. It is the staple of many native people in other parts of the world. There are several varieties; some are high in fat like the Hass or Fuerte, and some are high in water and starch. They vary in size and can weigh from a few ounces to a few pounds. Avocado is a great meat substitute, rich in proteins and fat, and more easily digestible than meat. In Brazil and Mexico, it is made into an ice cream because of the high oil and fat content. Unfortunately, the oil turns rancid quickly and is difficult to preserve. It is important to eat this fruit when ripe and when soft to the touch.

Energy: Moisturizing, Slightly Warm

Taste: Sweet

Post Digestive: Sweet

Indications. Weak muscles, tissue, lungs, liver, skin, baldness

Systems: Endocrine, Epithelial, Circulatory, Muscular

Dosha Affected:

Vata: Excellent

Pitta: Moderation (due to high oil content, Fuerta is best)

Kapha: Use in very small amounts due to high fat content

Mixes Well With: Sweet fruits, green leafy vegetables

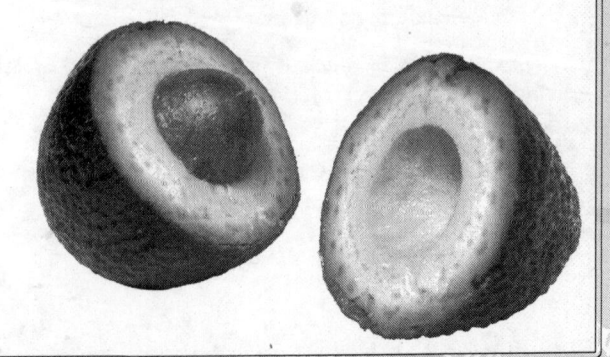

Avocado a la Mexicana

Serves 2

- 1 tablespoon cumin seeds
- 1 tablespoon olive oil
- ½ cup green onions, chopped
- 1 cup red or yellow pepper, chopped
- 1 cup celery, chopped
- 1 bunch cilantro, chopped
- 2 tablespoons mild salsa
- 3 avocados

Sauté cumin seeds in wok or frying pan, then add olive oil, onions, peppers, and celery, and continue cooking for 15 minutes until vegetables are soft. Mix cilantro with salsa (saving a small amount of cilantro for garnish), then stir in cooked vegetables.

Cut avocados in half and remove pits. Place portion of vegetable mixture in center of each avocado; garnish with leftover cilantro.

Avocado Dressing

Serves 4

- ¼ cup sunflower seeds
- 2 avocados, cut in half (remove pit)
- 2 tablespoons lemon juice
- ½ cup water
- ¼ cup cilantro, well chopped
- 2 tablespoons olive oil
- ¼ cup chopped celery
- 1 tablespoon churna or mild curry powder
- Bragg's or salt

Grind the sunflower seeds in a coffee grinder. Blend all ingredients together in blender; refrigerate.

Serve on salad or vegetables.

Cold Avocado Soup
Serves 4

3 avocados, skin and pit removed
1 small onion, chopped
1 medium tomato, chopped
2 tablespoons lemon juice
1 tablespoon olive oil
5 cups water
¼ cup dillweed, chopped
1 cup cilantro, chopped
Bragg's

Put all ingredients in blender, and blend until smooth. Add Bragg's to taste.

Serve chilled with cilantro garnish.

Healthy Guacamole
Serves 2

3 avocados
1 tablespoon fresh lime juice
½ cup green onions, chopped
1 tomato, well chopped
1 clove garlic, well chopped (for Kapha only)
2 tablespoons salsa (mild for Pitta, medium for Vata, hot for Kapha)
1 teaspoon cumin, ground
salt

Mash avocados, and add lime juice. Stir in remaining ingredients; add salt to taste.

Serve with salad or steamed vegetables, or as appetizer with chips.

Banana

Botanical Name: Musa paradisiaca Musa cavendishii

The banana has made history around the world, because it is shipped globally at any time of the year. Over 70 million bananas are imported into the United States and Canada yearly and approximately 3 million into Europe. In Central and South America, bananas represent what grains are to the Western Nation. The green fruit is very starchy and when ripe turns into an easily digestible concentrated sugar and carbohydrate. There are many varieties. The Plantain is one of the largest and can be boiled or baked when unripe (like a potato) or fried when ripe (for a dessert). Bananas provide a high-energy boost due to a high sugar content. They are high in vitamin B-5 and have the ability to clear waste. Best eaten ripe unless using plantains. High in phosphorus and potassium.

Energy: Cooling

Taste: Sweet, Astringent

Post Digestive: Sweet

Indications: Anemia, ulcers, convalescence, diarrhea, weak children, to gain weight. However can also be difficult to digest due to high starch content and the lack of water compared to other fruits

Systems: Excretory, Muscular, Urinary

Dosha Affected:

Vata and **Pitta**: Excellent when ripe

Kapha: Avoid due to too much starch and muscle building

Mixes Well With: Green leafy vegetables, sweet fruits

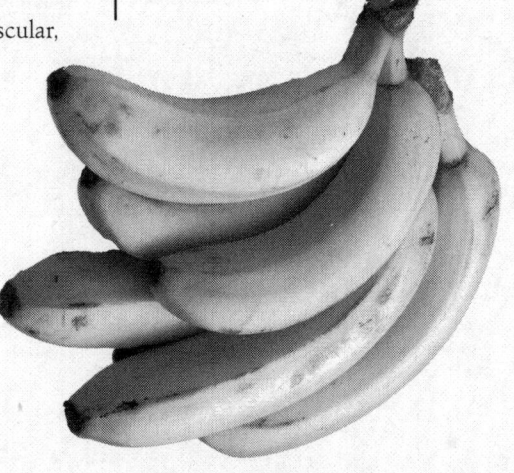

Tropical Banana Bread
1 large loaf

- 4 very ripe bananas
- 1 tablespoon lemon juice
- 1 teaspoon cinnamon
- 1 teaspoon cardamom
- 1 egg, well beaten
- 1 tablespoon ghee
- 1 tablespoon vanilla
- 1 cup yogurt
- 1 teaspoon sucanat or jaggary
- 2 cups pastry flour
- 2 teaspoons baking powder
- ½ teaspoon baking soda
- 1 cup raisins
- ½ cup nuts

Preheat the oven to 350°.

Mash bananas and lemon juice together; set aside. In large bowl, mix egg, ghee, vanilla, yogurt and spices. Then add sucanat, flour, baking powder and soda, raisins, and nuts. Fold in mashed bananas. Oil a loaf pan, pour in batter, and bake for 1 hour (or until done).

Plantain Casserole

Serves 4

- ½ cup of spinach or chard, chopped
- 1 carrot, grated
- 1 sweet onion, chopped
- 4 green plantains
- ½ cup olive oil
- 1 tablespoon Bragg's
- 1 cup cheese, grated

Steam spinach, carrots, and onion; set aside. Boil plantain until soft; remove skin when cool. Mash well, then add olive oil and Bragg's. Grease baking pan with oil and layer half of the mashed plantain, then the vegetables, then the remaining plantain. Spread grated cheese on top. Bake 10 to 15 minutes until cheese melts. Cut into squares and serve.

Plantains a la Coconut

Serves 2-4

- 2 tablespoons ghee
- ¼ teaspoon cinnamon
- ¼ teaspoon cardamom
- 1/8 teaspoon nutmeg
- 2 ripe plantains, cut into ½-inch round slices
- 2 tablespoons maple syrup or rice syrup
- ¼ cup (2 ounces) coconut rum.

Sauté spices in ghee for 30 seconds. Add plantain slices and sauté on both sides until brown. Add maple syrup or rice syrup and rum, and flambé for 10 seconds, until flame is gone.

Serve with greens.

Blackberry

<u>Botanical Name: *Rubus nigrobaccus*</u>

Blackberries belong to the same family as raspberries, and are an ovate fruit. One of the most valuable fruits of North America, there are over 100 species. It has highly medicinal properties, both the leaves and the fruit, especially for diseases of the eyes and the mouth.

Energy: When ripe they are warming; when unripe they are cooling

Taste: Sweet, Sour, Astringent

Post Digestive: Sweet

Indications: Excellent for circulation, varicose veins, sexual vitality, and aids in the building of the blood

Systems: Circulatory, Reproductive, Urinary

Dosha Affected:

Vata and **Pitta**: Good but can increase Kapha

Kapha: Very small amounts

Mixes Well With: Sweet and sub-acid fruit and other berries

Season: Summer & Fall

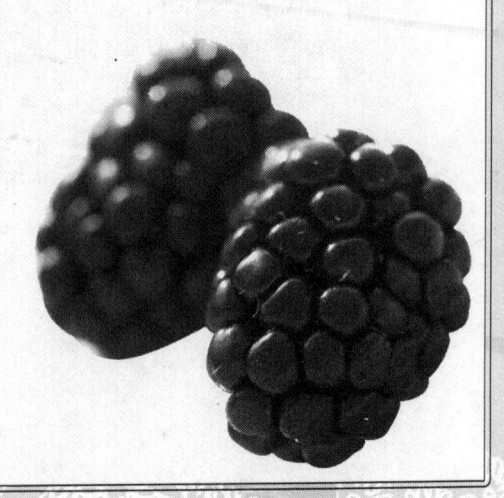

Blackberry Pie

Serves 6

- 1 cup dried orange peel
- 2 cups graham crackers (divided)
- ¼ cup apple juice
- ½ cup sucanat
- 2 tablespoons ghee
- 1 pint blackberries
- 1 cup orange juice
- 2 tablespoons cardamom
- 2 tablespoons ginger, freshly grated

Grind orange peels and 1½ cups of the graham crackers into powder. Mix with apple juice, sucanat, and ghee, to make dough. Oil pie pan with a little ghee, and spread dough in pan to form crust. Bake for 15 minutes at 250°, and remove from oven.

Crush remaining graham crackers, and mix in bowl with blackberries, orange juice, cardamom and ginger. Spread evenly in baked crust, and bake for another 15 minutes.

Blackberry Corn Muffins

Serves 2

- 1 cup blackberries
- 2 cups yellow corn flour, organic
- ½ cup pastry flour
- 2 tablespoons baking powder
- 1 cup milk
- 1 cup raw sugar
- 2 eggs, well beaten
- 1 teaspoon vanilla
- ½ teaspoon salt

Mix flour, eggs, and ghee together. Add milk, vanilla, sugar, and baking powder. Fold in blackberries. Pour batter into oiled muffin pan. Preheat oven for 5 minutes at 375. Bake for 20-30 minutes.

Blueberry

Botanical Name: Vaccinium angustifolium, Vaccinium corymbosum

Blueberries are not botanically related to any other family. They are best eaten raw, as they lose vitamin C when cooked. They are native to North America. In ancient times the root was used to relieve pain during childbirth. Blueberries are extremely high in antioxidants, used to support the immune system. They contain elegiac acid that prevents high sugar levels. They strengthen the blood and capillaries. Blueberries support all tissues in the body.

Energy: Cooling, Moisturizing

Taste: Astringent, Sweet

Post Digestive: Sweet

Indications: Diabetes, high blood sugar, high cholesterol, fevers, rheumatoid arthritis, bruising, excellent for circulation

Systems: Endocrine, Digestive, Circulatory

Dosha Affected:
Good for all body types

Mixes Well With: All fruits

Season: Spring & Summer

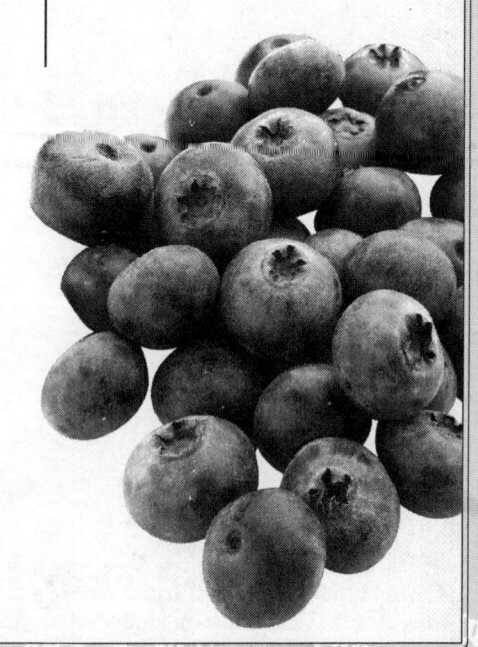

Blueberry Divine

a liver flush

- 1 cup blueberries
- 2 tablespoons fresh aloe vera, chopped
- 1/4 cup ginger, chopped
- 2 tablespoons olive oil
- 1/4 teaspoon milk thistle, ground
- ½ teaspoon cinnamon
- ½ teaspoon cardamom
- 1 clove garlic (for Kapha only)
- 2 tablespoons lemon or lime juice

Prepare aloe vera leaf: remove spines, cut leaf into small pieces. Mix all ingredients in blender; blend until smooth.

Drink first thing upon waking; do not eat or drink for 2 hours to allow time for the oil to be digested. Then resume normal life!

Blueberry Smoothie

- 1 cup blueberries
- 1 cup yogurt
- ½ tablespoon cinnamon
- ½ tablespoon nutmeg
- 1 teaspoon sucanat, jaggary, maple syrup, or honey
- ½ teaspoon fennel, ground

Place all ingredients in blender; blend until smooth.

Breadfruit

Botanical Name: Artocarpus communis

Breadfruit is not commonly known in North America, yet it is one of the staples for many people in the South Pacific Islands and Southern India. The fruit is quite large and starchy with a green or yellow color. It is best eaten when unripe, prepared by baking or cooking. The flavor and texture is of a sweet potato. The tree is huge with large, heavy leaves. Sometimes the fruit is roasted and served in the huge leaves. Many native people eat the fruit when it is ripe, even though it is extremely sweet then and not really desirable. The ripe fruit is fermented and used as a cheese sauce. A particular variety, called Bretnut, is very high in protein and contains seeds that can be roasted. Highly nutritious; high in minerals and fat.

Energy: Heating, Warming

Taste: Sweet

Post Digestive: Sweet

Indications: To gain weight, anorexia, bulimia, nervous disorders, anxiety

Systems: Muscular, Reproductive, Endocrine

Dosha Affected:

Vata: Excellent because of high nutrition and starch

Pitta: Good

Kapha: An occasional small amount, baked

Mixes Well With: Green leafy vegetables

Season: Winter Tropical Fruit

Breadfruit Casserole

- 1 medium breadfruit
- 2 tablespoons ajwan seeds
- 2 tablespoons ghee
- 1 medium onion, well chopped
- 1 bunch kale, thinly sliced
- ½ bunch parsley, chopped
- 2 tablespoons olive oil
- Bragg's

Peel breadfruit and cut into small cubes; steam until soft (approximately 20 minutes). In saucepan, roast ajwan seeds for 10 minutes. Add ghee and onions to pan; caramelize onions at low heat. Add kale, parsley, olive oil, and softened breadfruit cubes to saucepan, mixing well with other ingredients. Add Bragg's to taste, and simmer for about 10 minutes.

Baked Breadfruit

- 1 medium breadfruit
- ½ bunch parsley, chopped
- 1 onion, well chopped
- 2 cloves garlic, minced
- 2 tablespoons olive oil

Cut breadfruit into small cubes. Mix all ingredients together in baking dish, and bake at 350° for 45 minutes. Garnish with parsley.

Carambola (Star Fruit)

<u>Botanical Name:</u> *verrhoa carambola*

Native to China and India. In these countries it is eaten unripe as a vegetable; when ripe, it is eaten as a fruit. Today, the fruit grows in many tropical areas. The fruit is very fragrant, yellow-orange in color, oval in shape, with fine angles. When it is cut, the slices look like stars. Very high in vitamin C and potassium, low in carbohydrates, and has a citrus taste.

Energy: Warming
Taste: Sweet Sour
Post Digestive: Sweet
Indications: Infections, jaundice, alcoholism
Systems: Endocrine, Digestive, Urinary Tract, Circulatory.

Dosha Affected:
Vata: Good
Pitta: Moderation
Kapha: Only when green
Mixes Well With: Sub-acid & acid fruits
Season: Spring Tropical Fruit

Carambola (Star Fruit) Tropical Salad

<u>Serves 4</u>

3 carambola, cut horizontally into "stars"
1 sunrise papaya, cut in cubes
1 banana, sliced
1 teaspoon fennel, ground
1 teaspoon cardamom
1 teaspoon nutmeg
1 tablespoon lemon juice
1 teaspoon maple syrup

Mix all ingredients in salad bowl; let sit for a half hour before serving.

Carob

Botanical Name: Ceratonia siliqua

Also known as St. John's Bread or Honey Locust. The tree is a handsome evergreen that can be as high as 40 to 60 feet and can live 100 to 200 years. The fruit is used today for livestock and is not commonly sold in the market because of the tough fiber of the fruit. It grows well in milder climates and is cultivated in many parts of the United States. The fruit looks like a large bean pod and, when ground and roasted, is an excellent substitute for chocolate. Commonly sold in health food stores as carob powder. Emulcent, stimulating, good for debilitating conditions and weaknesses. The carob pod is very high in B vitamins. A great replacement for chocolate. Not high in fat. It contains a good amount of protein. The Bible talks about sages that fasted on this fruit, sustaining themselves for 40 days. It is also low in sodium and high in calcium and magnesium.

Energy: Warming

Taste: Sweet, Astringent

Post Digestive: Sweet

Indications: Pancreatic disorders, menopause, PMS, weight gain, sugar cravings, weak children, for fasting

Systems: Good for all systems.

Dosha Affected:

Vata: Be careful because it is roasted and dry; need to take as a warm drink

Pitta: Great

Kapha: Good

Mixes Well With: All sweet fruits and milk products

Season: Fall Tropical Fruit

Ayurvedic Curative Cuisine for Everyone

Carob Tonic – For Vigor & Strength
Serves 1

- 1 cup carob powder
- 1 tablespoon shatavari powder
- 1 tablespoon ashwagandha
- 8 dates, soaked
- ¼ teaspoon mint
- 1 teaspoon vanilla
- 2 tablespoons ghee
- 1 cup water

Put all ingredients in blender and blend well until smooth.

Carob Sauce or Topping
Serves 4

- 2 tablespoons carob powder
- 2 tablespoons of a nut butter of your choice
- 2 tablespoon honey
- ¼ teaspoon vanilla
- ¼ teaspoon cardamom
- 2 teaspoons ghee

Mix all ingredients together in a bowl until smooth. Add this topping to fruit or ice cream.

Cherimoya

Botanical Name: Annona cherimola

Better than honey! A gift from the Gods! One of the finest fruits in the world! It is native to the Andes and today is cultivated in Central America, Africa, India, and many other countries. The taste is similar to a mixture of custard, apples, and pineapples with vanilla (the fruit is also known as "custard apple"). It grows well in high, cool climates. The fruit can be round or cone shaped. It can weigh between several ounces and several pounds. It is light green in color, contains sweet, juicy, white meat inside, and is filled with numerous brown seeds. High in minerals. Excellent for digestion. Builds bulk. Tonic.

Energy: Cooling, Moisturizing

Taste: Sweet

Post Digestive: Sweet

Indications: For gaining weight, infections, fevers, inflammations, constipation, hemorrhoids

Systems: Muscular, Digestive, Circulation

Dosha Affected:

Vata and **Pitta**: Good

Kapha: A very small amount

Mixes Well With: All sweet and sub-acid fruit

Season: Summer of Fall Tropical Fruit

Cherimoya Custard

- 2 ripe cherimoyas, peeled and seeds removed
- 1 cup apple juice
- 1 teaspoon cinnamon
- 1 teaspoon cardamom

Blend all ingredients until smooth. Pour into cups and refrigerate; serve chilled.

Cherimoya Fruit Salad

- 2 ripe cherimoyas
- 2 apples
- ½ pineapple
- ¼ cinnamon
- ¼ cardamom

Peel and cut all fruit into small pieces. Mix in spices. Serve.

Cherimoya Sauce

Serves 2

- 3 cherimoya, peeled, chopped
- 1 tablespoon jaggary
- ½ teaspoon nutmeg
- 2 tablespoons almond milk
- ½ cup water
- ¼ cup water
- ½ teaspoon vanilla
- 2 teaspoons arrowroot

In small pan, simmer cherimoya on low heat with ¼ cup water until soft. Then add almond milk, ½ cup water, vanilla, nutmeg, and arrowroot. Stir well, so it does not clump, until pudding consistency. Whisk is best

Cherry

Botanical Name: Prunus avium, Prunus cerasus

This wonderful fruit is a native of Asia and has traveled all over the world. There are approximately 100 varieties of cherries, some of which are sour, some sweet. The cherry orchards of America produce 250 tons each season. Cherries are excellent for the blood, a tonic which is good for the heart, helps build plasma, good for varicose veins and kidneys. Like all berries they are high in elegiac acid, which blocks cancer cells. They are high in anthrocyanins, which are rich in antioxidants.

Energy: Warming

Taste: Sweet, Sour

Post Digestive: Sweet

Indications: Varicose veins, heart disorders

Systems: Circulatory, Urinary

Dosha Affected:

Vata: Excellent

Pitta: Need to avoid sour cherries; better with yellow cherries

Kapha: Can eat sour and sweet cherries in very small amounts

Mixes Well With: Sub-acid, sweet fruits

Season: summer

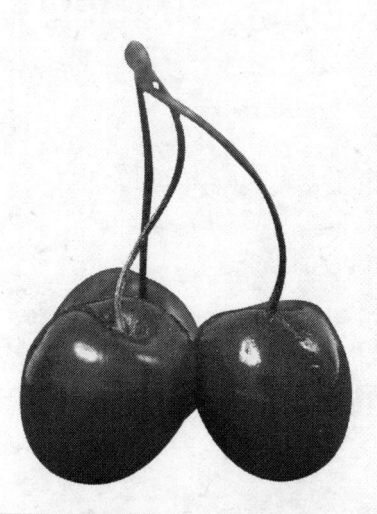

Cherry Pie

Serves 6

- 1 cup dried lemon peel
- 2 cups graham crackers (divided)
- ½ cup apple juice
- ½ cup sucanat (divided)
- 1 tablespoon ghee
- 3 cups cherries, pitted
- ½ cup water
- 2 tablespoons lecithin
- 2 tablespoons arrowroot

Grind lemon peel and 1½ cups of the graham crackers into powder. Mix with apple juice, ¼ cup of the sucanat, and ghee, to make dough. Oil pie pan with a little ghee, and spread mixture in pan to form crust. Bake for 15 minutes at 250°, and remove from oven.

Crush remaining ½ cup graham crackers. In a saucepan, cook cherries in water with lecithin, arrowroot, and remaining ¼ cup of sucanat until thick, about 10 minutes. Mix in crushed graham crackers, pour into pie crust, and bake for another 20 minutes at 350°.

Graham Cracker Crust

Makes 1 pie shell

- 24 graham crackers
- 2 tablespoons jaggary, well ground – or sucanat
- ½ teaspoon cinnamon
- ½ teaspoon cardamom
- ½ pound butter

In bowl, crush crackers into a powder. Melt butter and add spices and sugar. Then add to graham crackers and mix well.

Pour into pie pan to form a pie crust, using spoon or fingers. Let sit to cool down so that the butter hardens again. Bake for 5 minutes at 350. Cool. Fill with your desired filling. You may need to bake again, depending upon what filling you use.

Cranberry

Botanical Name: Vaccinium macrocarpon

Cranberries are grown in swampy, sandy meadows and mossy environments. The fruit of the shrub in ancient times grew wild and today is highly cultivated. The berries are bright red and the size of a small marble. They are high in malic acid and benzoic acid. Cranberries are best eaten when cooked with added sweeteners. They are diuretic and alterative. The juice is good for conditions of infection, skin rashes, and blood poisoning. Best mixed with other juices. Cranberries are a great immunity booster for colds and flu, and support kidney and adrenal functions.

Energy: Warming

Taste: Astringent, Sweet

Post Digestive: Sweet

Indications: Bladder infections, kidney stones, cystitis, blood poisoning

Systems: Urinary Tract, Circulation, Muscular

Dosha Affected:

Vata and **Pitta**: Use with lots of sweetener

Kapha: Good as a diuretic

Mixes Well With: Other acid fruits

Season: Fall or Winter

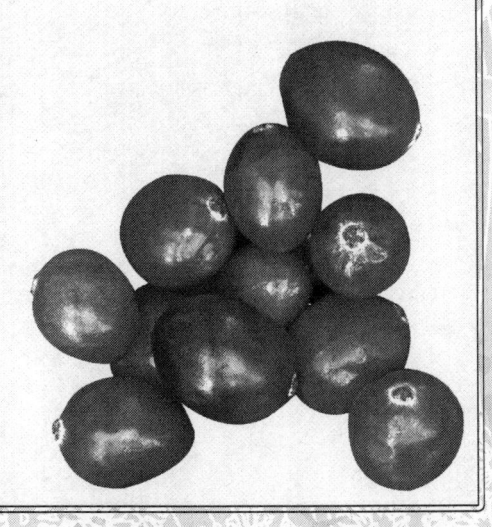

Cranberry Bread

Serves 4

- 2 cups cranberries
- 1 cup orange juice
- 2 tablespoons grated orange peel
- 1½ cups flour, whole wheat or unbleached
- 2 teaspoons baking powder
- 2 eggs, well beaten
- ½ cup sunflower seeds
- ¼ cup coconut
- ¼ cup sucanat or jaggary
- 1 tablespoon ghee

Chop cranberries in blender with orange juice and peel. In large bowl, mix flour, baking powder, and eggs. Fold in cranberries, sunflower seeds, coconut, and sucanat. Oil loaf pan with ghee, spoon in batter, and bake at 250° for 45 minutes.

Cranberry Sauce

Serves 4

- 2 cups cranberries, fresh
- ½ cup orange juice
- ¼ cup water
- 3 tablespoons orange peel, grated
- 1 tablespoon maple syrup
- 1 teaspoon cardamom (optional)
- 1 teaspoon cinnamon (optional)

Place all ingredients in saucepan, and simmer at low heat about 20 minutes (until a smooth gel). Cover, cool, and serve.

Currant

<u>Botanical Name: *Ribes sativum*</u>

Often this fruit is confused with grapes but, as you might notice, it has its own botanical name. It looks like a small grape and is similar in taste, yet is in a whole different category. It is a little hardier than grapes and is mainly cultivated for drying. It is higher in minerals than grapes are.

Energy: Warm

Taste: Sweet, Sour

Post Digestive: Sweet

Indications: Anemia, blood clotting, varicose veins

Systems: Digestive, Endocrine, Circulatory

<u>**Dosha Affected:**</u>

Vata: Good (if soaked overnight)

Pitta: If sweet

Kapha: Only dried

Mixes Well With: Sub-acid and acid fruits

Season: Summer

Ayurvedic Curative Cuisine for Everyone

Currant Energy Bars

Serves 4

2 cups currants

1 cup golden flaxseed

½ cup psyllium seeds

1 teaspoon cinnamon

1 teaspoon slippery elm

grated coconut

Soak currants, flaxseeds, and psyllium seeds overnight, in water that covers them. The next day, grind all ingredients together. Place in pan, and let set for 2 hours in refrigerator. Cut into bars. Sprinkle coconut on top.

Currant Sauce

Serves 2

1 cup currants, dried

2 cups water

¼ teaspoon cardamom

¼ teaspoon ginger

¼ teaspoon cinnamon

Soak dried currants overnight in water. Next day blend currants and water into smooth sauce along with spices.

Can be added to fruit salad or bread.

Fresh Currant Juice

Serves 2

1 pound currants, fresh

1 cup water

1 cup apple juice - best if organic

Remove currents from the vine (like grapes) – Place in blender with water. Liquify. Strain through a colander. Add apple juice.

Date

Botanical Name: Phoenix dactylifera

Dates are one of the oldest foods of the desert. Date palms are famous with many of the scriptures of the world. Another gift from the Gods! These palms are active both as shelter and nutrition. A date palm has to be at least five years old before it can produce fruit and can then give 150 to 200 fruits per year. There are over 7,000 varieties. A mature date can be as large as one to three inches. Unfortunately, most of the dates we get in the market, like bananas, are ripened artificially. Dates are highly nutritious. Tonic. Aphrodisiac. Laxative. Restorative. Good for convalescence, lung diseases, asthma, and fevers. Excellent to add to herbal formulas.

Energy: Cooling, Moisturizing

Taste: Sweet

Post Digestive: Sweet

Indications: Anemia, female problems

Systems: Reproductive, Epithelial, Respiratory

Dosha Affected:

Vata: When dry can aggravate; best soaked

Pitta: Good

Kapha: Avoid

Mixes Well With: All sweet fruits, sub-acids, non-starchy, leafy green vegetables

Date Coconut Malt

<u>Serves 2</u>

8 dates
2 cups coconut milk
2 tablespoons barley malt
1 tablespoon ashwagandha
1 teaspoon vanilla
½ teaspoon cardamom
¼ teaspoon cinnamon

Put all ingredients in blender and blend until smooth

Date Chutney

2 tablespoons ajwan seeds
2 teaspoons coriander
1 tablespoon grated ginger
1 tablespoon grated turmeric
2 tablespoons ghee
½ bunch green onions, well chopped
2 cups dates
½ cup water
3 tablespoons lemon juice
½ bunch cilantro, well chopped
1 teaspoon sea salt

In saucepan, sauté ajwan, coriander, ginger, and turmeric in ghee. Add onions, date, and water, and simmer for 20 minutes. When everything is soft, add lemon juice, cilantro, and salt.

Serve with vegetables and meats.

Raw Tip: Place all ingredients into blender & mix until smooth sauce.

Fig

<u>Botanical Name: Ficus</u>

Fig trees are natives of the Persian Gulf and perfectly adapted to all warm temperate climates, especially that of the Mediterranean. There are about six hundred varieties of fig trees, and very few of these produce fruit. The ficus carica produces the fruit commonly found in the marketplace; it is pear shaped, and usually swollen and hollow. Figs are highly nutritious, and of a similar composition as that of human milk. There are many varieties of figs; Black Mission, Scaimyrna, White Figs, Turkish Smyrna, Adrianic, and the Greek Strings.

Energy: Cooling

Taste: Sweet, Astringent

Post Digestive: Sweet

Indications: Toxic blood, to gain weight, diarrhea, infertility, anti-cancer agent, restorative for the ill, hemorrhoids, juice is good to destroy parasites, indigestion

Systems: Excretory, Immune, Digestive, Respiratory, Urinary Tract

Dosha Affected:

Vata: Moderation (best cooked or in pudding)

Pitta: Good

Kapha: Avoid or reduce

Mixes Well With: Sweet and sub-acid fruits, non-starchy vegetables

Season: Summer & Fall

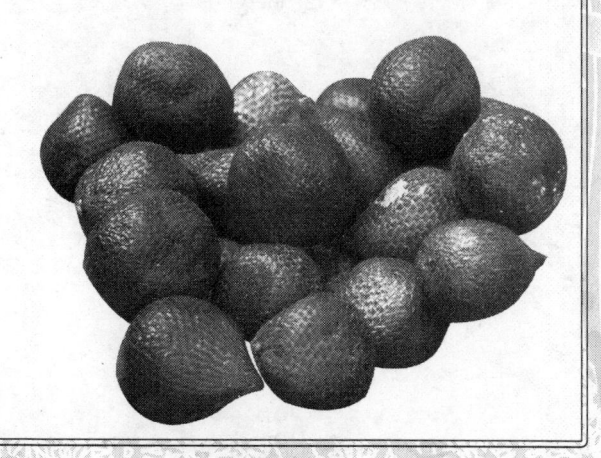

Ayurvedic Curative Cuisine for Everyone

Fig Pudding

Serves 4

- 2 cups figs
- 2 cups water
- 1 teaspoon cardamom
- 1 teaspoon nutmeg
- 1 teaspoon agar agar
- 1 teaspoon arrowroot powder

Soak figs overnight. The next day, blend figs and spices in water until smooth. Place in saucepan and bring to a boil. When boiling, slowly stir in agar agar and arrowroot powder. Refrigerate; serve chilled.

Fig Shake

Serves 4

- 4 figs
- 2 cups almond milk
- 1 tablespoon flax seed
- 1 tablespoon pumpkin seeds
- 1 cup water
- 1 teaspoon of jaggary or black strap molasses

Blend all ingredients in blender. Drink.

Grape

Botanical Name: Vitis

There about 1,500 varieties of grapes cultivated around the world; they are considered to be an ancient fruit. The origin of the grape is somewhat indefinite, because it seems to be from Central Asia but was also found growing wild in Argentina and near the Caspian Sea. It was also seen in Central, South and North America, but failed to grow well in North America until grafting was used. Once planted, grapes need much care and pruning; production is ongoing for as much as fifty years. Other regions where grapes were found growing wild were New York, Michigan, Missouri, and the shores of Lake Erie. Currently, South America is one of the largest exporters in the world. The most important varieties of grapes in the United States are the Concord, Catawba, Salem, Delaware, Jessica, Muscadine, Malaga, Muskat, Sultana, Thompson, and Tokay. One must be very careful when eating grapes due to the high use of pesticides; best to eat organically grown, or at least unsprayed. Eighty-five percent of wine is made from grapes. Because of the concentrated sugar in grapes, they should only be eaten on an empty stomach. Raisins are dried grapes. In Ayurveda, they are used as a tonic. They can also be used as a sweetener substitute and can be added to many medications. When grown without pesticides, they are the best food for cleansing the liver. Grapes are high in elegiac acid, which supports the immune system. High in vitamins B-6 and B-3, biotin, potassium, zinc, and anthrocyanins.

Energy: Cooling

Taste: Sweet, Sour

Post Digestive: Sweet

Indications: Arthritic joints, jaundice, gall bladder problems

Systems: Circulation, Endocrine, Respiratory, Digestive, Urinary Tract, Excretory

Dosha Affected:

Vata: Grapes are good; soak raisins overnight

Pitta: Grapes good if sweet; avoid sour grapes; raisins are good

Kapha: Can have raisins; avoid or reduce grapes

Mixes Well With: Sub-acid and sweet fruits

Season: Summer

Ayurvedic Curative Cuisine for Everyone

Grape and Apple Salad

Serves 2

- 1 pound grapes, pitted
- 2 apples, sliced
- ½ cup raisins, soaked
- 2 tablespoons mint
- 2 tablespoons cilantro

Drain water from raisins. Put all ingredients in salad bowl and mix well.

Grape Liver Flush

Serves 2

- 1 cup grapes
- 2 tablespoons olive oil
- ¼ thumb size fresh ginger, chopped
- 1 teaspoon manjistha powder
- 1 teaspoons guduchi
- 2 tablespoons aloe vera gel – or from fresh leaf
- 1 teaspoon milk thistle
- ¼ teaspoon cardamom
- ¼ teaspoon coriander

Chop the fresh ginger well. Place all ingredients in blender until smooth. Do not eat anything for 2 hours.

Oil must be thoroughly digested.

Draksha Digestive Herbal Wine

- 1 bottle red table wine (sulfite-free) or non-alcoholic red wine
- 1 teaspoon of the following herbs: cinnamon, cardamom, clove ginger, fennel
- ½ teaspoon of following herbs: cumin, coriander, nutmeg, mace, black pepper

Heat wine in pot to 200 degrees or slightly less than boiling. Remove from heat. Add herbs. Cover and steep for 10 minutes.

Strain herbs. If powdered herbs were used, strain through cloth. Serve warm.

Grapefruit

Botanical Name: Citrus paradisi

    Grapefruit is a native of the continent of Asia and the Malaysian Archipelago. All of the species of citrus were brought to the Mediterranean during the period of Alexander in Western Asia. Christopher Columbus planted the first citrus in American soil. Shortly after the introduction into Europe, citrus were used almost exclusively in rituals and medicine. As their reputation grew, people started putting them in seasonings, and it became a common fruit. But for many years, only the wealthiest were able to eat this wonderful fruit. There are many varieties of grapefruit: Washington Navel, Jaffa, Marsh, and pink grapefruit. The Duncan is superior to any other variety in flavor and is delicious; it is called honey sweet grapefruit. Eating the fruit 15 minutes before a meal reduces appetite. It acts as a powerful detoxifier which inhibits cancer cells. The pulp is high in pectin, which prevents cholesterol buildup. The seeds contain anti-parasitic and anti-fungal properties, but it is best to use the extract of grapefruit seeds.

Energy: Warm

Taste: Sour, Astringent

Post Digestive: Sour

Indications: Obesity, diabetes, high cholesterol, colds, flu

Systems: Circulatory, Respiratory, Digestive, Endocrine

Dosha Affected:

Vata: Good

Pitta: Moderation

Kapha: Moderation (even though it assists in weight loss, it can be aggravating and sour-producing in the body. Long use of grapefruit can aggravate Kapha)

Mixes Well With: Acid and sub-acid fruits, greens

Season: Tropical Fall & Winter

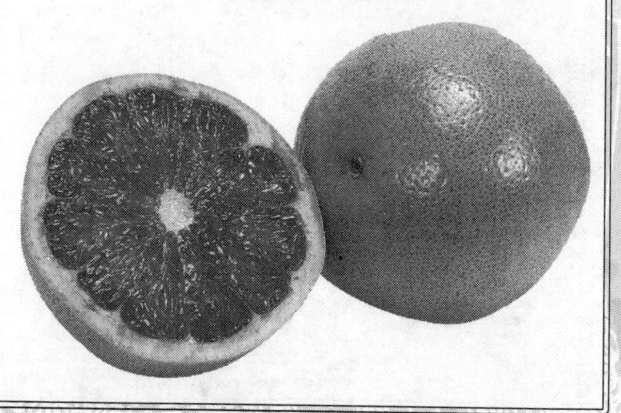

Selene's Grapefruit and Fennel Salad

Serves 4

- 3 pink grapefruit
- ½ cup olive oil
- 2 tablespoons balsamic vinegar
- ¼ ounces Juniper berries
- 1 whole bulb fennel, thinly sliced
- ½ bunch chives
- 1 tablespoon dillweed, well chopped

Take one grapefruit and juice well. Remove skins of two grapefruits and cut them in sections. Place juice, grapefruit sections, and remaining ingredients in bowl, and mix well. Cover and marinate overnight.

Stuffed Grapefruit

- 2 grapefruits
- ½ avocado, chopped
- 2 tablespoons maple syrup
- 1 cup rolled oats
- 1 tablespoon ghee
- ¼ cup cilantro or mint
- ½ cup sunflower seeds, ground
- 1 tablespoon grated ginger

Cut grapefruits in half. Remove sections with spoon and cut into small pieces. Mix with avocado and agave, and set aside. Roast oats in skillet. After oats are roasted, add ghee, cilantro, ground sunflower seeds, and ginger. Remove pan from heat, and stir in grapefruit mixture. Fill grapefruit shells with mixture.

Guava

Botanical Name: Psidium cattleianum

The guava is a native of Central and South America and dispersed throughout tropical climates. It is often seen in Florida and California. When a freeze occurs, however, there is no crop. Fortunately, within a few months, it will grow again. The guava is a very handsome small tree, similar to the mulberry, with very fragrant flowers. It is known as the apple of the tropics. It is filled with a multitude of tiny seeds, smaller than those of a tomato, only hard instead of soft. They can sometimes be troublesome to the teeth and intestines due to being difficult to chew. Some fruits are round and some are shaped like a small pear; some have yellow skin, others are white. They range in size from that of a large cherry to that of an apple. They are high in vitamins A and C, rich in fiber, and help the body detoxify to fight autoimmune disorders.

Energy: Warming

Taste: Sweet, Sour

Post Digestive: Sweet

Indications: Infections, colds, flu, fevers, asthma, bronchitis, fights bacteria, cndida, virus infection, parasites

Systems: Digestive, Circulatory, Respiratory, Immune

Dosha Affected:
Good for all doshas (Pittas must be sure it is ripe and sweet)

Mixes Well With: Sub-acid and sweet fruits

Guava Paste

- 10 ripe medium guavas, well washed
- 2 cups water
- ¼ cup lemon juice
- ¼ cup sucanat or jaggary
- 2 teaspoon arrowroot

Cut guavas in half and place in blender. Add water, lemon juice, and sucanat, and blend well. Place mixture in saucepan; bring to a boil and then add arrowroot, stirring well. Simmer for 45 minutes until mixture gels. Put in a baking pan and refrigerate to let it gel further.

Serve as a jelly substitute on crackers or sandwiches, or with fruit salad.

Guava Amaranth Pudding

- 1 cup amaranth
- 4 ripe guavas
- 1 tablespoon ghee
- ¼ cup water
- 1 teaspoon cardamom
- 1 teaspoon cinnamon
- 1 tablespoon honey

Soak amaranth overnight; drain the next day.

Scoop out guava pulp, and sauté in ghee for 10 minutes. Add water and cook for 25 minutes, to reduce liquid. Add spices and soaked amaranth; cook for 15 minutes more. Stir in honey; serve after cooling.

Guava Ghee

- 2 cups fresh ghee
- 4 guava, fresh -or- 2 ounces of guava paste

Chop guava into small pieces. When using fresh, you will need to blend in a food processor, blender, or a Vita-Mix. Serve on bread or crackers.

Kiwi

Botanical Name: Actinida chineusis

The kiwi is a native of China and sometimes called "Chinese Gooseberry." It was introduced into New Zealand in 1906 where cultivation was improved, and now NZ monopolizes kiwi production. Kiwis grow on a vine and are egg-shaped, 3 inches long, green in color, with the flesh and juice being sweet/sour in taste. They contain acetic and bromic acids. The vitamin content of kiwis keeps up to 6 weeks if refrigerated. They are high in vitamins C, B-3, and beta-carotene. The fruit is slightly tart and is best eaten when ripe. The Chinese have experimented with this fruit for esophageal cancer and found that high levels of nitrates were reduced in patient. Very high in vitamin A and potassium.

Energy: Warming

Taste: Sweet, Sour, Astringent

Post Digestive: Sour

Indications: Bronchitis, asthma, colds, fevers, heart, high blood pressure

Systems: Respiration, Excretory, Circulation

Dosha Affected:

Vata: Good

Pitta: Avoid

Kapha: Moderation

Mixes Well With: Sub-acid and acid fruits

Season: Tropical Winter

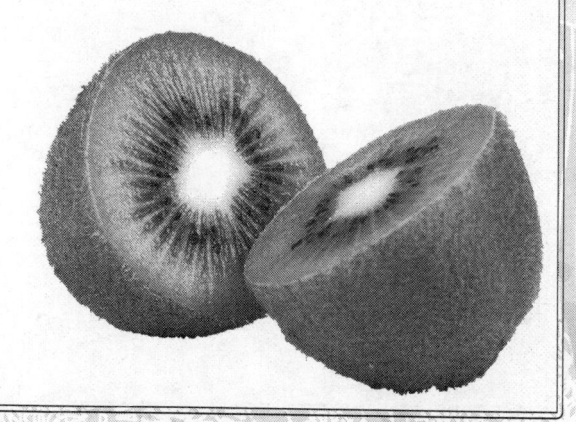

Kiwi Gel

- 3 cups water
- 1 lime
- 2 tablespoons agar agar, flakes or powder
- ¼ cup sucanat or jaggary
- 6 kiwis, peeled and sliced into rings

Boil water; add lime juice, agar agar, and sweetener. Place kiwi rings in a baking dish, and pour mixture over them. Let it gel, then refrigerate. Serve as a gelatin.

Kiwi Shake

Serves 4

- 4 kiwi
- 1 teaspoon vanilla extract
- 1 cup pineapple juice
- 1 cup coconut milk
- ¼ teaspoon cinnamon

Peel kiwi. Blend until smooth. Drink.

Kumquat

<u>Botanical Name: Fortunella margarita</u>

The kumquat resembles a tiny, golden orange. Originating in China, the tree grows to 16 to 20 feet high. It was introduced in Europe in 1846. The size of the fruit is approximately one to two inches in length, and it is covered with an edible rind. The rind is sweet, but the fruit is not so sweet. It is often an ornamental tree in Florida and Southern California.

Energy: Warming

Taste: Sour, Astringent

Post Digestive: Sour

Indications: Jaundice, infections, diabetes

Systems: Circulatory, Respiratory, Urinary, Excretory, Lymphatic

Dosha Affected:

Vata: Good

Pitta: Avoid

Kapha: Moderation

Mixes Well With: Sub-acid and acid fruits, green leafy vegetables

Season: Tropical Spring & Summer

Kumquat Dressing

- 1 cup kumquats, cut in half
- ½ bunch cilantro, chopped
- 1/3 cup olive oil
- 2 tablespoons Bragg's
- 2 tablespoons coriander
- 1 teaspoon fennel
- 1 tablespoon lemon juice, fresh

Mix all ingredients in blender until smooth. Serve on salad, on top of steamed leafy green vegetables, or on grilled vegetables.

Kumquat Ice Cream

Serves 4

- 2 cups almond milk, frozen
- 2 pounds frozen kumquats
- 1 cup jaggary or raw sugar
- 1 teaspoon vanilla
- ½ teaspoon almond extract

Freeze kumquats for 2 or 3 days. When well frozen, remove from freezer along with frozen almond milk. Add all ingredients together, except the almond milk. Blend very slowly on low setting. Add the frozen almond milk slowly and blend with kumquat mixture. Blend - Do not liquefy (or you will get a juice).

Lemon

Botanical Name: Citrus limonia

The lemon is a native of China and India, introduced to Palestine during the 10th century, and brought into Europe by the Franciscan Monks. It was introduced to the Americas by Christopher Columbus. Lemons are not cultivated nearly as much as oranges but have the greatest commercial value of the entire citrus family. The tree and flowers are faster growing and larger than those of an orange tree. The fruit has more commercial uses.

Energy: Cooling

Taste: Sour, Astringent

Post Digestive: Sour

Indications: Sore throats, appetite stimulant, liver/gall bladder disorders, age spots

Systems: Good for all systems

Dosha Affected:

Vata: Good

Pitta: Moderation (must take with sweetener)

Kapha: Moderation

Mixes Well With: Sub-acid and acid fruits, great on fish or in ceviche (raw fish marinated in lemon juice)

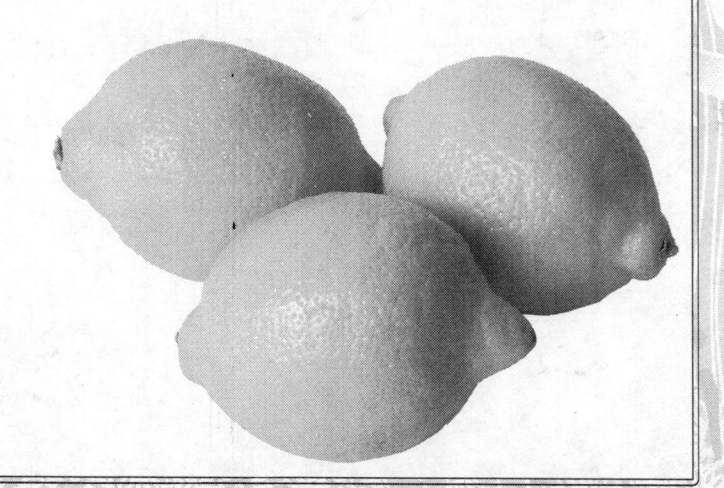

Ayurvedic Curative Cuisine for Everyone

Lemon Ginger Blast

Makes ½ gallon

- Juice of 3-4 lemons
- 2 quarts water
- 2 teaspoons fennel seeds
- ¼ cup chopped ginger
- honey or maple syrup

Blend lemon juice, water, fennel, and ginger in blender. Strain through colander and discard solids. Add honey or maple syrup to taste.

Lemon Kale

Serves 4

- 2 ½ cups kale, thinly sliced
- ½ cup olive oil
- 2 teaspoons cumin seeds
- 1 tablespoon ghee
- 1 bunch green onions, chopped
- 2 teaspoons coriander
- 2 teaspoons ground cumin
- ½ cup lemon juice
- Bragg's, salt or Nama Shoyu tamari
- ½ cup cilantro, well chopped
- Soak kale in olive oil for 2 hours.

Roast cumin seeds in skillet for 5 to 10 minutes, then add ghee, green onions, coriander, and ground cumin. When onions are soft, add the soaked kale, lemon juice and Bragg's to taste. Just before serving, add cilantro.

Lemon Three-Layer Cake

- 1 box yellow cake mix (purchase at health food store)
- 2 cups sucanat or jaggary
- 1 cups lemon juice
- 1 tablespoon ghee
- 2 tablespoons lemon zest (grated lemon peel)

Follow instructions on cake mix box, but pour batter equally into three round cake pans. When cakes are done, let them cool.

In blender, mix lemon juice, sweetener, and ghee until it becomes a syrup. Place first layer of cake on a plate and saturate it with one third of the syrup while poking holes into each cake with chopstick or other utensil so that lemon sauce will penetrate cake well. Stack on the second layer and saturate it, and finally repeat with the remaining layer. Sprinkle lemon zest on top, and enjoy!

Lemon Ice

Serves 2

- 1 cup lemon juice
- ½ cup mint
- 1 teaspoon fennel powder
- 2 cups water
- 4 cups crushed ice cubes
- ¼ cup suganat

Place the lemon, mint, fennel, sugar, and water together and blend in a blender until well blended. Then make ice cubes out of this mixture. When frozen, place cubes into blender to slowly crush the cubes. Do not mix too long or it will liquefy – you want it to be like an ice cone. If more ice is need add more.

Ayurvedic Curative Cuisine for Everyone

Lime

Botanical Name: Citrus aurantifolius Citrus latifolia

The lime is a native of the Malaysian Archipelago. The least acidic of all citrus fruits, it grows on a small, thorny, tropical evergreen. The flowers are smaller than all other citrus. The skin is thinner, and the fruit weighs less than a lemon. Limes are extremely sensitive to frost and grow best in tropical climates. The two kinds of limes typically found in U.S. markets are the larger Persian (or Bears) limes, and the smaller Key (or Mexican) limes. Lime juice makes an excellent addition to seafood, as it will destroy any toxins. Also, the sour taste stimulates hydrochloric acid, which helps with assimilation of proteins.

Energy: Cooling

Taste: Sour, Bitter

Post Digestive: Sour

Indications: Sore throat, obesity, liver/gall bladder disorders

Systems: Circulatory, Endocrine, Digestive

Dosha Affected:

Vata: Good

Pitta: Good

Kapha: Moderation

Mixes Well With: Acid fruits

Season: Tropical Late Summer - Early Fall

Mint Limeade

½ cup fresh lime juice

¼ cup mint leaves

1 tablespoon fennel seeds

4 cups water

sucanat or jaggary

Blend lime juice with mint leaves and fennel seeds in blender, then strain, and discard pulp. Put back in blender with water and sucanat to taste; blend well. Serve chilled.

Bucerias Key Lime Pie

Serves 6

4 egg yolks

2½ teaspoons key lime zest (grated lime peel)

2 cups thick cashew or almond milk (unstrained)

1/3 cup key lime juice

3 tablespoons sucanat or jaggary

1 teaspoon vanilla

graham cracker crust

Preheat oven to 300°. In mixing bowl, beat egg yolks and zest together. Slowly add nut milk and mix until well combined. Add lime juice, sweetener, and vanilla. Pour into crust and bake 30 minutes, or until center of pie is done. Cool, and then refrigerate.

Loquat

Botanical Name: Eriobotrya japonica

The loquat plant is native to Japan and is also called "Japanese Plum." It is used as an ornamental plant and is closely related to the apple and pear. The fruits grow in clusters like grapes, yellow-orange in color, and each has a large seed with a firm covering. The flavor resembles that of a cherry. The loquat tree is often seen in Florida and Southern California, where it is often wasted because its owners are not aware of its sweet taste.

Energy: Warm

Taste: Sweet

Post Digestive: Sweet

Indications: Liver/gall bladder disorders, colds, flu

Systems: Endocrine, Digestive, Immune, Respiratory

Dosha Affected:

Vata and **Pitta**: Good

Kapha: Moderation

Mixes Well With: Sub-acid and acid fruits

Season: Tropical Late Spring, Summer

Loquat Apple Smoothie

- 1 cup loquats, pitted
- 2 cups apple juice
- ½ cup orange juice

Blend all ingredients together until smooth.

Loquat Cough Syrup

- 8 loquats, fresh
- ½ cup water
- 1 tablespoon raw honey
- ½ tablespoon lime juice
- ¼ thumb size fresh ginger

Pit the loquats. Mix all ingredients in blender until smooth. Drink. Can keep in refrigerator for a while.

Loquat Preserves

Makes 8 ounces

- 12-16 loquats, fresh, pitted
- ½ cup water
- 1 tablespoons jaggary
- 1 teaspoon honey

Grate jaggary. Add loquat, water, & jaggary into a pan. Simmer on very low for 15-20 minutes. When water evaporates, cool down and add honey. Place in a jar and refrigerate.

Lychee

<u>Botanical Name: *Litchi chinensis*</u>

The lychee (or litchi) is a rare, exotic, delicious delicacy from China. It is often found in U.S. markets in Chinatown. This fruit is not well known in the U.S. but has been cultivated in Asia for over 2000 years, where it has become part of the Chinese New Year celebration. It is served in Chinese restaurants in a preserved form. In the U.S., it can also be found dried and similar in taste to a raisin. It can be seen in many Florida yards as an ornamental tree. The fruit is red in color, the size of a large grape, with a firm skin, and contains a large seed surrounded by delicious, succulent, white, gelatinous flesh.

Energy: Cooling

Taste: Sweet

Post Digestive: Sweet

Indications: Ulcer, female tonic, to gain weight, constipation

Systems: Digestive, Excretory, Reproductive

Dosha Affected:

Vata and **Pitta**: Good

Kapha: Normally avoid – but because it is such a delicacy it should at least be experienced in small quantities

Mixes Well With: Sweet fruits

Lychee Ambrosia for the Gods

- 1 cup raisins
- ½ cup dates, quartered
- 2 cup water
- 1 pound lychees
- ¼ cup maple syrup
- 1 teaspoon cinnamon

Soak raisins and dates overnight in water. The next day, remove skins from lychees, cut them in half, and remove pits. Place all ingredients in saucepan; simmer until lychees are soft and mixture is of a sauce consistency.

Serve with fruit salad.

Lychee Ice Cream

Serves 2

- 2 cups lychee, peeled, pitted
- 2 tablespoons raw sugar or sucanat
- 4 cups frozen cream made into cubes in ice cube tray
- 1 teaspoon, ginger, grated
- ½ teaspoon vanilla

Put all ingredients in the blender at a low speed. Slowly increase to a higher speed. Do not liquefy. Serve.

Ayurvedic Curative Cuisine for Everyone

Mango

Botanical Name: Mangifera indica

The mango is an ancient fruit which has been cultivated for over 4,000 years. It has been used by the Hindus for many medicinal uses. The fruit is grown in the tropics and available in many western markets. The tree can be as tall as 60 feet high. The fruit is oval to ovate in form and can weigh from 6 ounces to 3 pounds. Mangos can be used in chutneys, as fruit preserves, and in pies. There are approximately 500 varieties in the world. The juice is rich in flavor and is a high source of Vitamin C. The tree is in the Sumac family. The sap and skin of the fruit can cause itching and skin irritation. Over-consumption can cause Pitta fevers and skin swelling.

Energy: Warm

Taste: Sweet, Pungent

Post Digestive: Sweet

Indications: Constipation, dysentery, jaundice, hemorrhoids

Systems: Digestive, Endocrine, Excretory

Dosha Affected:

Vata: Excellent

Pitta: Moderation (can cause skin irritations – and must be eaten ripe)

Kapha: Moderation

Mixes Well With: Sub-acid fruits

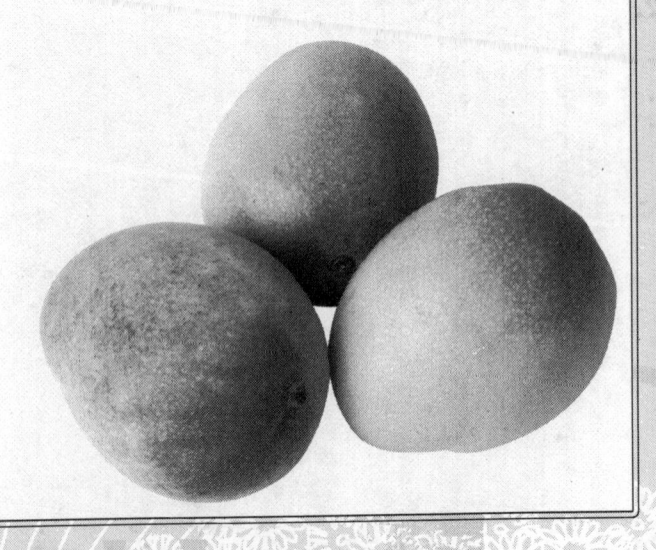

Mango Chutney

- 1 teaspoon cumin seeds
- 1 tablespoon ghee
- 1 medium onion, chopped
- 2 ripe mangos, peeled and chopped
- 1 teaspoon coriander, ground
- 1 teaspoon cloves, ground
- 2 tablespoons lemon juice
- 1 tablespoon sucanat or jaggary

Roast cumin seeds in skillet. Add ghee and onions, and cook until onions are caramelized. Add remaining ingredients, mix well. Store in refrigerator.

Raw tip: You can also pulse raw ingredients together in a food processor until blended but still chunky.

Mango Lassi

- 2 ripe mangos, peeled and chopped
- 2 tablespoons (1 ounce) rosewater
- 1 cup yogurt, unsweetened
- ½ teaspoon cardamom
- ¼ teaspoon sucanat or jaggary
- 1 teaspoon vanilla

Mix all ingredients together in blender.

Melon

<u>Botanical Name: *Cucumis melo*</u>

Melons are native to Asia and Africa. They were introduced to Europe and North America by the missionaries. There are many varieties today, including muskmelon, nutmeg melon, casaba or winter melon, honeydew, and cantaloupe. Watermelon is loosely considered a type of melon, but has a different botanical classification (*Citrullus lanatus*).

Energy: Cool

Taste: Sweet

Post Digestive: Sweet

Indications: Constipation, bladder infection, colitis

Systems: Urinary Tract, Endocrine, Excetory

<u>Dosha Affected:</u>

Good for all doshas

Mixes Well With: Other melons, papayas

Season: Summer & Early Fall

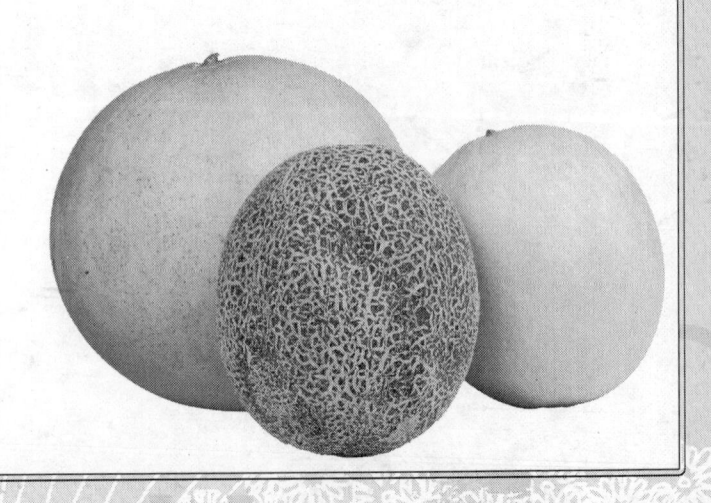

Melon Salad

Serves 4

- 2 slices watermelon
- 2 slices honeydew
- 2 slices cantaloupe
- 1 slice casaba melon
- 1 teaspoon cinnamon
- 1 teaspoon fennel
- 1 teaspoon ginger
- 1 teaspoon cardamom
- fresh mint

Cut fruit into cubes, add spices, and mix in mint.

Watermelon Juice

Makes approximately 1 quart

- ½ water melon, sliced
- 1 teaspoon lime juice

Remove the green & white portions of watermelon. Cut red portion into small pieces. Blend until smooth. Strain the pulp in a colander, pressing pulp to get more juice. Then add lime or lemon juice. Drink.

Nectarine

Botanical Name: Prunus persica

Nectarines are actually the same species as peaches, but with smoother skin. The nectarine is smaller in size than a peach, and its taste is sweeter and stronger than a peach. Those who do not like the fuzziness of peaches may prefer nectarines instead.

Energy: Warm

Taste: Sweet, Sour

Post Digestive: Sweet

Indications: Stomach disorders, infections

Systems: Digestive, Circulatory, Immune

Dosha Affected:

Vata: Good

Pitta and **Kapha**: Moderation

Mixes Well With: All fruits

Season: Summer

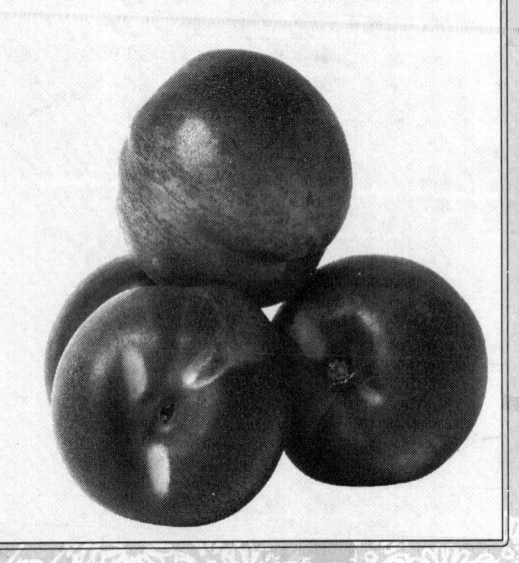

Nectarine Salad

Serves 4

4 nectarines, cut in small pieces
½ cup ground almonds
1 cup chopped celery
½ cup cilantro, chopped
2 tablespoons lemon juice
1 tablespoon jaggary or sucanat
½ teaspoon vanilla

Mix all ingredients in a bowl.

Nectarine Pudding

Serves 4

4 nectarines, sliced
¼ teaspoon nutmeg
¼ teaspoon cinnamon
¼ teaspoon ginger
3 tablespoon tapioca flour
1 ½ tablespoons ghee
2 tablespoons jaggary or raw sugar
3 tablespoons of quick oats

Cut nectarines into slices. Oil baking dish. In a bowl, place nectarines, ghee, tapioca, flour, and spices. Mix.

Bake at 350 for 25-30 minutes.

Orange

<u>Botanical Name:</u> *Citrus sinensis*

The orange is queen of the fruits, and one of the oldest fruits known to man. Its origin is from India and China; it has spread all over the subtropical and tropical parts of the world. This fruit has made history in many of the ancient texts, as in the Charaka Samhita. It was brought to the Americas by the Spanish Conquistadors. The Seminole Indians traded for the orange and took long journeys and vision quests carrying only this fruit. Along the way, they dropped the seeds, which was the beginning of the famous Florida orange groves. Originally, there were mostly sour oranges and less of the sweet variety. We now have mostly sweet oranges among the 10 to 15 varieties available on the market. It is very important to rinse the mouth after eating citrus, as the citric acid is known to erode dental enamel. Over-consumption will cause skin and arthritic symptoms. Best to avoid all citrus for arthritic or rheumatic conditions. Best to eat oranges when fully ripe. If green, may cause problems with joints due to the acid content.

Energy: Sweet, Sour, Cool

Taste: Sweet

Post Digestive: Sweet

Indications: Asthma, constipation, cellulite, colds, flu, varicose veins

Systems: Respiratory, Digestive, Circulatory

Dosha Affected:

Vata and **Pitta**: Good

Kapha: Moderation

Mixes Well With: Sub-acid and acid fruits, green leafy vegetables

Season: Tropical Fall & Winter

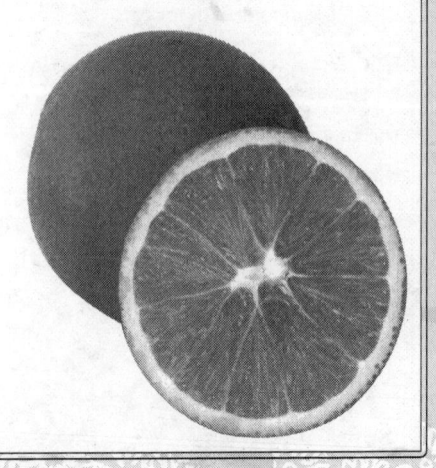

Orange-Kiwi Delight

Serves 6

- 3 cups orange juice, fresh
- 2 cups apple juice, fresh if possible
- ½ package agar flakes
- 2 cups kiwi slices, peeled

Put orange juice and apple juice in saucepan and cook until boiling. Add agar flakes, stirring until smooth. Layer kiwi slices in baking pan. Pour half of the juice mixture over the kiwi, add another layer of kiwi, and pour the remaining juice over it. Cool until gelled.

Orange-Almond Drink

Serves 3

- 2 cups orange juice, fresh squeezed
- 1 teaspoon vanilla
- 1 teaspoon slippery elm
- 1 cup almond milk

Mix all ingredients in blender. Drink quickly otherwise it will become Very thick and firm.

Papaya

Botanical Name: Carica papaya

The papaya is a native of Central America and was brought to Africa, Asia, and Polynesia by missionaries. It is one of the most important fruits in tropical climates, easy to grow, and bears fruit in nine months to one year. The tree has an appearance similar to a small palm tree. It grows vertically 3 to 4 feet per year; the fruit must eventually be picked with a long pole. It can produce fruit for ten to fifteen years. There are many varieties and sizes. The fruit is cylindrical, with soft smooth skin, and has a yellow-orange color when ripe. Many Asians prefer to eat the fruit unripe as a starchy fruit salad. This is wise, because the green fruit has more papain enzymes. Inside this delicious fruit, there are many black gelatin-like seeds about the size of small peas. Shipping of this fruit is often unsuccessful as it spoils easily; therefore, it is more common in the marketplaces of Florida, California, and Hawaii. Mexican papayas are often as large as a football. Hawaii has a small "sunrise" variety with very sweet red flesh.

Energy: Warm

Taste: Sweet

Post Digestive: Sweet

Indications: Indigestion, ulcers, constipation, psoriasis

Systems: Digestive, Excretory, Immune, Reproductive

Dosha Affected:

Vata: (decreases) – best eaten with a bit of lemon

Pitta: (increases) – reduce consumption

Kapha: Moderation

Mixes Well With: Sweet fruits and melons.

Season: Tropical, year round

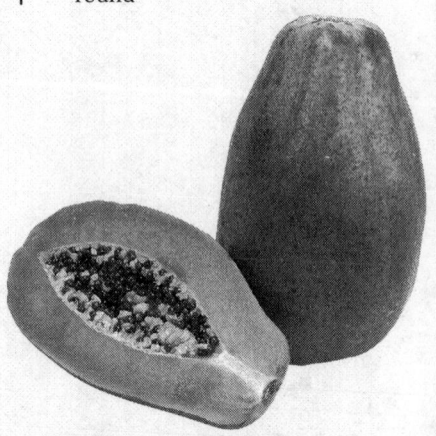

Green Papaya Salad

Serves 2

1 large papaya, green
¼ cup lemon juice
½ bunch green onions, chopped
¼ cup raisins, soaked
1 teaspoon sea salt
½ bunch cilantro, well chopped
½ bunch mint, well chopped

Grate fresh, green, firm papaya into a bowl; add lemon juice and chopped onions. Add soaked raisins and sea salt, and let marinate for about 45 minutes. Add cilantro and mint; serve on bed of lettuce.

Papaya Chutney

2 teaspoons cumin seeds
2 tablespoons ghee
1 medium onion, chopped
1 medium papaya
½ cup water
¼ cup apple cider vinegar
¼ cup sucanat or jaggary
1 teaspoon salt
1 teaspoon curry, mild
½ teaspoon cinnamon

In saucepan, roast cumin seeds until aroma is released. Add ghee and onions, and sauté until caramelized. Remove skin and seeds of papaya, chop well; add papaya and water to pan; simmer for 10 minutes. Add vinegar, sucanat, salt, and spices; cover pan and simmer on low for 15 minutes more. Store in jar in refrigerator.

Raw tip: Just pulse ingredients in a food processor instead of cooking.

Baked Papaya with Syrup

- 1 large papaya (or 3 small ones), cut in half and seeds removed
- 4 tablespoons ghee
- Juice of one lime or lemon
- 1 cup raisins or dried cranberries, soaked
- 1 tablespoon ginger, grated
- 1 tablespoon mint, chopped
- 2 tablespoons honey

Preheat oven to 250°. Place papayas in baking pan with skin side down and baste with some of the ghee and the lemon juice. Bake for 10 to 15 minutes, then remove from oven. Blend raisins with leftover ghee, ginger, mint and honey in a blender. Pour the mixture over baked papaya and garnish with mint.

Raw tip: Mix ingredients together and allow to marinate 20 minutes.

Papaya Shake

Serves 2

- 2 cups papaya
- ¼ cup dry elderberries
- ¼ thumb size piece of fresh ginger
- 2 cups coconut milk or water
- ¼ teaspoon ginger powder
- 1 teaspoon jaggary
- 1 tablespoon lemon or lime juice

Place all ingredients in blender. Blend until smooth. Drink.

Passion Fruit

Botanical Name: Passiflora edulis

The passion fruit is a vining plant native to Brazil. In various countries it goes by the names of granadilla, maracuja, lilikoi, chanola, parcha, and markisa. Brought to other tropical areas of the world by missionaries and is today highly cultivated in Malaysia. The skin is fibrous, but the jelly is a mass of orange seeds. It is flavorful eaten alone or blended, strained, and sweetened. Extremely high in vitamin C and potassium.

Energy: Cooling

Taste: Sweet, Sour

Post Digestive: Sweet

Indications: Fever, infection, colds, flu, asthma, bronchitis, insomnia

Systems: Immune, Respiratory, Nervous

Dosha Affected:

Vata: Good

Pitta and **Kapha**: Moderation

Mixes Well With: Sub-acid and acid fruits, honey-lemon drinks

Season: Tropical year round

Passion Lemon Drink

- 2 cups passion fruit pulp
- ½ cup lemon juice, fresh
- 4 tablespoons agave syrup
- 2 teaspoons fresh mint (or 1 teaspoon dried mint)
- 2 quarts water

Cut passion fruits in half and scoop out the pulp (seeds included). Place pulp & seeds in blender with lemon juice, agave, and mint; blend well on high speed. Strain through fine mesh strainer, add water, and garnish with fresh mint leaves before serving.

Aloha Shake

Serves 4

- 2 cups passion fruit, pulp
- 1 cup coconut milk
- ¼ cup pineapple chunks, fresh
- ½ teaspoon ginger, grated
- 1 cup pineapple juice

Blend all ingredients together until smooth. Serve.

Passion Fruit Coconut Drink

Serves 4

- 6 passion fruit
- 1 cup coconut water
- 1 cup coconut milk

Place all ingredients in blender until smooth. Serve.

Peach

Botanical Name: Prunus persica

This fruit can easily be called the national fruit of the United States because of its agricultural abundance. Its consumption is comparable with apples and oranges. One significant difference is that it does not have as long a shelf life. A native of Persia and China, it is another fruit brought to North America by the colonizers. The peach was known at one time as a Persian Apple. Today, there are hundreds of varieties cultivated throughout the world. In order to extend the life cycle, this tree requires very good soil with much care and pruning.

Energy: Warming

Taste: Sweet, Sour

Post Digestive: Sweet

Indications: Colds, constipation, liver/gall bladder disorders, blood purifier

Systems: Respiratory, Excretory, Reproductive

Dosha Affected:

Vata: Good

Pitta: Moderation (the peach skin can be a skin irritant)

Kapha: Avoid or reduce (Increases)

Mixes Well With: Sub-acid and sweet fruits

Season: Spring & Summer

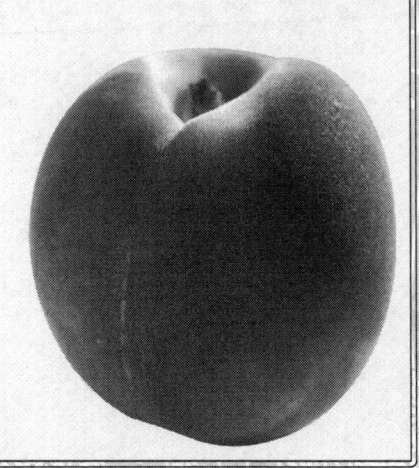

Peach Porridge

<u>**Serves 2**</u>

- 1 cup oat bran
- 1 tablespoon ghee
- 1 cup sunflower seeds, ground
- 1 cup almond milk
- 1 teaspoon grated ginger
- 1 teaspoon vanilla
- 4 peaches, peeled and sliced thin

In skillet, sauté oat bran in ghee. Then stir in sunflower seeds, milk, ginger, vanilla, and peaches. Cover and cook on low for 20 minutes. Serve warm or cold.

Peach Pie

<u>**Serves 6**</u>

- 6 peaches, pitted
- 12 ounces apple juice
- 3 tablespoons arrowroot
- ½ teaspoon baking powder
- ½ teaspoon cinnamon
- ½ teaspoon cardamom
- 2 tablespoons jaggary, grated

Cut peaches into small slices. In separate pan, mix apple juice, arrowroot, baking powder, and spices together. Simmer until slightly thickened. Fold in the peaches. Pour mixture into a pie crust. Bake at 325 for 30 minutes.

Pear

Botanical Name: Pyrus communis

The pear tree is older than the olive tree. Next to grapes, pears were originally used extensively for making fermented pear wines in Italy. The pear is indigenous to Europe and Asia and grows well in most temperate climates, although it is more limited in productivity than apples. There are a few hundred varieties of pears found around the world. The best flavor occurs when fruit is ripe. When purchasing pears unripe, store them at room temperature until soft (placing them next to a banana will actually hasten the ripening). The many different varieties of pears include Bartlett, Bosc, Comice, Concorde, Conference, d'Anjou, Passe-Crassane, and Seckel.

Energy: Cooling

Taste: Sweet

Post Digestive: Sweet

Indications: Stomach disorders, fevers, liver/gall bladder disorders, blood tonic

Systems: Digestive, Immune, Circulatory

Dosha Affected:

Vata: Avoid (unless cooked with spices)

Pitta and **Kapha**: Good

Mixes Well With: Sub-acid and sweet fruits

Season: Fall & Winter

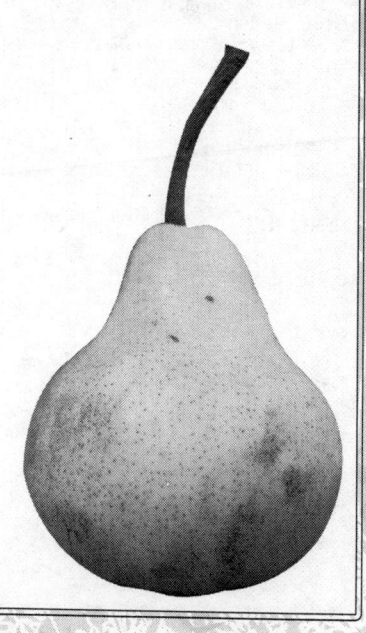

Bodhie's Poached Pears in Port Wine Sauce

Serves 3

- 1 12 ounce bottle port wine
- 1 cup sucanat
- 2 pieces of star anise
- 1 stick cinnamon
- 3 whole pears (Bartlett)

Cook wine, sucanat, and spices in a saucepan over low heat until it becomes a syrup. Add whole pears and simmer until soft but not broken. Cool both liquid and pears. Arrange pears on plates, pour syrup over them, and serve.

Pear Sauce

- 6 pears, peeled, cored, and chopped
- ½ cup water
- 1/3 cup lemon juice
- 1 teaspoon cinnamon
- 1 teaspoon cardamom
- ½ cup raisins, soaked

Put pears, water, lemon juice, raisins, and spices in a saucepan, and simmer on low heat until pears are soft. Blend until smooth.

Raw tip: This can also be simply blended in a blender until smooth.

Add this sauce to a fruit salad, spread on crackers, or eat by itself.

Persimmon

Botanical Name: Diospyros

Persimmon trees love the subtropical weather of Japan and China. Today, they are found growing wild in Florida, Louisiana, Texas, and California. The fruit is globular in form, with a thin skin, pink to orange in color, and can also be yellow inside. There are many species of persimmon. The astringent types, such as Hachiya, need to be eaten when very ripe and soft, or their enzymes will "turn your mouth inside out." The non-astringent types, such as Kaki or Fuyu (Fuju), can be eaten like an apple when still hard.

Energy: Cooling

Taste: Sweet, Sour, Astringent

Post Digestive: Sweet

Indications: Constipation, liver/gall bladder disorders, infertility, lung tonic

Systems: Excretory, Reproductive, Circulatory

Dosha Affected:

Vata and **Pitta**: Good

Kapha: Avoid or reduce (unless a Fuyu variety)

Mixes Well With: Sub-acid fruits, sweet fruits

Season: Fall & Winter

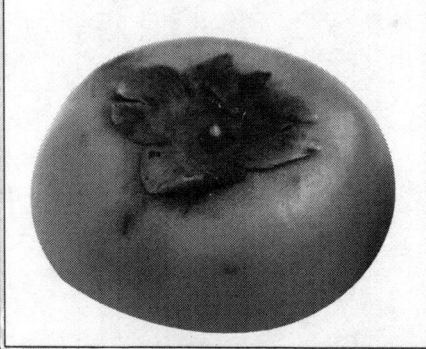

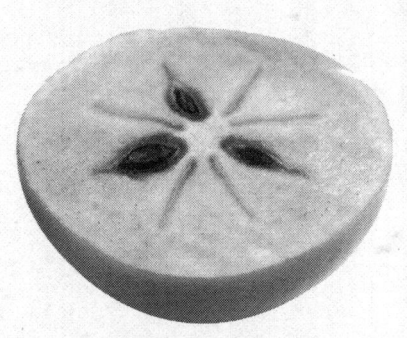

Persimmon Ginger Crisp

Serves 6

- ½ cup amaranth flour
- 2 tablespoons sucanat
- 1 cup rolled oats
- 1 cup ghee
- 2 tablespoons sucanat or jaggary
- 4 tablespoons pastry flour
- ½ teaspoon nutmeg
- 1 teaspoon cinnamon
- ¼ teaspoon ground ginger powder
- 1½ teaspoon fresh grated ginger
- 5 persimmons (fuyu), sliced

Preheat oven at 350°. To make topping, combine amaranth flour, sucanat, oats, and ghee in blender. Set aside. In a bowl combine sucanat, pastry flour, and spices. Add persimmon slices and fresh ginger, mix well. Pour into a buttered dish, and cover with the topping. Bake until the persimmons are soft, about 45 minutes.

Persimmon Pudding

Serves 2

- 3 persimmons, ripe
- 1 teaspoon cinnamon
- 1 cup coconut cream, fresh is best – Or if canned, drain water out.

Slowly blend into pudding consistency. If additional water is necessary, add some from canned coconut or use any good water.

Pineapple

<u>Botanical Name: *Ananas comosus*</u>

The pineapple plant looks like a tough, stiff grass with sharp pointed thorn-edged leaves, which can become as high as four feet. Even though many people experience the pineapple, very few in our part of the world have experienced its true flavor because the fruit is picked green for shipment. If picked when ripe, the taste is exquisite. Pineapples usually weigh 2 to 6 pounds, and are native to South America and Hawaii. At one time, Florida grew a large amount of pineapple but no longer does so, due to an unstable climate. The Philippines is the largest supplier for U. S. consumption now that Hawaiian production has fallen off. Green fruit and plants contain the proteolytic enzyme bromelain which, in high doses, can dissolve injured tissue, tumors, and clots. It also reduces inflammation.

Energy: Warming

Taste: Sweet, Astringent, Sour

Post Digestive: Sweet

Indications: Digestion, rheumatic joints, tumors, to lose weight, excellent cleansing diet

Systems: Lymphatic, Digestive

Dosha Affected:

Vata: Good

Pitta: Moderation* (eat only if sweet)

Kapha: Moderation

Mixes Well With: Greens, all acid fruits

Season: Tropical, year long

*Use caution if you have ulcers or high pitta digestion

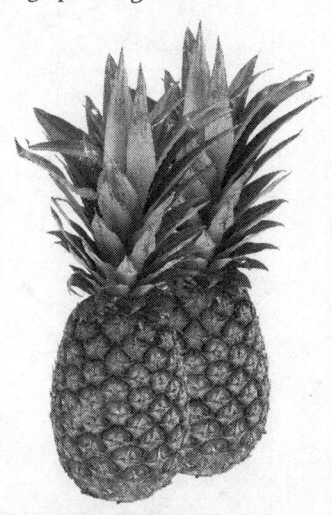

Pineapple Salad

Serves 4

- 1 ripe whole pineapple
- ¼ cup orange juice, fresh
- ½ bunch dill, chopped
- ½ bunch parsley, chopped
- Bragg's

Remove top and skin of pineapple, then remove core. Cut into small cubes and place in bowl. Add orange juice, parsley, dill, and Bragg's to taste.

Serve over greens.

Pineapple Pie

Serves 6

- 2 cups pineapple chunks, fresh
- ½ cup almond flour
- 1½ cup almond milk
- 3 eggs, well beaten
- ¼ cup jaggary or raw sugar
- ½ teaspoon vanilla
- 3/4 cup unsweetened coconut

Combine almond milk and flour. Beat eggs. Add eggs, vanilla, and coconut to almond milk blend. Pour into pie shell.

Preheat oven 325. Bake for 20 minutes.

Plum

Botanical Name: Prunus domestica

The plum is a native of South Eastern Europe, but has made its way around the world. The trees are small, and the fruit is usually easy to reach. Today, we have many varieties, some of which are also highly cultivated in desert areas. Many of these varieties have been cultivated in larger quantities in the past forty years. The fruit is high in sugar and contains approximately 30 minerals. Plums are also high in oxalic acid, so one should be careful with consumption.

Energy: Warming

Taste: Sweet, Sour

Post Digestive: Sweet

Indications: Constipation, flatulence

Systems: Excretory, Digestive

Dosha Affected:

Vata and **Pitta**: Good

Kapha: Avoid

Mixes Well With: Sweet and sub-acid fruits

Season: Summer

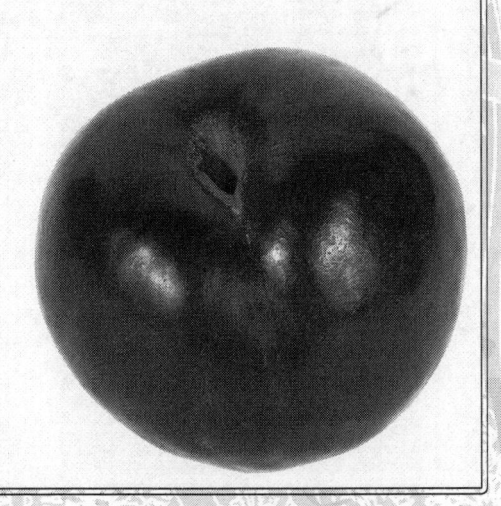

Plum Sauce

- 6 plums, pitted
- ½ cup apple juice
- 1 teaspoon agave syrup
- 1 teaspoon cinnamon
- 1 teaspoon fennel seeds
- 1 teaspoon fresh mint, chopped

Put all ingredients in blender, and blend until smooth. Serve on fruit salad or crackers.

Plum Pudding #1

Serves 4

- 1 pound ripe plums
- 1 cup dried coconut
- ¼ cup molasses
- 1 teaspoon vanilla
- 2 tablespoons lemon juice

Remove seeds and cut plums into small pieces. Place in food processor adding coconut slowly. Add molasses, vanilla, and lemon juice. Let sit. Serve at room temperature or place in refrigerator.

Plum Pudding #2

- 10 ripe plums
- 1 cup coconut cream, pouring off liquid at top
- ¼ cup jaggary, well ground - or sucanat
- 1 teaspoon vanilla
- 1 teaspoon fennel

In blender, put all ingredients together & blend until smooth. If it becomes too thick, add a bit of the coconut water left over. Make sure it is as creamy as a pudding

Raspberry

Botanical Name: Rubus idaeus, Rubus occidentalis

The raspberry is a native of Europe and known as a healing plant with the leaves being used medicinally for many ailments. It is also found growing wild in North America. Raspberries have a very distinctive flavor and come in many varieties and colors – red, black, purple, yellow, and white. Their short shelf life requires producers to rush them to the market immediately.

Energy: Warming

Taste: Sweet, Sour

Post Digestive: Sweet

Indications: Varicose veins, constipation, low blood sugar

Systems: Reproductive, Circulatory, Excretory

Dosha Affected:

Vata and **Pitta**: Good

Kapha: Moderation

Mixes Well With: All berries, sub-acid and sweet fruits

Season: Summer & Fall

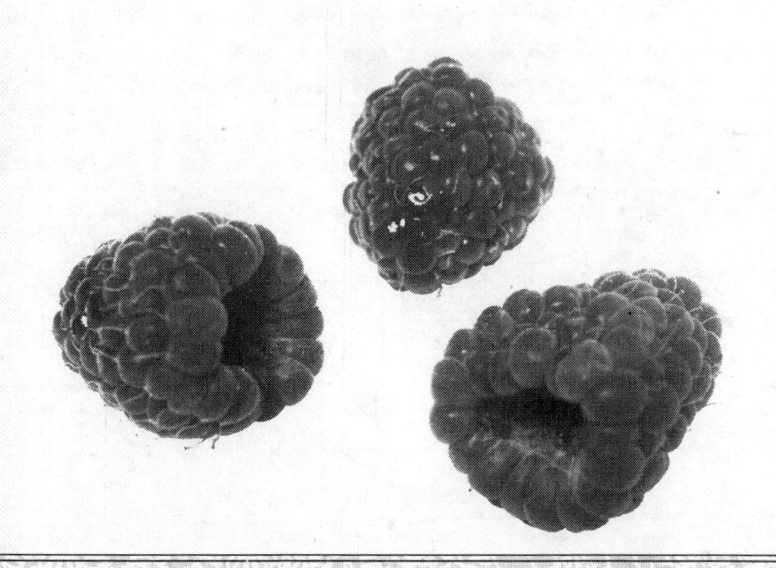

Ayurvedic Curative Cuisine for Everyone

Spicy Yogurt Raspberries

- 2 cups fresh raspberries
- 1 cup plain yogurt
- 2 teaspoons agave syrup
- 1 teaspoon vanilla
- ½ teaspoon cardamom
- ½ teaspoon nutmeg
- ½ teaspoon cinnamon

Stir all ingredients in a bowl; serve chilled.

Raspberry Cobbler

Serves 4

- 1 pound raspberries
- ¼ cup date sugar or jaggary
- ¼ cup quick oats
- 1 teaspoon cinnamon
- 1 teaspoon powdered ginger
- 1 teaspoon grated coconut
- 1 tablespoon arrowroot
- 1 cup water

Soak oats with 1 cup water for 1 hour. Add oats to berries. Simmer berries & oats with sugar, spices, arrowroot, and coconut. Stir well. Let sit 30-60 minutes. Serve. This recipe does not require baking.

Sapote

Botanical Names: Manikara zapota, Diospyros digyna, Casimiroa edulis, Pouteria sapota

Native to Mexico and Central America, the various fruits known as sapotes kept many of the Spanish settlers alive because of their nutritious vitamin content. There are actually several unrelated plants that are called sapote (which means "soft edible fruit" in Nahuatl, an indigenous Mexican language). They include Sapodilla (M. zapota), Black Sapote (D. digyna), White Sapote (C. edulis), and the Mamey Sapote (P. sapota). Any type of sapote may be used in the recipes below.

Energy: Warming

Taste: Sweet, Sour

Post Digestive: Sweet

Indications: Varicose veins, constipation, low blood sugar

Systems: Reproductive, Circulatory, Excretory

Dosha Affected:

Vata and **Pitta**: Good

Kapha: Avoid

Mixes Well With: Only with sweet fruits

Season: Tropical, Spring, Summer

Sapote Pudding

Serves 3

- 4 sapotes, skinned
- 1 cup coconut milk
- 1 teaspoon cinnamon
- 1 teaspoon cardamom, ground

Remove pits, and mash sapotes with potato masher. Add coconut milk and spices; refrigerate. Serve chilled.

Stuffed Mameys (this is a variety of Sapote)

Serves 4

- ½ cup dates
- 2 teaspoons cinnamon
- 2 teaspoons cardamom
- 2 mameys

Soak dates overnight in water to cover. The next day, blend dates and soaking water with spices until the consistency of butter. Cut mameys in half lengthwise, remove pits, and place a scoop of date mixture in center.

Strawberry

<u>Botanical Name: *Fragaria xananassa*</u>

Cultivation of the strawberry began in the sixteenth century. It is found in the forests of Europe, and has been extensively cultivated in the United States, Canada, and South America. The strawberry has become one of the most important summer fruits around the world. The plant grows well in any garden. It becomes more abundant and bears a larger crop if the fruit is picked as soon as it has ripened.

Energy: Warming

Taste: Sweet, Sour, Astringent

Post Digestive: Sweet

Indications: Varicose veins, constipation

Systems: Circulatory, Excretory

<u>**Doshas Affected:**</u>

Vata: Good

Pitta: Moderation

Kapha: Moderation

Mixes Well With: Acid fruits and other berries

Season: Sub-Tropical Winter, or Summer

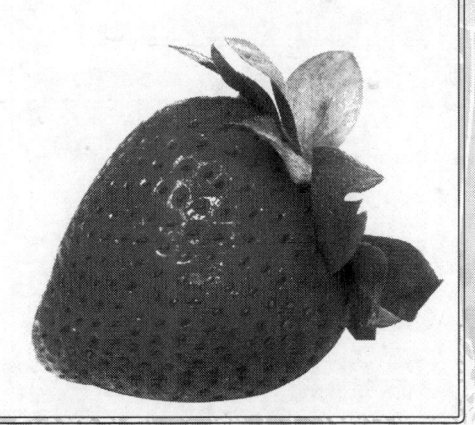

Strawberry Salad

- 1 cup strawberries
- 1 ripe mango
- 1 kiwi
- 1 tablespoon grated orange rind (may use the orange sections in salad)
- ½ cup raw cashews, ground

Mix all ingredients in a bowl; serve chilled.

Strawberry Parfait

Serves 6

- 2 cups strawberries, cut
- ¾ cup apple juice
- 3 tablespoons barley flour
- 2 tablespoons sucanat or jaggary
- ½ tablespoon fresh ginger, grated
- ¼ teaspoon fresh mint
- 1 tablespoon ghee

Cook the strawberries and apple juice in a pan on medium heat for 5 minutes. While cooking and stirring rapidly, slowly add barley flour, sucanat, ginger, and mint. When thickened, remove from heat stir in the ghee. Refrigerate. Garnish with strawberry and mint leaf, if desired, and serve chilled.

Strawberry Topping

- 3 cups pureed berries
- 1 ½ cups jaggary or raw sugar
- ¼ teaspoon cinnamon
- 1 tablespoon lime juice
- ¼ teaspoon cardamom
- ¼ teaspoon mint, dry or fresh, chopped
- ½ teaspoon arrowroot

Cook at low heat until desired thickness is reached. Arrowroot can be used to make it thicker.

Tamarind

Botanical Name: Tamarindus indica

The tamarind is native to tropical Africa and South Asia. It was brought to Brazil by the Portuguese Franciscan Priests. It is similar to the carob in shape, with a brown pod and a tough, rough skin that covers seeds encased in a sweet–sour membrane. It contains high amounts of sugar, acetic acid, lactic acid, and citrus acids. In the West Indies it is mashed, boiled, and blended into a beverage. In India it is made into chutneys and jams. Can be purchased at Indian, Spanish or Asian markets

Energy: Moisturizing, Cool

Taste: Sweet, Sour

Post Digestive: Sour

Indications: Constipation, kidney stones, digestive disorders

Systems: Excretory, Immune, Urinary

Dosha Affected:

Vata: Very Good

Pitta: Avoid

Kapha: Moderation

Mixes Well With: Acid fruits

Season: Tropical, year round

Tamarind Sauce

Makes approximately 1 cup

- ¼ cup tamarind pulp (concentrate)
- 1 cup water
- ¼ teaspoon cumin seeds
- 1/3 cup sucanat or jaggary
- 4 slices ginger, each 1/8 inch thick
- ¼ teaspoon salt
- 1/8 teaspoon garam masala

In 1-quart saucepan combine tamarind pulp and water and boil together for 5 minutes, stirring to break up tamarind; set aside. Meanwhile, in small frying pan over medium heat, roast cumin seeds until they brown and release their fragrance. Remove from heat and grind with a mortar and pestle; set aside.

Strain tamarind pulp through sieve into a bowl, pressing out all liquid. Discard pulp, and return juice to saucepan. Add ground cumin, sucanat, ginger, and salt, and bring to a boil. Turn down heat and simmer until mixture becomes a thin syrup (it will thicken as it cools). Remove from heat, remove ginger slices, and stir in garam masala. Serve at room temperature.

Tamarind Yogurt Dressing

Makes approximately 10 ounces

- 1 cup plain yogurt
- ½ cup tamarind paste (available at Indian groceries)
- 2 tablespoons water
- ¼ tablespoon olive oil
- 2 sprigs fresh mint
- 1 teaspoon salt
- 1 teaspoon ginger, well chopped
- 1 teaspoon maple syrup

Put all ingredients in blender, and blend until smooth. Dressing will keep for 2 weeks in refrigerator, and thickens to make a good dip.

Tangerine

<u>Botanical Name: *Citrus reticulata*</u>

The tangerine (also called mandarin orange) is native to China and India, and known for its fragrance and taste. Tangerines are similar to oranges, but the fruit is easier to peel than any other citrus fruit. They are delicious and easy to eat, and a good source of vitamin C, folate and beta-carotene.

Energy: Warming
Taste: Sweet, Sour
Post Digestive: Sweet
Indications: Colds, flu, constipation, arthritic joints, jaundice
Systems: Immune, Excretory, Circulatory

<u>**Dosha Affected:**</u>
Vata: Good
Pitta: Avoid
Kapha: Moderation
Mixes Well With: Acid fruits
Season: Tropical, summer, late fall

Tangerine Salad

Serves 4

- 2 teaspoon cumin seeds
- 2 teaspoon ghee
- ½ bunch chives, chopped
- 2 stalks celery, chopped
- 1 bunch baby spinach
- ½ bunch mint, chopped
- Bragg's to taste
- 6 tangerines, peeled (white "strings" removed)

Roast cumin seeds in saucepan until aroma is released. Add ghee, chives, and celery, and cook for 5 minutes. Add spinach, mint, and Bragg's, cooking for about 2 minutes more. Remove from saucepan and cool. Add tangerine segments, and serve on greens.

Citrus Delight

Serves 6

- 3 tangerines
- 2 nectarines
- 1 grapefruit
- 1 orange
- 1 kiwi
- ¼ cup sunflower seeds, ground
- 1 teaspoon nutmeg
- 1 teaspoon cinnamon

Peel all the fruit, separate sections or cut in pieces, and place in a bowl. Add the ground sunflower seeds and spices, and serve.

Tomato

Botanical Name: Lycopersicum esculentum

The tomato is an acid fruit. Even though it is usually served as a vegetable, it is botanically a fruit. Native to Central and South America, particularly Peru, there is evidence that tomatoes were brought to Europe by the Spaniards. The French called them pommes d'amour, or "love apples." Tomatoes were initially grown as ornamentals, and thought to be poisonous. They are related to the eggplant, potato, and chili peppers. There are hundreds of varieties of tomatoes, varying in size and shape. The tomato is low in calories (25 calories in a medium tomato), and rich in vitamin C and lycopene, a powerful antioxidant. Lycopene is good for the eyes

Energy: Warming

Taste: Sweet, Sour

Post Digestive: Sour

Indications: Circulation, blood builder, hypertension, cholesterol

Systems: Circulatory, Muscular

Dosha Affected:

Vata: Good

Pitta and **Kapha**: Avoid (unless cooked)

Mixes Well With: Proteins, greens

Season: Summer

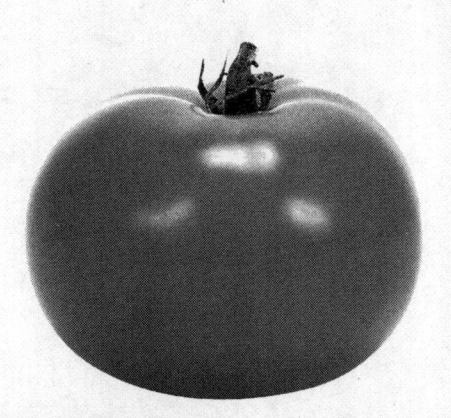

Tomato Delight Soup

Serves 8-10

- 5 large tomatoes, chopped
- 3 cups water (divided)
- 1 bunch Italian parsley, chopped
- 2 tablespoons fresh rosemary, cut in pieces
- 2 cups sweet potato peelings (sweet potatoes served for lunch)
- 1 large sweet onion, chopped
- 2 cubes vegetable bouillon **or** 1 teaspoon miso
- 2 tablespoons Bragg's **or** 1 teaspoon celtic salt
- 2 cups soy milk, rice milk or almond milk

Gradually blend tomatoes with one cup of water in blender. Add parsley and rosemary, and pour into saucepan. Cook sweet potato peelings and onion in two cups of water; blend until smooth, then add to tomato mixture. Add bouillon cubes and Bragg's; cook for 20 to 25 minutes. Add milk, and serve warm.

Stuffed Tomatoes

Serves 5

- 10 firm medium tomatoes
- 2 cups cashews, ground
- 2 cups celery, well chopped
- 1 cup grated carrots
- 1 cup chopped onions
- 1 cup fresh cilantro, chopped
- 2 tablespoons sesame oil
- 1 tablespoon Italian seasoning
- Bragg's

Scoop out centers of tomatoes, and chop. Set tomato shells aside. In a bowl, mix together the chopped tomatoes, ground cashews, celery, carrots, onions, cilantro, oil, and Italian seasoning; add Bragg's to taste. Stuff the mixture into the center of the tomato shells.

Serve with salad or steamed vegetables.

Summer Tomato Soup

Serves 6

- 6 ripe tomatoes, chopped
- ½ bunch cilantro, chopped
- 2 tablespoons Bragg's
- 1 bunch green onions, chopped
- 1 tablespoon Italian seasoning
- 3 cups water
- 1 tablespoon kelp
- 1 tablespoon sesame oil
- ¼ bunch parsley

Set a little cilantro aside for garnish.

Put the rest of the ingredients in a blender and blend until smooth. Refrigerate for 15 minutes; serve chilled, garnished with cilantro.

Serve with bread or crackers.

Tomato Mushroom Skewers

Serves 4

- 24 cherry tomatoes
- 1 onion, large, cut into cubes
- 24 mushrooms
- 24 olives, large
- 24 pieces mozzarella cheese, cut into cubes
- 3 tablespoons olive oil
- 2 tablespoons lemon juice
- 1 tablespoon Italian seasoning
- 1 tablespoon aminos

Use 12 wooden skewers. To each skewer, add 1 tomato, 1 cube onion, 1 mushroom, 1 mozzarella cube, 1 olive, and Continue filling skewer until full. Do all 12 skewers. Mix olive oil, lemon juice, Italian seasoning, and aminos. With a basting brush, baste each of the skewers. If any mixture is left, pour over skewers and let soak for a few hours in the refrigerator serve raw or broiled for a few minutes.

Ayurvedic Curative Cuisine for Everyone

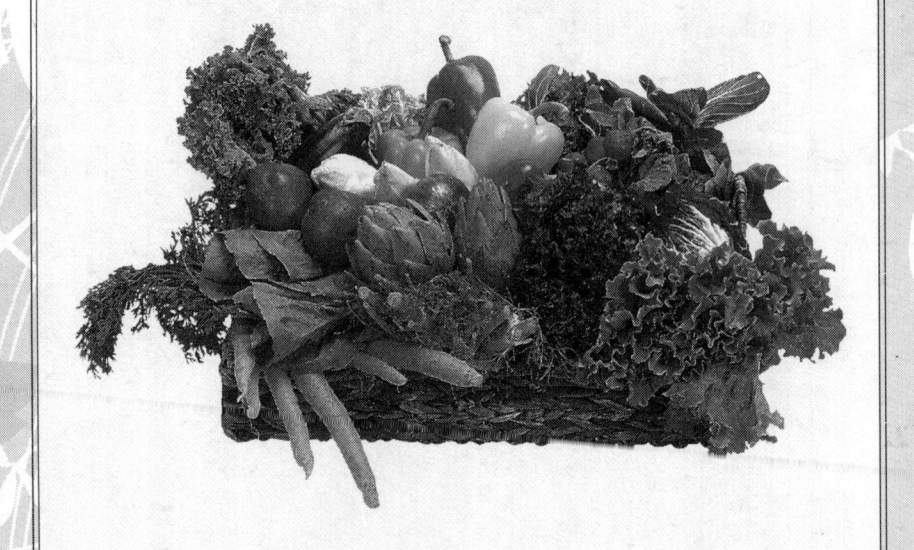

Vegetables

Vegetables

General Considerations

The definition of a vegetable is "any plant grown for edible food." This loosely describes all roots, stems, leaves, flowers, buds, heads, and seeds (like corn).

Vegetables play a very important role in nutrition because of their high content of essential vitamins and minerals. Various nutritional studies show that many Americans have significant vitamin deficiencies. A diet of protein and carbohydrates will not be sufficient for a healthy body. Today, Western society is paying more attention to the intake of vegetables, and vegetarianism is growing. Yoga practices encourage a more sattvic (pure) lifestyle. This way of eating keeps the mind clear and is karma free.

Eating vegetables that are in season, and organically grown, is always best. Our soils have been depleted by hundreds of years of use. The mineral content in commercial vegetables is low. Organic soils yield higher mineral contents in vegetables, and oceanic seaweeds are rich in macro and trace minerals.

Leafy green vegetables combine well with starches, starchy vegetables, and protein. Starchy vegetables do best with leafy green vegetables and starches.

Vegetable Juice: When vegetables such as carrots, celery, beets, broccoli and greens are juiced, the nutrients are more easily assimilated. Due to the concentrated vitamin and mineral content, fresh vegetable juice is highly nutritious, particularly when there are nutritional deficiencies. The juices detoxify and speed the healing process. Many vegetables, particularly green vegetable, detoxify the organs, have the potential to decrease tumors, assist in the cleansing process, and enhance immunity. Because of the concentration, some people prefer to add some water.

Use 1 cup juice & ¼ cup water.

# Artichoke

<u>Botanical Name: *Cynara scolymus*</u>

The Globe artichoke is a thistle-like perennial distinguished by its edible flower-like scales and bottoms with young succulents which, when blanched, are eaten like asparagus. It belongs to the thistle family and is considered the aristocrat of the vegetable kingdom. Artichokes require rich soil and careful cultivation. When harvesting, they must be cut while the flower is young, before it has begun to open, otherwise it will be tough and fibrous. The Jerusalem artichoke (Helianthus tuberosus) and the Chinese artichoke (Stachys sieboldii) are actually not artichokes at all, but tubers belonging to the sunflower and mint families, respectively. (See page 174 for Jerusalem artichokes.)

Energy: Cooling

Taste: Sweet, Astringent

Post Digestive: Sweet

Indications: Kidney stones, liver cleanser, PMS, blood disorders

Systems: Reproductive, Endocrine, Digestive, Circulatory

<u>**Dosha Affected:**</u>

Vata: Moderation (can be eaten with a creamy spiced dressing and lemon)

Pitta and **Kapha**: Good

Mixes Well With: Starches or proteins

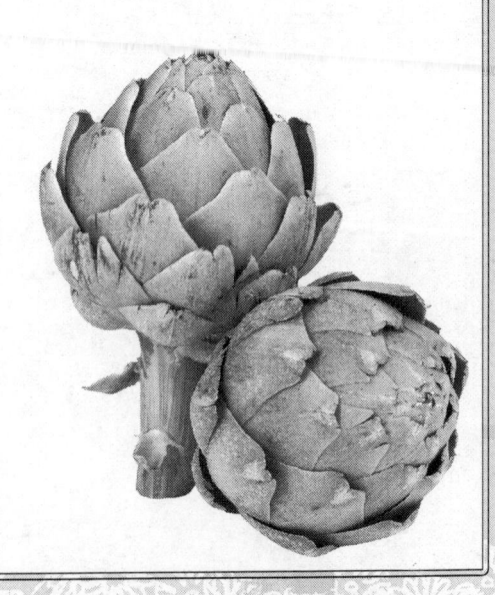

Marinated Artichoke Hearts

Serves 2

- 8 pieces of marinated artichoke hearts
- 2 tablespoons balsamic vinegar
- 2 tablespoons black olives, chopped
- 1 bunch green onions, chopped
- 1 chayote or yellow squash, chopped
- 1 teaspoon mustard (powered)
- ¼ teaspoon thyme
- 2 tablespoons lemon juice
- 3 tablespoons of cilantro, chopped
- 2 tablespoons parsley, chopped

Mix artichokes, vinegar, olives and let sit for 15 minutes. In a pan sauté onions and squash until soft. Add spices and lemon juice. When cooked, add cilantro, parsley, and artichoke-olive mixture.

Steamed Artichokes

Serves 4

- 4 artichokes
- ¼ cup ghee
- 2 tablespoons lemon
- Salt or Bragg's to taste

Place artichokes in large steamer for 35-50 minutes, depending upon their size, until they are soft. The leaves can be eaten by dipping them in melted ghee, lemon, and Salt or Bragg's mixture.

Artichoke Dip

Makes approximately 1 cup

- 4 artichoke hearts
- ¼ cup grated goat cheese
- 1 tablespoon lemon juice
- ¼ cup cilantro or parsley
- 1 tablespoon olive oil

Place all ingredients in blender until smooth. Serve with vegetables or crackers.

Arugula

<u>Botanical Name: *Eruca sativa*</u>

This annual pungent-smelling vegetable, sometimes called "rocket," is native to Europe and western Asia. It is particularly popular in the South of France, Italy, and Egypt. The Romans used its leaves and seeds. Arugula is a member of the cabbage family and is related to watercress, mustard, and radishes. It can grow to 20 inches, and has tender, smooth, sharply indented, irregularly shaped leaves (similar to those of a dandelion). The flavor is similar to that of watercress.

Energy: Warming

Taste: Bitter, Pungent

Post Digestive: Pungent

Indications: To lose weight, stimulates digestion, blood purifier, edema

Systems: Digestive, Circulatory

<u>**Dosha Affected:**</u>

Vata and **Pitta**: Avoid excessive use

Kapha: Good

Mixes Well With: Proteins, starches

Season: Spring & Summer

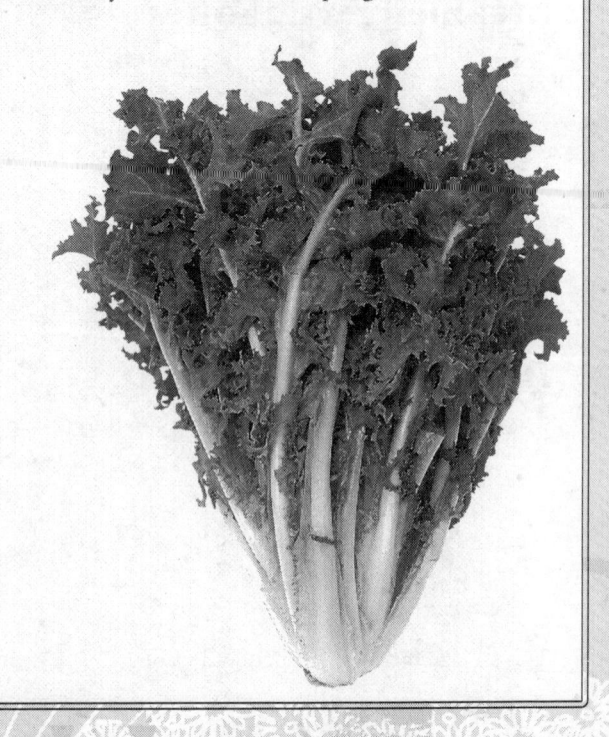

Arugula Salad

Serves 2

- 1 bunch arugula
- ½ jicama, peeled and grated
- 2 small carrots, grated
- 4 stalks of celery, well chopped
- ½ cup raisins, soaked
- 2 tablespoons olive oil
- 2 tablespoons balsamic vinegar
- 1 teaspoon rosemary
- 1 teaspoon thyme
- Bragg's to taste

Tear arugula greens into bite-size pieces. Add jicama, carrots, celery, and raisins. Mix oil, vinegar, herbs, and Bragg's together, pour over salad and toss.

Stir Fry Arugula

Serves 4

- 6 cups arugula
- 1 cup water
- ¼ cup cilantro, chopped
- 1 cup green onions, chopped
- 1 tablespoon ghee
- 1 teaspoon cumin powder
- 1 teaspoon coriander

Melt ghee in skillet. Add onions and cook for 2 minutes on low flame. Add arugula and wilt for 1-2 minutes.

Asparagus

<u>Botanical Name: *Asparagus officinalis*</u>

Asparagus is native to Europe and Southern Russia, Siberia, and Poland. There are approximately 50 species, many of which have strong medicinal properties and grow better in temperate climates. Some varieties are used as ornamentals rather than as a vegetable and are often seen in Florida and California yards. Many commercial fertilizers are used in order to meet the high demand; therefore, the asparagus found in our markets is usually inferior to that grown on a small farm. Generally, it takes 2–3 years to begin harvesting. Once the plant is established, it requires less attention than any other vegetable, and produces every spring for ten years or more. Asparagus must be carefully prepared by steaming for approximately three minutes in order to preserve the large quantity of vitamins and minerals. Wild asparagus is a tender delicacy.

Energy: Cooling

Taste: Sweet, Astringent, Bitter

Post Digestive: Sweet

Indications: Kidney stones, bladder infections, urinary tract infections, PMS, edema, blood purifier, venereal disease, herpes, gout, arthritis

Systems: Urinary, Immune, Endocrine, Circulatory, Muscular

Dosha Affected:

Vata: Moderation (eat well cooked; lots of oil)

Pitta: Excellent

Kapha: Good

Mixes Well With: Protein, grains, starches

Season: Early Summer

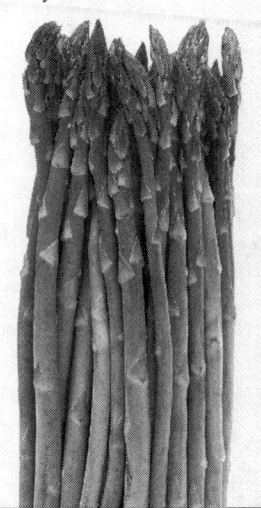

Cream of Asparagus Soup

Serves 4

- 1 bunch asparagus (cut woody stem ends off)
- ½ fennel bulb, thinly sliced
- 2 tablespoons ghee
- 2 sweet onions, chopped
- ¼ cup dill
- 4 cups soy milk
- 2 teaspoons mild curry powder
- 2 teaspoons coriander
- Bragg's

Set aside 3 stalks of asparagus for garnish. Steam fennel and asparagus for 10 to 15 minutes; set aside. Sauté onions and dill in ghee, then add soy milk and cook for 10 minutes. Add curry and coriander; turn heat to low. In blender, blend asparagus and fennel, 1 cup of water from steaming them, and the onion mixture. Add Bragg's to taste. Ladle into soup bowls; garnish with the 3 stalks of asparagus, chopped well.

(This soup can also be made using broccoli, spinach, or cauliflower.)

Asparagus Salad

Serves 4

- 1 pound asparagus, slightly steamed
- ½ cup arugula
- 1 head romaine lettuce
- ¼ cup olives
- 1/3 cup goat cheese, grated
- ½ cup chives or green onion tops

Mix all ingredients together in a bowl. Serve with your favorite dressing.

Bamboo Shoots

Botanical Name: Bambusa vulgaris, Phyllostachys edulis

Bamboo is native to China. In this part of the world fresh bamboo shoots are not often available – even in Chinese restaurants they are often the canned variety. Fresh bamboo shoots can be found in Asian stores; they are usually refrigerated. The young shoots of the bamboo plant are cut as soon as they sprout to the surface, which encourages continual production of new shoots. They can be eaten cooked or raw.

Energy: Cooling
Taste: Sweet, Astringent
Post Digestive: Sweet
Indications: Toxemia, Ama conditions, chronic illnesses, blood purifier
Systems: All systems

Dosha Affected:
Vata: Moderation (well cooked in a spiced, sweet/sour sauce)
Pitta and **Kapha**: Good
Mixes Well With: Proteins or starches
Season: Late Summer

Bamboo Shoots and Tomatoes

Serves 4

- 2 cups bamboo shoots
- 1 cup lotus roots, cut in halves
- 1 head of romaine, torn in pieces
- 2 tomatoes (or 6-8 cherry tomatoes)

Cut the bamboo shoots into rounds; mix with lotus root in a salad bowl. Add romaine and half the tomatoes, and toss together.

Make Dressing:

- 1 tablespoon sesame oil
- ¼ cup grated ginger
- 1 green onion, well chopped
- 1 teaspoon fennel, ground
- 1 teaspoon coriander, ground
- 2 tablespoons lemon juice
- soy sauce

In blender, blend all the ingredients with other half of the tomatoes.

Serve with proteins or grains.

Beans, Green and Yellow

<u>Botanical Name: *Phaseolus vulgaris*</u>

The name "bean," although applied to various trees and shrubs, like the tamarind and coffee, is usually applied to the common garden, snap, string, and stringless green beans - the immature pods of which are a delicious and valuable food. Certain terms are used to indicate special uses of certain beans. "Snap bean" refers to those varieties whose freshly gathered, immature pods, while thick and meaty, will break cleanly across when bent without leaving a "string" across the back. String beans as well as the yellow and green varieties, when fresh, are very rich in potassium and contain good amounts of sulphur, chlorine, calcium, magnesium, phosphorus, and sodium. As with all fresh beans, they are alkaline in reaction. In the fresh state, beans may be combined with any other vegetable and both protein and carbohydrate foods.

Energy: Cooling

Taste: Sweet, Astringent

Post Digestive: Sweet

Indications: Kidney disorders, infectious diseases, bleeding disorders, fevers, edema, rheumatism and arthritic joints, inflammations

Systems: Urinary, Immune, Circulatory

Dosha Affected:

Vata: Avoid or reduce

Pitta: Excellent

Kapha: Good

Mixes Well With: All vegetables or proteins

Season: Summer, Late Fall

Breaded String Beans

Serves 4

1 pound string beans

2 eggs, beaten

2 cups breadcrumbs

1 tablespoon ghee

1 medium sweet onion

2 teaspoons dried oregano

1 teaspoon dried rosemary

1 teaspoon dried sage

1 teaspoon dried basil

1 cup tomato sauce

2 tablespoons tomato sauce

Cut ends from string beans and steam them (whole) until soft. Dip the beans first into the beaten egg, then into breadcrumbs. Remove beans with spatula and sauté or stir-fry in ghee. Add onions, and cook until soft. Then add herbs and tomato sauce; stir well.

Elizabeth's Green Beans

Serves 4

3 cups green beans, fresh, steamed

1 large clove Elephant size garlic, chopped very small or 3-4 regular size garlic cloves

¼ thumb size fresh ginger, grated

3 tablespoons olive oil

1-2 tablespoons balsamic vinegar

Optional - 1 medium onion, sliced, steamed

Remove tips & strings from green beans. Steam until beans are tender & firm, but not mushy. (Add sliced onions to beans if desired). When cooked, place in bowl, add grated ginger, and chopped garlic. Then add olive oil. Mix until beans are well coated with oil. Let sit for 10 minutes or longer. Lastly, add the balsamic vinegar and mix well. The beans should be mildly flavored with balsamic vinegar, not overpowered by the vinegar. Serve at room temperature, lightly warmed, or cold.

Green Bean Salad #1

- 2 cups green beans
- 2 cups chopped jicama
- 1 cup pineapple chunks
- ½ bunch green onions, chopped
- 2 tablespoons cumin, ground
- 1 teaspoon coriander, ground
- ½ cup lemon juice
- 1 tablespoon olive oil
- Bragg's

Steam green beans until soft; cool. Add jicama, pineapple, onions, and spices. Mix lemon juice and oil together, and add to salad. Season with Bragg's to taste.

Raw tip: Slice beans thin, add remaining ingredients and allow to marinate 20 minutes before serving.

Green Bean Salad #2

Serves 2

- 2 cups green beans
- 1 onion, medium, well chopped
- 2 tablespoons mayonnaise
- 1 ¼ cup sunflower seeds
- Salt to taste

Remove green bean ends and strings. In a food processor, chop raw green beans. Grind sunflower seeds into powder in a bowl. Mix all ingredients together. Salt to taste. Serve with crackers, salad, or bread.

Punjab-Style String Beans and Kale

Serves 8-10

- 4-5 cups fresh string beans
- 2 bunches lacinato kale
- 2 tablespoons sunflower oil (divided)
- 2 teaspoons cumin seeds
- ½ teaspoon mustard seeds
- 1 teaspoon turmeric
- ¼ teaspoon hing
- ¾ teaspoon sea salt
- 1 cup water (divided)
- 2 tablespoons coriander, ground
- 5-6 whole black peppercorns
- 1 teaspoon rice syrup
- 1 teaspoon Bombay curry powder, mild cilantro leaves for garnish

Wash and dry string beans and kale. Slice kale into strips; cut beans lengthwise and then cut into 1- or 2-inch pieces, about 4 or 5 cuts per bean. Heat 1 tablespoon oil in large saucepan and add cumin and mustard seeds. When they pop, add turmeric, hing, salt and string beans. Stir, mixing well. Add ½ cup water and the kale. Cover and cook over medium heat for 15 to 20 minutes.

While beans and kale are cooking, heat 1 tablespoon oil in small frying pan, add coriander and peppercorns.

Sauté for about 3 minutes. Cool, then blend in blender with ½ cup of water. Add this mixture plus rice syrup and curry powder to cooked beans and kale; cook for an additional 5 minutes uncovered. Garnish with fresh cilantro.

Beets

Botanical Name: Beta vulgaris

The common garden beet, sugar and foliage beets, Swiss chard and amagelwarzel all spring from the same progenitor and have been cultivated for centuries. There are two classes of garden beet varieties, the long and turnip rooted. The sugar beet is grown largely for the manufacture of sugar in France, Belgium, Germany, America, and other countries. When grated raw and added to salad, it forms a colorful and delicious addition. Young beets may be steamed for 12-15 minutes or may be baked for approximately 30 minutes. They should never be peeled or cut before cooking, and the beet tops have great nutritional value and should be used.

Energy: Warming

Taste: Sweet

Post Digestive: Sweet

Indications: Blood purifier, anemia, varicose veins, constipation, menstruation disorders, amenorrhea (delay or absence of menstruation)

Systems: Circulatory, Reproductive, Excretory

Dosha Affected:

Vata: Excellent

Pitta and **Kapha**: Avoid or reduce

Mixes Well With: Green vegetables, starches

Season: Late Fall

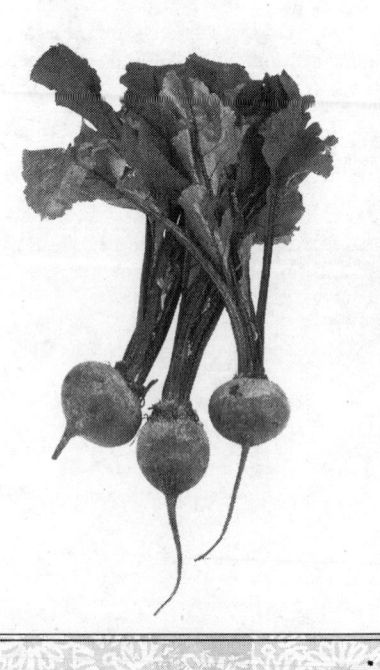

Beet Medley

Serves 4

3 beets, peeled and cubed small

2 turnips, peeled and cubed small

2 sweet potatoes (Vata and Pitta only), peeled and cubed

1 cup cabbage, thinly sliced

2 tablespoons ghee

1 teaspoon coriander, ground

1 teaspoon juniper berries, ground

1½ teaspoon cumin, ground

Put beets, turnips, and sweet potatoes in baking pan with 1 tablespoon ghee; bake at 350° for 30 minutes. Stir in cabbage, cover, and bake for 10 more minutes. Blend the ghee, coriander, juniper berries, and cumin until smooth. Pour over entire mixture; stir well.

Serve with grains or salad.

Beet, Carrot, and Apple Juice

Serves 2

2 beets, medium

2 carrots, medium

2 apples

¼ thumb sized ginger

Must have juicer or Vita-Mix. Slice all vegetable, blend in juicer, drink.

Beets in Lemon or Lime

Serves 2

- 3 beets, cut into cubes
- ½ cup lemon juice – Kapha only
- ½ cup lime juice – Vata and Pitta
- 2 cups water
- ½ bunch parsley, chopped
- 1 teaspoon coriander, ground
- ½ teaspoon fennel, ground
- ½ teaspoon ginger, ground

Place beets in bowl, add lemon or lime juice (according to dosha) and water; soak for 2 hours. Then place in saucepan and bring to a boil (or bake for 30 minutes). Add parsley and spices; cover and steep for 10 minutes. Drain and serve.

Raw tip: Grate beets finely and add remaining ingredients and allow to marinate 20 minutes before serving.

Beet Greens

Makes 2 cups

- 2 cups beet greens
- 2 tablespoons ghee or olive oil
- 1/3 cup water left over from steaming greens
- 1 tablespoon coriander
- 1 teaspoon fennel
- ¼ cup cilantro

Steam greens lightly until soft – do not overcook. Mix in remaining ingredients. Stir. Serve.

Bitter Melon

Botanical Name: Momordica charantia

Bitter melon (sometimes called bitter gourd) is highly recommended in Ayurveda to balance blood sugar. Polypeptide-p is the phytochemical in the plant that produces this effect. Bitter melon also helps accelerate the healing process of the pancreas when inflamed. It can be found in Asian markets.

Energy: Heating

Taste: Bitter

Post Digestive: Pungent

Indications: Diabetes, pancreatitis, constipation, malaria

Systems: Digestive, Endocrine

Dosha Affected:

Vata: Moderation* (eaten with sweet potatoes)

Pitta and **Kapha**: Excellent

Mixes Well With: Sweet vegetables, salads, grains

Season: Winter

Use caution if you have ulcers or colitis

Bitter Melon Casserole

Serves 4

- 6 medium bitter melons, sliced into rings
- 1 tablespoon fennel seed (divided)
- ¼ bunch cilantro, chopped
- ½ cup fresh mint, chopped
- 2 sprigs of curry leaves *(or 1 teaspoon curry powder)*
- 1 tablespoon whole mustard seed
- 1 tablespoon ajwan seed
- 1 tablespoon ghee
- 3 diced green onions, or ½ cup chopped yellow onions
    (green onions for less fire, yellow onions for more heat)
- 2 tablespoons coriander, ground
- 1 tablespoon fennel, ground
- 1 tablespoon Bragg's

Boil or steam the melon until soft, adding half of the fennel seeds to the cooking water to sweeten the bitterness. Drain the water. Add cilantro and mint. If you have fresh curry, add that too.

In a wok or skillet, roast the rest of the fennel seeds with the mustard and ajwan seeds, on low heat for 5 minutes while gently stirring or shaking the pan. Add ghee and green onions to pan. Sauté for 5 minutes, then add the soft bitter melon. Stir in coriander, ground fennel, curry powder, and Bragg's.

Broccoli

Botanical Name: Brassica oleracea, Italica group

Broccoli is a "green twin" to the cauliflower but has a longer neck, grows in milder climates with a longer growing season, and matures in the spring. The stems can be peeled and sliced for salads or soups; otherwise, they are hard to digest. This plant is the most common vegetable eaten in the west today, next to head lettuce.

Energy: Cooling

Taste: Astringent, Sweet, Pungent

Post Digestive: Pungent

Indications: Jaundice, osteoporosis, arthritis, anemia, diarrhea, kidney stones, urinary tract infections

Systems: Urinary, Endocrine, Circulatory,

Dosha Affected:

Vata: Moderation when in balance (well cooked, creamy dressing with butter, salt and spices; or in soups)

Pitta: Excellent

Kapha: Good

Mixes Well With: All starches or proteins

Season: Late Summer, Summer, Fall

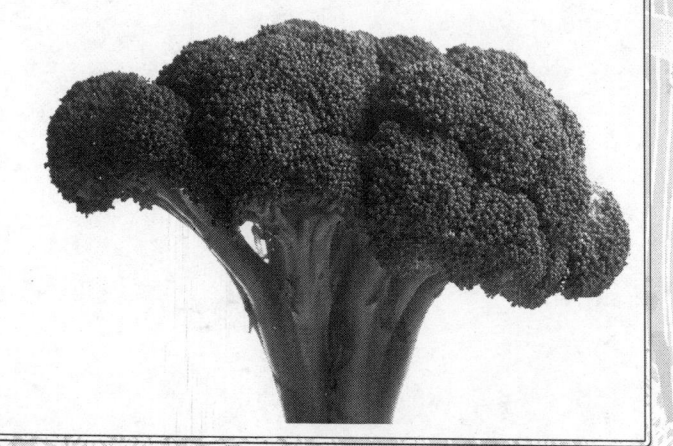

Broccoli or Cauliflower Subzi
(pronounced *sub-jee*)

Serves 6

- 1 large onion, finely chopped
- 3-4 garlic cloves, chopped – Kapha only
- 1 teaspoon cumin seeds
- 3 tablespoons ghee or olive oil
- ½ teaspoon fennel – Kapha only
- 1 teaspoon red chili powder – Kapha only
- ½ teaspoon turmeric
- 1 teaspoon salt (or to taste)
- ¼ cup water
- 1 head of broccoli or cauliflower, cut into flowerets
- 2 potatoes, cubed (optional – can add these for bulk if desired)
- 2 medium tomatoes, chopped
- ¼ cup cilantro

Sauté onions, garlic, and cumin seeds in ghee until light brown. Stir in spices and salt. Add water, broccoli or cauliflower (and potatoes if desired), cover pan, and slowly sauté for 10 minutes. Add tomatoes, and continue cooking. When vegetables are soft, add cilantro leaves to garnish and serve with rice or chapattis (Indian flatbread).

Brussels Sprouts

Botanical Name: Brassica oleracea, Gemmifera group

Brussels sprouts are a member of the cabbage family, having developed from the original wild cabbage. The plant has a stalk which is covered with many tiny compact head cabbages, and which can be kept in a warm cellar with a small amount of soil where it will continue to sprout all winter. They are the most delicious and delicate of all the members of the cabbage family. The cabbage family, as a whole, is known to be gas-producing due to its coolness. In order to remove the pungent odor, make a small hole with a knife point in the bottom of each Brussels Sprout

Energy: Cooling

Taste: Pungent, Astringent

Post Digestive: Pungent

Indications: Jaundice, ulcers, acidity, blood purifier, anemia, gout, diarrhea

Systems: Circulatory, Endocrine, Digestive

Dosha Affected:

Vata: Avoid or reduce

Pitta: Moderation

Kapha: Good

Mixes Well With: Vegetables, starches, proteins

Season: End of Summer, Fall

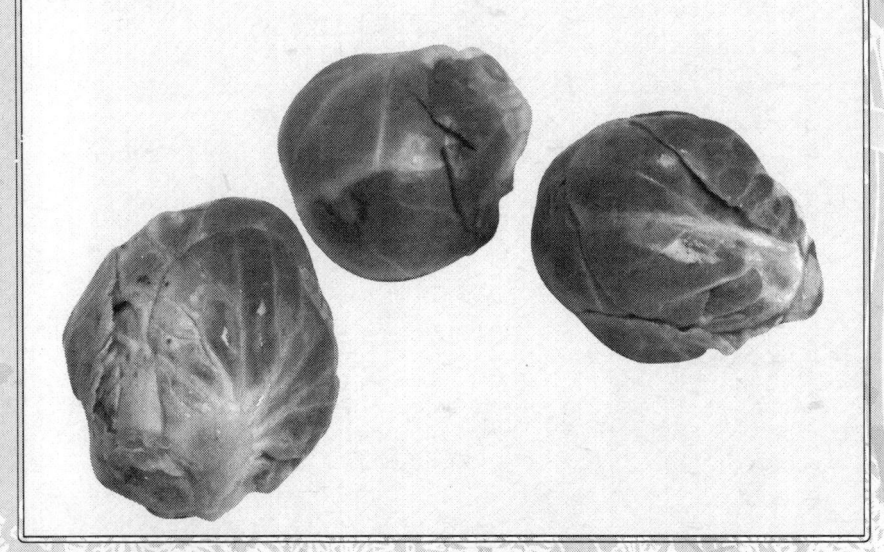

Brussels Sprouts

½ pound brussels sprouts, cut in halves
4-5 inch piece of burdock root, thinly sliced
1 medium onion, sliced into thin rings
2 tablespoons ghee
1 red or green pepper, chopped
1 tablespoon ginger, grated
½ cup almonds, slivered
2 teaspoons coriander, ground
2 teaspoons fennel, ground
Bragg's

Steam brussels sprouts and burdock until soft; set aside. Caramelize the onions in ghee; add peppers and ginger and continue cooking. Add brussels sprouts and burdock, coriander and fennel. Stir well; add Bragg's to taste.

Brussels Sprouts Soup

Serves 6

12 Brussels Sprouts, cut in half
1 cup bok choy, chopped
1 cup kale, well chopped
12 inches wakame seaweed, cut in small pieces
5 cups water
2 tablespoons olive oil
½ tablespoon juniper berries
1 tablespoon coriander
1 teaspoon fennel
¼ cup lemon juice, fresh
1 cup vegetable broth, organic

In a large pot, add water and Brussels sprouts. Add vegetable broth, onions, and wakame - bring to boil for 5 minutes. Cover, lower heat and add spices, lemon juice, bok choy, kale, and aminos. Cook for another 10 minutes on low heat.

Brussels Sprouts Endive

Serves 4

- 8 Brussels sprouts
- 2 endives, chopped
- 1 cup Arugula, chopped
- 1 green onion, chopped
- 1 leek, sliced thin
- 1 tablespoon fennel, ground
- 1 tablespoon coriander, ground
- 1 cup bamboo shoots (optional)

Steam brussels sprouts (can also be used raw, if marinated in olive oil overnight). Slice 7 of the sprouts, and set one aside for sauce (below). Toss all the ingredients together, add spices.

Top with the following dressing:

Brussels Sprout Sauce

- 1 brussels sprout, chopped
- ¼ cup chopped tomato
- ¼ cup pine nuts
- 2 tablespoons balsamic vinegar
- 1 tablespoon Italian seasoning
- Bragg's to taste

Blend until smooth, pour over salad above.

Serve with protein or grains.

Burdock

Botanical Name: Arctium lappa

Burdock (also known as gobo) is a native of Japan, where it is cultivated as a root vegetable. It is added to soups and used in other meal preparations. This highly nutritious vegetable can be found in many natural food stores and Asian markets. In the west, we only know this long, thin, starchy vegetable as an herb, which has recently become well-known as an anti-cancer food and preventative. It also purifies the blood. This food is high in minerals and B vitamins. Grated it can easily be added to salads. It can also be steamed and mashed with potatoes. Cut into slices, burdock can be added to stir-fry and subji.

Energy: Cooling

Taste: Astringent, Pungent

Post Digestive: Pungent

Indications: Lymphoedema, rashes, sore throats, skin conditions

Systems: Immune, Endocrine, Circulatory

Dosha Affected:

Vata: Avoid

Pitta and **Kapha**: Good

Mixes Well With: All vegetables, starches and Green Vegetables

Season: Fall

Burdock Soup

Serves 4

- 4 medium burdock roots, chopped
- 2 medium white potatoes, cut into cubes
- 6 cups water (divided)
- 1 tablespoon ghee
- 2 tablespoons coriander, ground
- 1 tablespoon ginger, grated
- 2 tablespoons ajwan seeds
- ½ bunch green onions, chopped
- ½ bunch cilantro, chopped
- 4 stalks celery
- ¼ pound shiitake mushrooms
- 1 package cellophane rice noodles
- 4 tablespoons rice miso

Bring the chopped burdock and potatoes to a boil in 3 cups of water. Roast ajwan seeds in a large pan, then add ghee, coriander, ginger, onions, cilantro, and mushrooms. When the burdock and potatoes are done, add them, the cooking water, and 3 more cups of water to the pan. Bring to a boil, then break the noodles in half and add. Simmer covered on low heat for 10 minutes. Remove from heat and stir in miso just before serving.

Cabbage

Botanical Name: Brassica oleracea

There are numerous varieties of cabbage cultivated around the world. This bi-annual plant is grown for its thick, round, large heads. The leaves may be smooth, wrinkled, round, flattened, oblong, or conical. Chinese cabbage or celery cabbage (Brassica rapa) is similar to the Western cabbage, and its usage is identical. The main variety is called Petsay cabbage and even though it has been around for 2,000 years, it is not a favorite because of its smell and the gastric distress it can produce. It needs to be cooked for only a short time, because it breaks down rapidly; ten minutes should be sufficient. It is delicious when cooked with seasonings.

Energy: Cooling

Taste: Sweet, Astringent

Post Digestive: Pungent

Indications: Kidney stones, ulcers, diarrhea, inflammations

Systems: Urinary, Excretory, Digestive

Dosha Affected:

Vata: Avoid

Pitta and **Kapha**: Good

Mixes Well With: Proteins or starches

Season: Fall

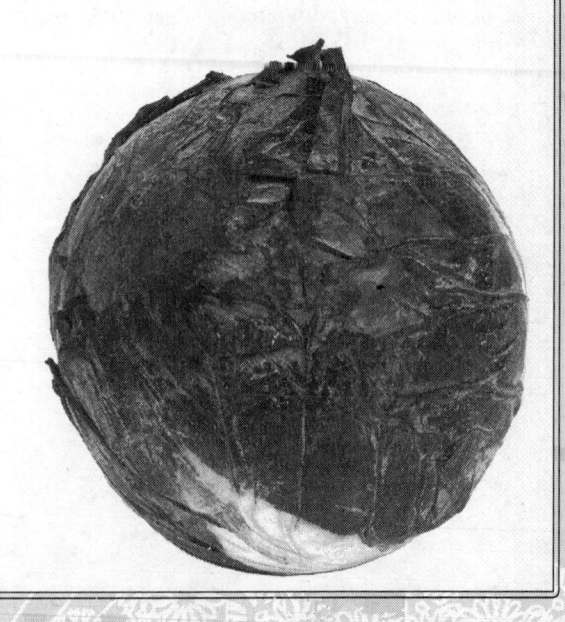

Sauerkraut

- ½ cup juniper berries
- 1 large onion, well chopped
- 1 large cabbage, grated
- 2 carrots, grated
- 4 tablespoons apple cider vinegar
- 2 ounces hiziki, crushed
- 1 tablespoon salt
- 2 tablespoons lemon juice

Put all ingredients in a ceramic crock. Cover, and let sauerkraut and vegetables ferment for a few days. Drain the liquids off, and transfer sauerkraut to container. Refrigerate.

Serve with proteins.

Vegetarian Cabbage Rolls

Serves 8

- ⅓ cup pearl barley
- 12 inches kombu, sliced
- 1 cup water
- 8 large cabbage leaves
- 1 green pepper, finely chopped
- 1 medium onion, finely chopped
- 1 cup string beans, finely chopped
- ¼ cup tomato sauce
- 2 tablespoons rosemary, fresh
- 2 tablespoons oregano, fresh
- Bragg's to taste

Cook barley with kombu in one cup of water until soft, about 30 to 40 minutes. Blanch cabbage leaves. Remove from water and lay leaves flat. Mix remaining ingredients together, and place about 2 tablespoons of mixture on each cabbage leaf. Roll cabbage leaves as if rolling up a burrito. Can be heated if desired. If necessary, insert toothpick into each roll to close.

Carrots

Botanical Name: Daucus carota

The carrots we eat today have been cultivated from the wild carrot, which was once a weed. Although indigenous to Europe, there is no evidence as to where it originated. Holland was given much credit for its cultivation, and from there it spread throughout Europe. The carrot is one of the most important vegetables due to its high nutritional balance of vitamins and minerals. It can be baked similar to potatoes. It is delicious when juiced by itself, or its sweetness can be added to other juices to make them taste more palatable.

Energy: Warming

Taste: Sweet, Pungent

Post Digestive: Sweet

Indications: Chronic fatigue syndrome, high cholesterol, night blindness, cataracts, bursitis, bruising, edema, infections, cancer sores

Systems: Circulatory, Endocrine, Urinary

Dosha Affected:

Vata: Good (best cooked)

Pitta: Avoid or reduce

Kapha: Good

Mixes Well With: Leafy green vegetables, starches

Season: Fall

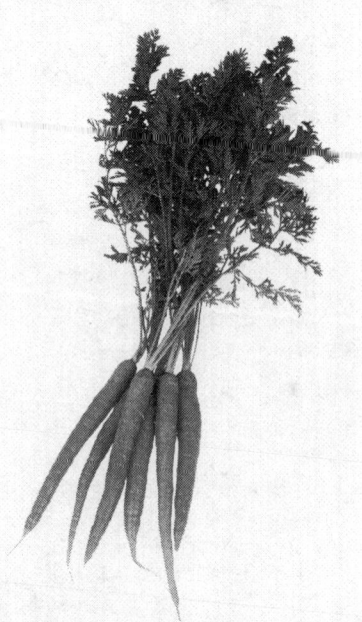

Carrot Halvah

Serves 6-8

- ½ cup raw cashew pieces
- 2 tablespoons ghee
- ½ cup raisins
- 1 lb. carrots, grated
- 1 pint soy milk
- 1 teaspoon cardamom, ground
- ½ cup sucanat or jaggary

In skillet, roast cashews in ghee until golden brown, then add raisins to pan for few seconds. Add carrots and sauté. Add soy milk and cardamom; heat for about 1 hour, stirring. Lower heat after mixture starts boiling; cook until almost dry. Mix in sucanat, and continue to cook until halva is semi-dry. Remove from heat, and stir in cashews and raisins.

Carrot Sauce

- 6 carrots, well steamed
- ½ cup water
- ½ cup lemon juice
- 2 tablespoons ghee
- 1 tablespoon coriander, ground
- 1 teaspoon fennel, ground
- 1 teaspoon mild curry powder

Cut up steamed carrots, and place in blender with other ingredients. Blend until smooth and creamy.

Serve over grains.

Raw tip: Ingredients can also be blended until smooth, without steaming.

Cauliflower

<u>Botanical Name: Brassica oleracea, Botrytis group</u>

The cauliflower is a native of West Asia, and was brought to Europe in 540 B.C. The cultivation of this vegetable was popular during the Christian era and also with the Moors of Spain around the 12th century. The cauliflower is another development of the wild cabbage, and is the hardiest member of the cabbage family. Most cabbage are rajasic; the cauliflower, however, is an exception. Because of its sweet taste, it's found to be a bit sattvic.

Energy: Cooling

Taste: Sweet, Pungent

Post Digestive: Pungent

Indications: Blood purifier, bruises, nervousness, insomnia, diarrhea

Systems: Circulatory, Excretory, Nervous

<u>Dosha Affected:</u>

Vata: Moderation (well cooked)

Pitta: Good

Kapha: Moderation

Mixes Well With: All proteins or starches

Season: Fall

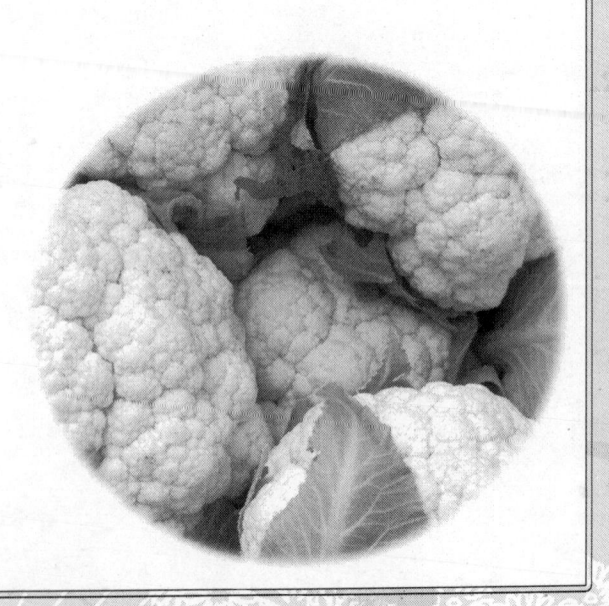

Cauliflower Loaf

- 2 medium heads of cauliflower
- 2 eggs, beaten – OR – 1 tablespoon lecithin
- 2 tablespoons brewer's yeast
- 2 tablespoon Italian seasoning
- 2 cups almonds, well ground
- 1 bunch green onions, chopped
- 1 tablespoon olive oil
- 1½ tablespoons Bragg's

Cut cauliflower into pieces and steam until soft. While steaming, grind almonds. Drain cauliflower and mash like mashed potatoes. Add brewer's yeast and eggs (or lecithin) into mixture. Sauté onions and add with Italian seasoning and Bragg's; stir well. Place in oiled loaf pan. Bake at 350° for 15 minutes. Garnish with parsley or cilantro.

This recipe can also be served raw for Pitta and Kapha.

To prepare: Grind cauliflower in champion juicer or food processor, and follow above instructions using lecithin (not eggs) and using more olive oil. Put into loaf pan, but do not bake. Cool before cutting. Serve with salad.

Cauliflower – Dill - Fennel Soup

Serves 4

- 3 cups cauliflower, chopped
- 2 cups fennel, cut into small pieces
- 1 onion, chopped
- 1 cup cream
- 2 tablespoons fennel seed powder
- 2 tablespoons coriander
- ½ cup dill, fresh, well chopped
- 6 inch piece of Kombu, cut into small pieces
- 5 cups water
- Salt to taste

Put water and all ingredients in a large soup pot except for the fresh dill and the cream. Cook for 25 minutes. Then add cream and dill – save a little dill for garnish. Blend until smooth.

Celeriac

<u>Botanical Name: *Apium graveolen*</u>

Celeriac is in the same family as celery, and some say it originated from the root of the celery plant. It is used for flavoring or eaten as a vegetable. This plant is more familiar to people in countries outside the U.S. When picked, this vegetable is muddy and needs to be soaked in fresh water until clean. The taste is quite delicious and can be a great substitute for mashed potatoes for those who avoid the nightshades. High in minerals, phosphorus, and potassium. Low in fat.

Energy: Warming

Taste: Sweet

Post Digestive: Sweet

Indications: Acne, rashes, nervous conditions, insomnia

Systems: Circulatory, Nervous, Muscular, Lymph

Dosha Affected:

Vata and **Pitta**: Good

Kapha: Moderation

Mixes Well With: Green leafy vegetables, starches

Season: Fall

Mashed Celeriac Root

- 2 celeriac roots, peeled and chopped
- ½ potato, peeled and chopped (optional– do not add if you have joint pain or arthritis)
- 2 tablespoons ghee
- ½ cup soy milk, unsweetened – or almond milk
- ¼ cup parsley or cilantro, chopped
- Bragg's or salt

Steam or boil vegetables until soft. Drain and mash; add ghee, soy milk, and parsley. Add Bragg's to taste.

Celeriac Root & Greens

Serves 4

- 2 celeriac roots, medium
- 1 cup kale
- 1 cup chard
- 1 onion, medium, chopped
- 2 cups water
- 1 tablespoon ghee
- 2 tablespoons Churna – either Vata or Pitta

Peel celeriac & cut into small cubes. Add to water & boil until tender. In skillet or wok, add ghee & onion. While cooking the onions, cut chard & kale into small pieces. Add churna to greens. Drain water from celeriac. Mix all together. Add Bragg's to taste.

Celery

<u>Botanical Name: *Apium graveolens*</u>

There is almost no trace of history for this vegetable until the Middle Ages, and celery later became well known in the 1800's. This vegetable requires a rich sandy soil with plenty of moisture. It is one of the most sattvic vegetables due to its tryptophan content. Celery is a great source of all the B vitamins, A, C, E, calcium, and potassium. Excellent for adrenal function and weight loss. Cut into small pieces, can be added to salads, soups, or juices.

Energy: Cooling

Taste: Astringent, Sweet, Salty

Post Digestive: Pungent

Indications: Infections, mental illnesses, ulcers, insomnia, kidney stones, edema

Systems: Nervous, Urinary, Immune

Dosha Affected:

All Doshas: Good (for Vata, is best well-cooked)

Mixes Well With: All proteins, vegetables, starches

Season: Summer & Fall

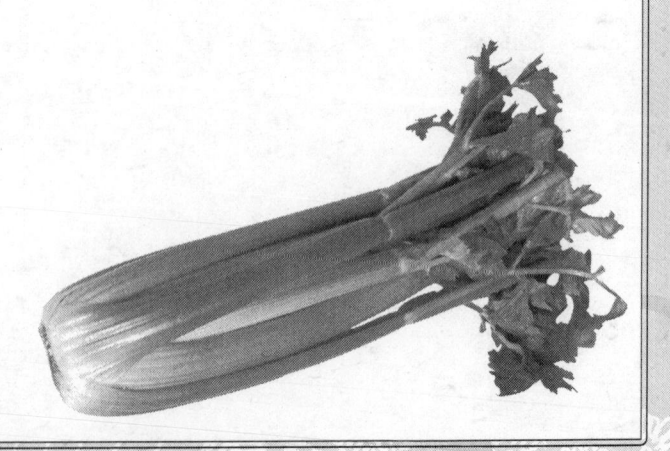

Baked Celery

Serves 4

- 10 celery sticks cut into thirds
- 1 sweet onion, sliced into rings
- 2 tablespoons ghee
- ½ cup vegetable broth
- 2 tablespoons coriander, ground
- 1 tablespoon ajwan seeds
- 2 tablespoons cumin, ground
- 1 cup almond milk
- 1 tablespoon Bragg's
- 2 cups millet breadcrumbs (see page 339)
- ¼ cup mozzarella cheese (optional)

Layer celery and onions in baking pan oiled with ghee. Mix broth, coriander, ajwan, cumin, almond milk, and Bragg's. Toss ingredients, and pour over vegetables. Add breadcrumbs (and cheese, if desired). Bake at 350° for 30 to 40 minutes.

Celery-Carrot Juice

Serves 2

- 3 carrots
- 6 celery stalks
- ¼ bunch cilantro
- ½ bulb celery

Slice all vegetables into pieces. Put into juicer or Vita-Mix. Drink.

Chard

<u>Botanical Name: Beta vulgaris</u>

Chard, a native of Asia, has been cultivated for over 2,000 years, and is now known throughout the world. Chard is sometimes called "leaf beet" – it is actually the same species as the beet, used for its leaves rather than the root. There are many varieties, with leaves of green, red, yellow, or white. The young leaves can be used in salad. When leaves are mature, they are best cooked. Chard is high in minerals.

Energy: Warming

Taste: Bitter, Sour, Sweet

Post Digestive: Sweet

Indications: Blood and circulation, varicose veins, anemia, weak heart

Systems: Circulatory

Dosha Affected:

Vata: Good (well cooked)

Pitta: Moderation (green variety is better than the red; young leaves are best)

Kapha: Good

Mixes Well With: Proteins and starches

Season: Spring & Summer

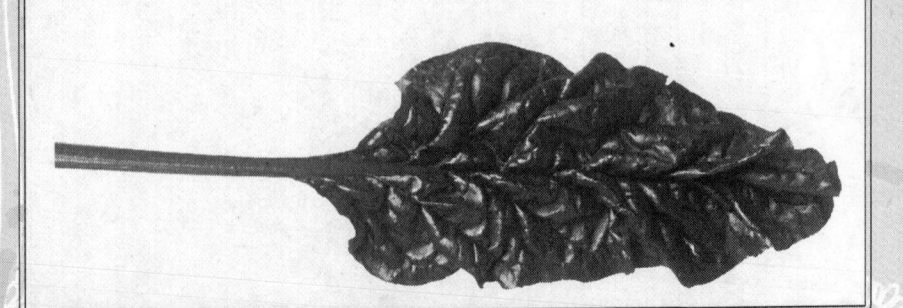

Chard Veggie Combo

Serves 2

- 1 tablespoon ghee
- 4 green onions, chopped
- 1/3 cup fresh ginger root, grated
- 1/4 cup fresh turmeric, peeled and grated
- 12 large leaves and stems of chard, thinly sliced
- 1/2 cup kale, thinly sliced
- 1 bulb fennel, chopped
- 1/4 cup cilantro, chopped
- 1/4 cup basil
- 1/4 cup unsweetened vanilla almond milk

In large wok or skillet, melt ghee. Sauté green onion, ginger, and turmeric until aromas are released (1 to 2 minutes). Add chard, kale, fennel, cilantro, and basil, and sauté for 10 minutes. Add almond milk and cook 2 more minutes.

Serve with Green Tara Dressing (see page 384).

Rainbow Chard Pepper Combo

Serves 4

- 1 teaspoon cumin seeds
- 1 tablespoon ajwan seeds
- 1 tablespoon ghee
- 1 red pepper, chopped
- 1 onion, chopped
- 2 bunches of chard, chopped
- 1/4 cup water
- 1 tablespoon coriander, ground
- 1/2 tablespoon ginger powder
- Bragg's or salt to taste
- sunflower seeds or pine nuts (optional)

Roast cumin and ajwan seeds for 5 to 10 minutes, stirring constantly; then add ghee. When warm, add peppers, onions, and chard. Then add the water, and cook on low heat, covered, for 10 to 15 minutes. Stir in the coriander, ginger and Bragg's to taste; cook for 15 minutes more.

Serve with proteins or grains.

ium edule for Everyone

Chayote

Botanical Name: *Sechium edule*

Chayote (pronounced chai-O-tay) is a native of tropical America and belongs to the same family as squash, cucumbers, and melons. It is grown for its large, green-skinned, pear-shaped fruit. It can be grown anywhere that it does not freeze more than one inch or so deep. The roots can survive in the winter if given protection. The young leaves of the plant can be eaten in salads or steamed. The fruit does not need to be peeled and can be eaten raw in salads. It can also be boiled, stuffed, mashed, baked, or pickled. Both the fruit and the seed are rich in amino acids and vitamin C. High in potassium and low in calories

Energy: Warming

Taste: Sweet

Post Digestive: Sweet

Indications: Kidney disorders, varicose veins, edema, inflammations

Systems: Circulatory, Urinary

Dosha Affected:

Vata: Good

Pitta: Moderation

Kapha: Excellent

Mixes Well With: All vegetables, starches

Season: Tropical, year round

Stuffed Chayotes

- 3 chayotes
- 1 tablespoon sunflower oil
- 2 cups cauliflower
- 3 tablespoons sunflower seeds
- 2 tablespoons almonds, ground
- 1/3 cup rose petals
- 1/2 sweet onion, chopped
- 1 yellow pepper, chopped
- 1/2 cup fresh basil, finely chopped
- 1 bunch cilantro, finely chopped
- 1 tablespoon mild curry powder
- 1 cup fresh mozzarella cheese, grated (optional)

Cut chayotes in half lengthwise, and scoop pulp into a large bowl. Baste shells with oil; place in baking dish, and bake at 350° for 20 minutes. In a food processor, grind cauliflower, sunflower seeds, almonds, and rose petals. Add to chayote pulp, then mix in onions, peppers, basil, cilantro, and curry powder. Fill the chayote shells with this mixture; sprinkle on grated cheese (if desired), and bake for 10 minutes more.

Chayote & Rice

Serves 6

- 3 cups chayote, sliced lengthwise like avocado
- 1 onion, chopped
- 1 green pepper, chopped
- 1 cup rice, cooked
- 1 cup tomato sauce
- 2 tablespoons ghee
- 1 tablespoon oregano, well chopped
- 1 tablespoon rosemary, well chopped
- 2 cups water
- 1 cup cheese, grated

Steam the chayote until tender. In a skillet, add ghee, onions, peppers, oregano, rosemary, and tomatoes. Mix well. Serve chayote and rice together in a bowl. Sprinkle cheese on top.

Chicory

Botanical Names: Cichorium intybus (Wild Chicory),
Cichorium endivia (Curly Endive and Escarole)

Chicory is presumed to have originated in the Mediterranean and was originally used by the Greeks and Romans for its medicinal properties. Chicory and escarole have been consumed as a vegetable since the fourteenth century in Europe. Wild chicory grows throughout North America, Europe and the temperate regions of northern Africa. Its short stems consist of green, tooth-edged leaves, similar to those of the dandelion, and are very bitter tasting. Young and tender chicory leaves are used in salads. Curly endive is a very full, thick, voluminous plant with slender, pointed leaves, used primarily in salads. Escarole is also a voluminous plant but has broad, less curly leaves than the curly variety and is not as bitter tasting.

Energy: Cooling

Taste: Bitter

Post Digestive: Bitter

Indications: Slow digestion, obesity, Ama buildup

Systems: Urinary, Digestive, Muscular

Dosha Affected:

Vata: Avoid

Pitta and **Kapha**: Excellent

Mixes Well With: Protein or starches

Season: Early Summer

See "Endive" for recipe, page 173.

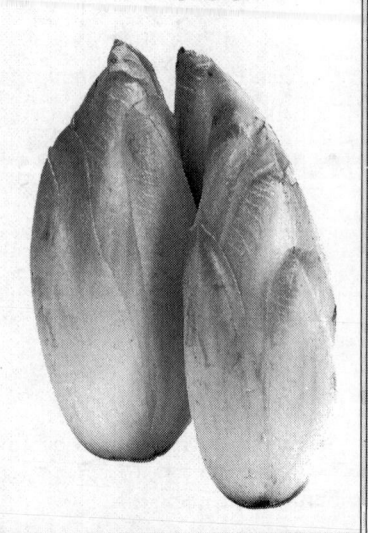

Collards

<u>Botanical Name: Brassica oleracea, Acephala group</u>

The collard plant can reach a height of 2 to 4 feet and closely resembles kale; unlike kale, it does not form a head. It is higher in minerals than any other member of the cabbage family, turnip greens, or spinach. A very hardy plant, it is easy to grow and can be planted in spring where it will grow through late fall. When lightly touched by frost, the flavor improves. Collard greens should be cooked for only 3 to 5 minutes to maintain the nutritional value.

Energy: Cooling

Taste: Bitter, Astringent

Post Digestive: Pungent

Indications: Varicose veins, anemia, boils, gallstones, liver disorders

Systems: Nervous, Endocrine, Circulatory, Epithelial

Dosha Affected:

Vata: Avoid

Pitta and **Kapha**: Excellent

Mixes Well With: All vegetables, starches or proteins

Season: Spring (depending on climate) & Summer

Stuffed Collard Greens

Serves 5

- 1 cup black-eyed peas
- 4 cups water
- ½ teaspoon hing
- 2 tablespoons ajwan
- 2 tablespoons cumin seeds
- 6 bay leaves
- 1 bunch green onions
- 10 large collard leaves
- 1 tablespoon tamarind pulp
- 1 cup baby spinach, chopped
- ¼ cup grated carrot
- 1 tablespoon coriander, ground
- 2 tablespoons Bragg's

Soak black-eyed peas overnight, in water to cover. The next day, drain water, add 4 cups fresh water and cook beans with hing, ajwan, cumin seeds, bay leaves, and onions. Bring to a boil, lower heat, and cook for 45 minutes, until beans are soft.

Lightly steam collard greens, keeping the leaves whole (and not mushy). Remove the stems. Blend the cooked beans to a smooth consistency. Add tamarind, spinach, grated carrots, coriander, and Bragg's.

Place 2 tablespoons of mixture on each leaf; fold in the corners and wrap like a burrito.

Serve with your choice of sauces: Tamarind (page 112), Spinach (page 211), and/or Carrot (page 147).

Corn

Botanical Name: Zea mays

Corn has been known for a hundred thousand years. Recent discoveries found a fossilized ear of corn in Peru, which provides evidence of its historic significance. It was grown and used in North America by the Native American Indians, who then introduced it to the first settlers. Corn is the leading cereal crop in the United States. This is not a common grain in Europe except for livestock feed, yet it is the main food of Central America where it is made into tortillas. The corn silk, or thread, can be used as a diuretic tea. Fresh corn needs to be chewed very well; there is a tendency to swallow before it is thoroughly masticated. Chewing is very important in order to assist in the digestion and assimilation of the starch content. It is best to eat young kernels, cooked for only two minutes. Serving it roasted or boiled can also be very palatable.

Energy: Warming

Taste: Astringent, Sweet

Post Digestive: Sweet

Indications: Jaundice, hepatitis, dispels phlegm, kidney stones

Systems: Endocrine, Urinary, Circulatory

Dosha Affected:

Vata: Moderation (lots of butter or ghee)

Pitta: Moderation

Kapha: Good

Mixes Well With: Green vegetables, starches

Season: Summer

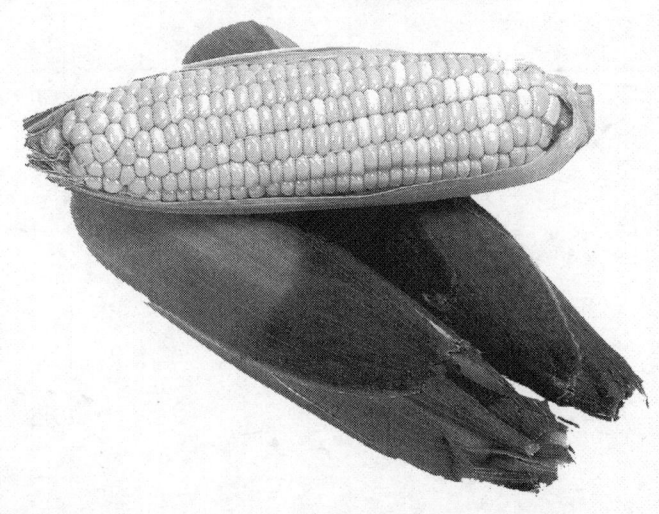

Cream of Corn Soup

Serves 4

- 6 ears of corn, shucked
- 4 tablespoons coriander, ground
- 2 tablespoons fennel, ground
- 2 cups soy milk or rice milk
- 2 cups cream (for Vata only)
- ½ bunch cilantro, chopped
- Bragg's or salt

Remove corn kernels from ears. Add to boiling water and cook until soft (about 5 minutes). Remove from stove; drain water, saving 1 cup. Blend corn and water with coriander, fennel, and milk until smooth. Heat until warm; add cilantro, and Bragg's to taste.

Polenta

Serves 6

- 1 roll polenta (made from corn)
- 1 red or yellow pepper, chopped
- 1 large sweet onion, chopped
- ½ bunch cilantro, chopped
- 1 bunch basil, chopped
- 2 tablespoons mild salsa
- Bragg's or salt

Cut polenta into small cubes. Saute onion at very slow heat until caramelized (soft and sweet). Add peppers and cook until soft. Stir in polenta cubes. Add cilantro and basil, salsa and Bragg's to taste.

Serve with salad or greens.

Cress

Botanical Name: Nasturtium officinale (Watercress) Lepidium sativum (Garden Cress)

Cress is believed to have originated in the Middle East, and has been known for its medicinal properties since ancient times. The Latin name for this plant, nasturtium, is derived from "nasus tortus" ("twisted nose") in reference to the effect on the nasal passages of eating the pungent, peppery-tasting plants. There are several types of cress, with the most popular being watercress and garden cress (or pepper grass). Watercress, a low trailing European perennial, is the variety most familiar to Americans. It is an aquatic plant that roots in fresh cold-water streams. It has thin stalks with dark green, glossy, compound leaves, either round or oval in shape. The variety known as Garden Cress grows more rapidly and easily than most other greens. It is grown in soil, and can also be grown hydroponically.

Energy: Warming

Taste: Bitter

Post Digestive: Bitter

Indications: Infections, low appetite, low agni, constipation, anemia, blood purifier, bursitis, tendonitis

Systems: Immune, Digestive, Excretory, Circulatory

Dosha Affected:

Vata and **Kapha**: Good

Pitta: Avoid or reduce

Mixes Well With: All vegetables, proteins or starches

Season: summer (depending on climate)

Ayurvedic Curative Cuisine for Everyone

Watercress Salad

Serves 2

- 2 cups water cress, cleaned and cut in pieces
- ½ head romaine lettuce, torn into bite-size pieces
- 1 sweet onion, sliced into rings
- ½ bunch cilantro
- 1 cup celery, chopped
- 2 tomatoes, chopped
- ¼ cup almonds, ground
- ¼ cup olive oil
- 2 tablespoons fennel, ground

Place vegetables in a large bowl. Toss together. Mix almonds, oil, and fennel, and pour over salad.

Watercress Soup

Serves 2

- 2 large bunches watercress, chopped
- 4 cups sesame milk
- 1 sweet onion, large
- 2 tablespoons ghee
- 2 tablespoons coriander
- 1 tablespoon fennel powder
- Aminos to taste

In a skillet add ghee with onions and caramelize at very low heat, stirring them to release the sugar. Put all ingredients in the blender and blend until smooth. Add aminos to taste.

Cucumber

Botanical Name: Cucumis sativus

The cucumber is one of the oldest vegetables known to man, cultivated before the Greek and Egyptian civilizations, and is referred to in earlier literature. It is native to Northern India and grown in England for two hundred years. Many varieties are now cultivated around the world. It is a wild offspring of the Persian melon. Most people are familiar with cucumbers in the form of pickles. The Burr cucumber is primarily used for pickling. The English variety is long and slender. Cucumbers are green when mature and have a 95% water content.

Energy: Cooling

Taste: Sweet

Post Digestive: Sweet

Indications: Skin infections, kidney stones, seizures, inflammations, fevers, indigestion, muscle cramps, ulcers

Systems: Urinary, Muscle, Digestive, Epithelial, Nervous, Immune

Dosha Affected:

Vata: Moderation, best pickled or in raita (an East Indian yogurt dish)

Pitta: Good

Kapha: Avoid or reduce

Mixes Well With: Vegetables or proteins

Season: Summer & Early Fall

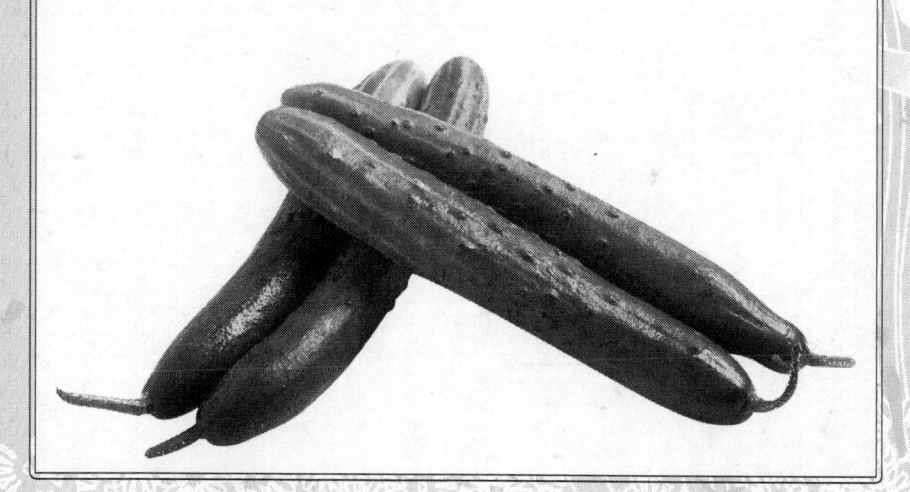

Raita

Serves 8

- 1 cup minced white onion
- 2 medium cucumbers, peeled, seeded and coarsely grated (about 2 cups)
- ½ teaspoon minced green chili (serrano, Thai or jalapeno)
- 2 cups plain yogurt
- ½ teaspoon ground cumin
- 1/16 teaspoon cayenne pepper
- 1/16 teaspoon ground black pepper
- 1 teaspoon salt

In a bowl combine all ingredients. Set aside for 20 minutes before serving. Consistency of raita should be slightly runnier than yogurt. Serve cool or at room temperature.

Stuffed Cucumber Boats

Serves 4

- 2 medium cucumbers, seeds removed
- 1 cup celery, chopped
- 1 cup red peppers, chopped
- ¼ cup ground sunflower seeds
- ¼ cup almonds
- 2 tablespoons olive oil
- ¼ cup chives or top of green onions
- 1/3 cup dill, finely chopped
- 1/3 cup mint, finely chopped
- 1 teaspoon kelp flakes

Slice cucumbers in half lengthwise. Scoop seeds out. In a food processor - add cucumber seeds, celery, red peppers, sunflower seeds, and almonds. Mix everything in processor. Empty into bowl, then add chopped dill & mint. Salt to taste or use Bragg's to taste. Then take mixture and place into cucumber shells. Serve with meat or green salad.

Eastern Salad

<u>Serves 4</u>

- 3 cucumbers, well washed
- 2 carrots
- ½ cup plain yogurt (divided)
- ¼ bunch parsley
- 1 bunch chives
- ¼ cup chopped olives
- 1 teaspoon agave syrup or honey
- 1 teaspoon lemon juice
- 1 teaspoon salt
- 1 teaspoon black pepper
- 1 teaspoon cardamom
- 1 teaspoon coriander
- 1 teaspoon ajwan seeds
- 1 tablespoons olive oil
- 1 head romaine lettuce

Peel the cucumbers and set aside the peels. Grate the cucumbers and carrots into a bowl. Add ¼ cup of yogurt, parsley, chives, and olives.

Dressing: In blender, put ¼ cup of yogurt, cucumber peels, agave, lemon juice, salt, pepper, cardamom, coriander, ajwan, and olive oil; blend until smooth.

Put romaine in salad bowl, top with grated veggies, then dressing. Empty into bowl, then add chopped dill & mint. Salt to taste or use Bragg's to taste. Then take mixture and place into cucumber shells. Serve with meat or green salad.

Eggplant

<u>Botanical Name: Solanum melongena</u>

The eggplant is said to be native of South America or the West Indies and was first cultivated in England in 1596. This vegetable is known by different names, among them Aubergine and Guinea Squash. In cultivation, this plant needs much attention and a soil rich in minerals. The color is dark or light purple, and it is a member of the nightshade family. For preparation, it should be boiled or baked no more than 15 minutes.

Energy: Cooling

Taste: Sweet, Astringent

Post Digestive: Sweet

Indications: Fevers, skin disorders, low blood sugar, constipation, uterine disorders

Systems: Circulatory, Reproductive, Excretory

Dosha Affected:

Vata: Moderation (add warming spices or seeds or oil)

Pitta: Good

Kapha: Avoid or reduce

Mixes Well With: Vegetables, starches or proteins

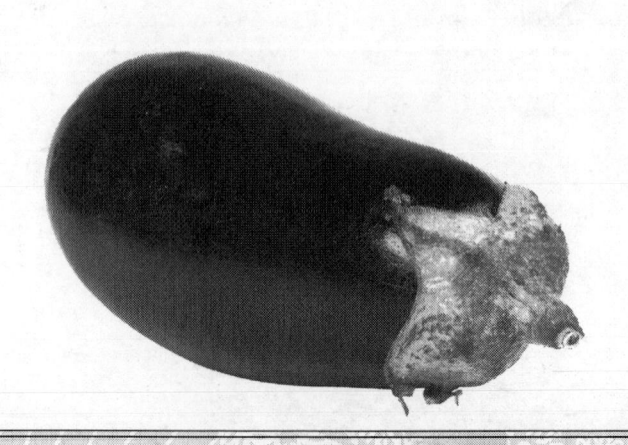

Eggplant Subzi

Serves 4

- 2 eggplant, peeled and chopped
- 2 potatoes, cut into cubes
- 2 green chilis, split – Kapha only
- 2 tablespoons sesame oil (divided)
- ½ cup water
- 1½ teaspoon cumin seeds
- 1 teaspoon mustard seed – Kapha only
- 2 medium onions, sliced
- 2 small red chilis, whole
- ½ cup coconut, grated
- ⅛ cup sesame seeds
- 10-15 almonds, chopped
- ¼ teaspoon turmeric
- salt to taste
- 1 tablespoon tamarind pulp mixed with 1 cup water
- 1 tablespoon sucanat or jaggary
- 1 sprig curry leaves, sautéed

Sauté eggplant, potatoes, and green chilis until light brown in 1 tablespoon sesame oil and water; set aside. Roast cumin and mustard seeds in another pan, then add 1 tablespoon oil and onions, and sauté until light brown. Add red chilis and coconut, and continue cooking for 10 minutes. Add sesame seeds, almonds, and sauté. Add turmeric, salt and tamarind water. Mix in eggplant-potato mixture and sucanat. Garnish with sautéed curry leaves.

Serve with rice.

Eggplant Supreme

Serves 4

1 large eggplant, peeled and chopped
3 tablespoons nut butter (cashew or almond)
1 teaspoon fennel, ground – for Kapha
1 tablespoon cumin seed
2 tablespoons olive oil
1 clove garlic – for Kapha
2 teaspoons cardamom
1 onion, well chopped
1 bunch basil, chopped
Bragg's

Steam chopped eggplant well. When soft and tender, mash with potato masher. Add nut butter; set aside. Roast fennel and cumin seeds. In blender, blend roasted seeds with olive oil, garlic, cardamom, onions, and basil. Blend well, then add to the eggplant mixture. Add Bragg's to taste. Serve it as a dip, over rice, or as a spread.

Serve as a dip, over rice, or as a spread.

Eggplant & Almond Sauté

Serves 4

2 eggplants, peeled, sliced
½ cup almonds, slivered
2 tablespoons ghee
¼ cup parsley

In a skillet, sauté ghee and eggplant. Cook until soft. Add almonds and parsley. Mix well. Serve.

Eggplant Bhurta

Serves 6

- 1 eggplant (8-10 inches long)
- ¼ teaspoon cumin seeds
- 3 tablespoons olive oil
- 2 cups onion, chopped
- 1 teaspoon minced ginger
- 1 teaspoon minced garlic
- 1 teaspoon minced green chili (Serrano, Thai, or jalapeño)
- 1 cup coarsely chopped tomatoes, fresh or canned, drained
- ⅛ teaspoon red pepper, ground
- ⅛ teaspoon black pepper, ground
- ½ teaspoon coriander, ground
- 1½ teaspoon salt
- 2 tablespoons chopped cilantro
- ¼ teaspoon garam masala

Preheat oven to 450°. Rub the eggplant skin lightly with a few drops of oil, and pierce in several places with a knife to prevent it from bursting. Put eggplant in pie pan or on cookie sheet and bake for 40 minutes, or until dark brown. It should yield readily when pressed with a spoon. Flesh will have shrunk considerably and possibly even have separated from the skin. Submerge eggplant in cold water for a few minutes. When cool enough to handle, peel off skin (which should come off readily if eggplant is cooked enough). Chop flesh into small pieces, and set aside in a colander to drain.

In a wok or large skillet, over medium-high heat, roast cumin seeds until slightly brown. Add oil and onion, and sauté until nicely browned. Add ginger, garlic, and green chili, and sauté for 1 minute, stirring constantly. Mix in tomatoes, spices, salt, and drained eggplant. Stir, still over medium-high heat, until eggplant is thoroughly cooked and all liquid has disappeared (see note). Consistency desired is like a lumpy paté. Stir in garam masala and remove from heat. Garnish with chopped cilantro.

Note: Keep temperature high enough and stir constantly to prevent eggplant from boiling in its own juices and becoming a paste.

Endive

Botanical Name: Cichorium endivia

Endive was accidentally "discovered" in 1850 by a Belgian who dug up wild chicory roots that resembled long, yellowish shoots. Later, a Belgian botanist named Brezier made numerous improvements to the endive, leading to what we enjoy today. The cultivation of endive is a complex process consisting of storing the freshly harvested roots for at least one month, during which time the cool temperatures stimulate the metabolism of the roots, making production of the endive possible. The roots are then "forced" (transplanted in a dark, warm environment to keep them from turning green and to preserve their mild flavor). They then develop into an endive and are harvested 3 to 4 weeks later. The crisp, creamy white (with a hint of yellow) leaves are 4 to 8 inches in length and approximately 2 inches in diameter with a slightly bitter taste.

Energy: Cooling

Taste: Bitter

Post Digestive: Pungent

Indications: Infections, Ama, to lose weight, colds, flu

Systems: All systems

Dosha Affected:

Vata: Avoid or reduce

Pitta and **Kapha**: Excellent

Mixes Well With: Proteins or starches

Season: Summer

Stuffed Endive

Serves 4

2 endives, medium size
½ cup pumpkin seeds, ground
½ cup sunflower seeds, ground
½ cup carrots, grated
1 bunch green onions, chopped
½ cup sunflower oil
1 tablespoon Bragg's
1 teaspoon coriander, ground
1 teaspoon rosemary, ground
1 tablespoon ginger, grated
3 endives, medium size

Mix all ingredients except endive in a bowl. Open the endive leaves and stuff each leaf individually. Mix all ingredients except endive in a bowl. Open the endive leaves and stuff each leaf individually.

Jerusalem Artichoke
(Sunchokes)

<u>Botanical Name: *Helianthus tuberosus*</u>

The Jerusalem artichoke, also called a "sunchoke," is neither an artichoke nor from Jerusalem! It is the edible tuber of a species of sunflower native to North America. The plant reaches a height of six feet, and has hairy foliage and yellow flowers. The tubers are gnarled, about 3" long, and look similar to ginger roots. They are very high in minerals, and are being made into tablets and sold in health food stores today. Sunchokes are harvested in the fall and are excellent when steamed. Good in salads either raw or steamed.

Energy: Warming, Moisturizing

Taste: Sweet

Post Digestive: Sweet

Indications: Female tonic, menopause, infertility, immune builder, emaciation, chronic diseases, to gain weight

Systems: Reproductive, Immune, Muscular

Dosha Affected:

Vata: Excellent (due to high mineral content)

Pitta: Good

Kapha: Avoid or reduce

Mixes Well With: All starchy vegetables, greens

Season: Late Summer & Late Fall

Sunchoke Soup

Serves 4

- 1 lb. Jerusalem artichokes, chopped
- 2 leeks, thinly sliced
- 1 large potato, cut into cubes
- 6 cups water
- 1 bunch basil, chopped
- ½ bunch cilantro, chopped
- 1 tablespoon cumin, ground

Boil vegetables in water until soft; add basil, cilantro and cumin. When cooked, put all ingredients in a blender, and blend until smooth. Garnish with cilantro, and serve.

Sunchoke (Artichoke) Stir Fry

Serves 4

- 2 cups sunchokes, sliced in small pieces
- 4 carrots, sliced in small pieces
- 1 cup cilantro
- 1 tablespoon ghee
- 1 thumb size ginger, fresh, grated
- 1 cup green onions, chopped
- 1 teaspoon ajwan seeds
- 1 teaspoon cumin seeds
- 2 cups spinach
- ½ cup water
- Bragg's to taste

In skillet or wok, roast cumin & ajwan seeds for 5 minutes, low flame. Add ghee, onions, sunchokes, carrot, grated ginger, and water. Increase fame to medium. When vegetables are tender, add cilantro and spinach. Cook briefly. Add Bragg's to taste.

Sunchokes, Tomatoes, and Celery Combo

Serves 4

- 8 ounces Jerusalem artichokes, sliced into rounds
- 8 slices sun-dried tomatoes
- 1½ cups water (divided)
- 1½ teaspoons ajwan seeds
- 1 tablespoon cumin seeds
- 1 tablespoon ghee
- 1 sweet onion, chopped
- 3 stalks celery, chopped
- Bragg's or salt

Steam sunchokes until soft but not mushy; drain and set aside. Place sun-dried tomatoes in one cup of warm water to reconstitute. In a sauté pan, roast ajwan and cumin seeds for 5 minutes on low heat, stirring constantly. Then add the ghee and onion, and cook onions until caramelized. Mix in celery and add ½ cup of water; cover and cook on low heat until soft. Drain the reconstituted tomatoes, and add with artichokes to celery-onion mixture, then add Bragg's or salt to taste.

Serve with proteins, grains, or vegetables.

Steamed Sunchokes With Carrots

- ½ pound sunchokes, steamed
- 4 carrots, medium, thin slices
- 2 stalks celery, steamed
- ¼ cup green onions
- 1 cup cilantro
- ½ teaspoon ajwan
- ½ teaspoon cumin
- ¼ cup parsley, chopped
- 1 tablespoon ghee

Steam carrots, sunchokes and celery. Roast ajwan and cumin seeds for 2 minutes, low flame. In skillet, add ghee & onions and sauté for few minutes. Drain water from steamed carrots, sunchokes, and celery. Add chopped parsley. Mix. Serve.

Jicama

Botanical Name: Pachyrhizus erosus

Jicama (pronounced HEE-kah-mah) is native to Mexico and Central and South America; the Aztecs used its seeds medicinally. Its name is derived from xicamalt, the Aztec term for this vegetable. The jicama plant was brought to the Philippines in the seventeenth century by the Spanish explorers and cultivation then spread throughout Asia and the Pacific. The jicama's tuberous root measures 4 to 6 inches, and resembles a turnip, with thin light brown skin and juicy white, crisp, sweet flesh (similar to a raw potato in texture). Jicama can be eaten raw or cooked; the delicate flavor is like that of a water chestnut or apple. Always make sure that you peel and remove the brown skin. This tubor is high in potassium and B vitamins. Great as a potato substitute. Can be eaten in a salad and as a snack with lemon and cayenne.

Energy: Cooling

Taste: Sweet

Post Digestive: Sweet

Indications: Rheumatic joints, fevers, to gain weight, anorexia

Systems: Immune, Nervous, Digestive

Dosha Affected:

Vata: Good (cooked)

Pitta: Good

Kapha: Avoid or reduce

Mixes Well With: Proteins or starches

Season: Tropical, Winter Season

Jicama Fries

Serves 2

- 1 large jicama, peeled
- 1 tablespoon olive oil
- 2 tablespoons lemon juice
- 1 tablespoon coriander, ground
- 1 tablespoon cumin, ground
- 1 tablespoon curry powder
- 1 tablespoon brewers yeast (optional)

Peel and cut jicama to look like French fries. (For Vata, steam the cut up jicama). Place in bowl, add olive oil, lemon juice, then add seasonings. (If you steam the jicama slices, make sure they are dry before you mix seasonings.)

Jicama Stir Fry

Serves 2

- 1 jicama, medium, sliced into cubes
- 1 onion, medium, cut into rings
- 2 tablespoons salsa
- 1 cup cilantro, chopped
- 1 tablespoon ghee
- 3 tablespoons water

In skillet or wok, add ghee and onions. Sauté for 5 minutes. Add Jicama And water until simmer until tender. Add salsa and cilantro before serving.

Kale

Botanical Name: Brassica oleracea

Kale is a hardy biennial plant that belongs to the cabbage family. Kale is sometimes grown as an ornamental. It is best grown during the fall and early winter, with flavor improving after the first light frost. It can also be used as a ground cover. There are many varieties of kale; Scotch Curled and Siberian are both very good. The young leaves can be eaten in salads or can be lightly cooked. Kale is considered to be one of the most highly nutritious vegetables, with powerful antioxidant and anti-inflammatory properties. It is high in minerals, especially calcium.

Energy: Cooling

Taste: Bitter, Astringent

Post Digestive: Pungent

Indications: Blood purifier, anemia, skin disorders, osteoporosis, muscle cramps, fevers, arthritis

Systems: Circulatory, Skeletal, Muscular

Dosha Affected:

Vata: Avoid or reduce

Pitta and **Kapha**: Excellent

Mixes Well With: All vegetables, proteins

Season: Spring, Summer

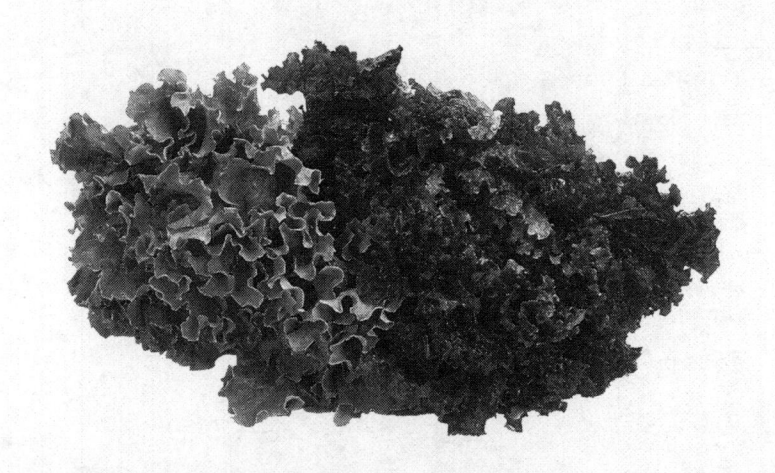

Ayurvedic Curative Cuisine for Everyone

Kale Ambrosia

Serves 2

- 10 large leaves and stems of kale, thinly sliced
- ¼ cup lime juice
- 1 teaspoon agave syrup
- 2 tablespoons olive oil
- 2 tablespoons juniper berries
- ½ cup pecans, chopped
- 2 apples, chopped
- 1 cup pineapple chunks

Place kale in a covered container with lime juice, agave, olive oil, and juniper berries, and let sit overnight. The next day, add pecans, apples, and pineapple to covered container.

Serve as salad with proteins and grains.

Kale a la Cream

Serves 2

- 1 onion, well chopped
- 1 tablespoon ghee
- 10 large leaves and stems of kale, chopped
- 2 tablespoons lemon juice
- 1 tablespoon coriander, ground
- 1 tablespoon fennel, ground
- 1 cup soy milk or almond milk
- Bragg's

Sauté chopped onion in ghee until caramelized. Add chopped kale, lemon juice, and spices; cover pan and cook for 5 minutes. Add milk and, stirring constantly, cook uncovered for another 5 minutes. Add Bragg's to taste.

Serve with protein or starches.

Kohlrabi

Botanical Name: (Brassica oleracea, Gongylodes Group)

Kohlrabi is a native of the Mediterranean region, particularly in Egypt where it was used in culinary and medicine. It is a member of the cabbage family, and is also called a turnip-rooted cabbage. Grown in spring, summer, and fall, the color ranges from green to purple. It takes 65 days from planting to harvest. The taste and texture of kohlrabi are similar to those of a broccoli stem or cabbage heart, but milder and sweeter. It can be eaten in salads, boiled, steamed or baked, and takes 15 to 20 minutes to cook. A good cancer preventative. This tubor is very high in vitamin A and is a great source of fiber. Can be eaten raw or cooked.

Energy: Warming

Taste: Sweet, Bitter

Post Digestive: Pungent

Indications: Skin infections, liver disorders, gallbladder, fevers, inflammations, cancer preventative, heart disorders, alcoholism, improves eyesight

Systems: Endocrine, Epithelial

Dosha Affected:

Vata: Moderation (well cooked with lots of spices and oils)

Pitta and **Kapha**: Excellent

Mixes Well With: All vegetables, starches, proteins

Season: Late Fall

Kohlrabi Mint Delight

Serves 4

- 3-4 kohlrabi (green or purple), peeled and cut into cubes
- ½ cup onions, chopped
- ½ cup mint leaves, chopped (divided)
- ⅛ cup olive oil
- ½ cup grapefruit juice
- 2 tablespoons Bragg's
- 1 tablespoon agave syrup
- 1¼ cups slivered almonds

Steam chopped kohlrabi and onion for 15 minutes, or until soft. Drain water, and mix the kohlrabi with ¼ cup fresh mint; set aside. In blender or food processor, combine onion with oil, grapefruit juice, Bragg's, and agave until it is a smooth sauce. Pour sauce over kohlrabi and toss well. Garnish with rest of mint and the almonds.

Kohlrabi Salad

Serves 4

- 2 kohlrabi, medium, peeled
- 2 carrots, grated
- 1 beet, medium, grated
- 1 bag baby greens, Spring mix
- ½ cup parsley
- ½ cup olives, black, without pits

Grate carrots, beets, & kohlrabi. Add grated vegetables, greens, olives, and parsley to bowl.

Dressing:
- 1 tablespoon olive oil
- 1 tablespoon lemon juice
- 1 teaspoon fennel
- 1 teaspoon mint
- ¼ teaspoon maple syrup

Mix ingredients together. Add dressing to salad just before serving.

Lamb's Lettuce

Botanical Name: Valerianella locusta

This annual, frost-resistant plant is believed to have originated in the Mediterranean. Europeans have enjoyed the delicate flavor of its tender leaves since the time of the Roman Empire. Also known as "corn salad" and "mâche," lamb's lettuce is closely related to valerian. Several varieties exist, all of which produce clusters of leaves at soil level with wide or narrow leaves, and come in various shades of green. Some varieties have a hazelnut flavor. Lamb's lettuce has a delicate flavor when fresh, and a bitter taste if wilted. This lettuce can be used as a spinach substitute

Energy: Cool

Taste: Bitter, Astringent, Sweet

Post Digestive: Pungent

Indications: Kidney infection, constipation

Systems: Urinary Tract

Dosha Affected:

Vata: Avoid or reduce

Pitta and **Kapha**: Good

Mixes Well With: Vegetables, grains or proteins

Season: Early Summer

Lamb's Lettuce Sauce

Serves 2

4 cups lamb's lettuce

1 tablespoon olive oil

¼ cup lemon juice

¼ cup water

1 teaspoon agave syrup

1 tablespoon coriander, ground

Steam lamb's lettuce just until wilted. Add with all other ingredients to blender; blend until smooth. Serve over eggs, or with proteins, vegetables, or salad.

Lamb's Lettuce Scramble

Serves 2

2 cups lamb's lettuce

4 eggs

1 tablespoon ghee

1 onion, chopped

½ cup mushrooms, sliced

¼ cup parsley

1 teaspoon Vata, Pitta, or Kapha Churna

Salt or Bragg's to taste

In a skillet add onions, mushrooms, and ghee and sauté for 5 minutes. Add Lamb's lettuce and simmer for 10 minutes.

Add well beaten eggs, and scramble in skillet. Add Vata, Pitta, or Kapha Churna for your body type.

Lettuce

<u>Botanical Name: *Lactuca sativa*</u>

Lettuce, a native of Asia and Africa, was first cultivated in the western world in 1562. Considered an herb, it is also a very important ingredient for salads in the West. Many varieties exist, including Bibb (also called Butterhead), Romaine, Looseleaf, Summer Crisp, and Iceberg. The iceberg variety has a 97% water content and little nutritional value. When fed to chickens, they may die within 24 hours or develop skin diseases. Cows fed surplus lettuce lost their hair. (Could there be any connection to all the baldness in America?!) We recommend eating non-iceberg lettuce.

Energy: Cooling

Taste: Astringent

Post Digestive: Pungent

Indications: Fevers, blood purifier, insomnia, lymphatic disorders, fevers, inflammations

Systems: Circulatory, Nervous, Lymphatic

Dosha Affected:

Vata: Avoid

Pitta: Excellent

Kapha: Good

Mixes Well With: All leafy greens, starchy vegetables, or proteins

Season: Late Spring & Summer

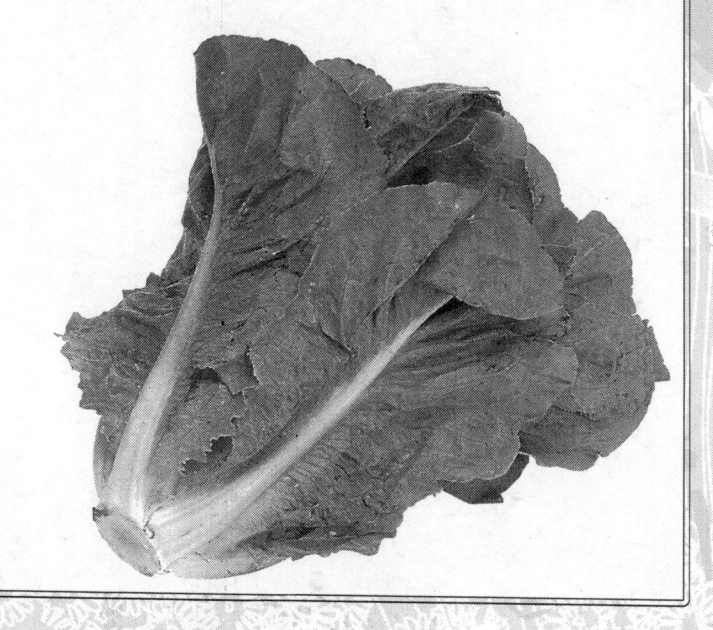

Nutty Lettuce Wraps

Serves 4-6

- ¼ cup almonds, ground
- ¼ cup cashews, ground
- ½ cup dill, finely chopped
- ½ cup parsley, finely chopped
- 4 green onions, well chopped
- 1½ tablespoons olive oil
- ⅛ cup lemon juice
- 1 tablespoon Bragg's
- 2 tablespoons mild curry powder
- ½ head romaine or curly lettuce

Mix nuts, dill, parsley, and onions in bowl; add olive oil, lemon juice, Bragg's, and curry powder. Mix into a paste. Trim the spine from the lettuce leaves. Spread the nut-spice paste on each leaf and roll like a burrito. Repeat until you have a collection of lettuce wraps. Serve alone, or with grains or salad.

Grilled Romaine Salad

- 1 head Romaine lettuce
- 2 Roma tomatoes
- 1 red onion, small – may not use entire onion
- 2 oz. Feta cheese
- 2 cups balsamic vinaigrette
- Salt & pepper to taste

Prep: Clean the Romaine leaves & trim off top. Lightly coat leaves with extra virgin olive oil. Do not drown leaves in oil. Once leaves are oiled, gently dab off excess oil if necessary. Salt & pepper leaves lightly.

Mark leaves: On grill or char broiler = place leaves on grill to mark. Be sure surface is hot - you only score leaves.

Once grill mark is noticeable, remove from heat source. Be sure leaves are grilled, not wilted. Tomatoes, slice lengthwise in half, place on sheet pan. Sprinkle with salt & pepper & EVOO - place in oven until roasted, approximately 20 minutes. Cool. Place on opposite corners of plate. Sautee red onion with EVOO and place on side...use salt & pepper to add flavor if necessary

Serve: Place leaves in middle of plate, lightly use balsamic vinaigrette reduction to add color and taste to leaves. Place Roma tomatoes on opposite corners of plate. Place red onions lightly on tomatoes to splash color. Sprinkle Feta cheese lightly on top. Serve.

Romaine Salad

Serves 4

- 2 heads romaine lettuce
- ½ head escarole
- 1 cup baby spinach
- ½ cup cucumber, sliced
- ¼ cup green onion, chopped
- ½ cup cilantro, chopped
- ½ cup parsley, chopped

Tear lettuce into bite-size piece; wash well. Put all ingredients into a salad bowl, and top with dressing just before serving: Serve with protein or starches.

Dressing:
- 2 tablespoons olive oil
- 1 tablespoon balsamic vinegar
- 1 teaspoon agave syrup
- Bragg's to taste

Lotus Roots
Botanical Name: Nelumbo nucifera

The plant known as blue lotus, Indian lotus, or sacred water-lily is an aquatic perennial, native to a large area from Southeast to Central Asia. It is the National Flower of India and Vietnam, and cultivated as both an ornamental and a food plant. Lotus roots are very nutritious, and have been used as food for many centuries. They are rich in dietary fiber, vitamin C, potassium, several B vitamins, phosphorus, copper, and manganese, while very low in saturated fat. Lotus roots can be purchased at Asian grocery stores.

Energy: Warming, Astringent

Taste: Sweet, Bittersweet

Post Digestive: Sweet

Indications: Heart, blood cleanser, prostate, amenorrhea

Systems: Reproductive, Immune, Nervous

Dosha Affected:

Vata: Moderation (add spices and ghee)

Pitta: Good

Kapha: Moderation

Mixes Well With: Proteins, starches

Season: Winter

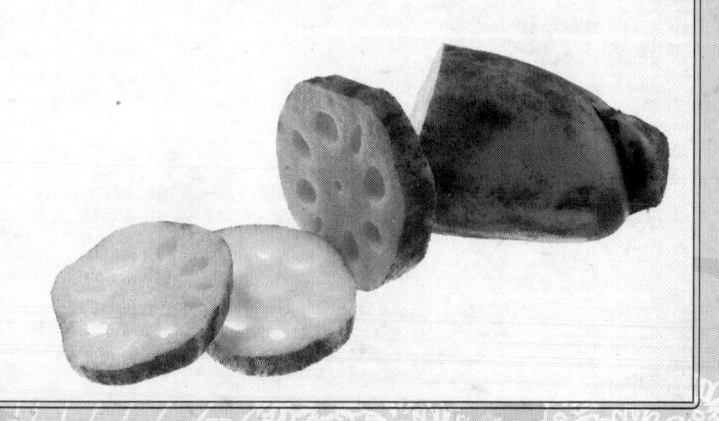

Lotus Root Stir Fry

Serves 4

- 1 tablespoon sesame oil
- ½ leek, sliced
- 2 tablespoons grated ginger
- 10 lotus roots, sliced into rounds
- 2 carrots, sliced diagonally
- 2 stalks celery, sliced diagonally
- ¼ cup water
- 1½ cups fresh bean sprouts
- 1 tablespoon soy sauce

In wok or sauté pan, sauté leeks and ginger in sesame oil. Add lotus roots, carrots, celery and water. While stirring, cook for 10 to 15 minutes on low heat, until cooked but still crisp. Add bean sprouts and soy sauce, and heat through.

Serve with grains (especially rice).

Lotus Saffron Rice

Serves 4

- 1 cup lotus seeds
- 1 cup basmati rice
- 10 threads saffron
- ½ cup green onions, chopped
- 1 tablespoon ginger, chopped
- 3 ½ cups water
- ¼ teaspoon cardamom powder
- 1 tablespoon Vata, Pitta, or Kapha churna

Soak lotus seed over night in one cup of water. Next day strain water. In a pot Bring water to boil add rice, lotus seeds , saffron, cardamom, and water and cook for 20 minutes. Then lower heat to simmer. In a small skillet, saute the ghee, onions, churna, and ginger. When the rice is done, add ginger, churna, and onions. Mix together. Serve.

Mushroom

<u>Botanical Name: Agaricus bisporus</u>

Mushrooms belong to the fungus family with many varieties, some of which are poisonous. Having a very simple structure, mushrooms grow close to the ground and prefers moist, dark, cool places. The creamy white Button mushroom is the most commonly cultivated variety found in U.S. grocery stores – and Portobello is a strain of this same species. Other edible mushrooms, such as Oyster (Pleurotus ostreatus) and Shiitake (Lentinula edodes), are becoming more available in U.S. stores. In Chinese medicine, mushrooms are used medicinally for their bitter and astringent properties as immune builders.

Energy: Cooling

Taste: Sweet, Astringent

Post Digestive: Sweet

Indications: Blood disorders, anti-tumor, anti-cancer, reduces cholesterol, promotes longevity

Systems: Muscular, Immune, Circulatory

Dosha Affected:

Vata: Moderation (cooked in oil, ghee or butter)

Pitta and **Kapha**: Good (avoid when imbalanced with pus or infection)

Mixes Well With: All vegetables, proteins

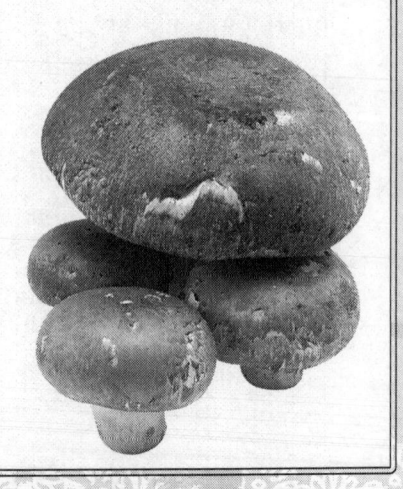

Shiitake and Spinach

- 1½ teaspoons ajwan
- 1½ teaspoons cumin seeds
- 2 tablespoons ghee or olive oil
- 1 cup green onions, chopped
- 2 tablespoons ginger, grated
- 2 large shiitake mushrooms, sliced
- ⅛ cup water
- 1 bunch spinach, thinly sliced
- 1 tablespoon Bragg's

Roast ajwan and cumin seeds in a wok or skillet. Add ghee, onions, and ginger to pan, and sauté.

When the seeds and the onions are soft, add mushrooms and cook until tender. Add the water and spinach leaves; cover and simmer 5 minutes. Stir in Bragg's.

Mushroom Tambay

Serves 4

- 1 tablespoon cumin seeds
- 1 teaspoon ajwan seeds
- 2 tablespoons ghee
- ½ onion, chopped
- 8 ounces mushrooms, sliced
- 1 yellow squash, chopped
- ½ eggplant, chopped
- ½ bunch cilantro, chopped
- ¼ cup water

In a skillet, roast ajwan and cumin seeds for 5 minutes; add ghee and onions. Keep stirring so the seeds do not burn. Add mushrooms and yellow squash; cook for 10 minutes more. Add eggplant, cilantro, and water; cover pan and cook on low heat for another 10 minutes. Take off heat and let it steep for about 10 minutes.

With a tambay cutter or a tiny cup, put the mixture in small mounds on the plate. Serve with grains (buckwheat is good) or proteins.

Rose Mushrooms

1 pound. mushrooms
1 cup rose petals
1½ cups rosewater
1 cup walnuts, finely ground
⅓ cup onion, chopped
1 cup sunflower seeds
2 tablespoons ghee
1 teaspoon thyme
2 teaspoons coriander
1 teaspoon rosemary
1 tablespoon dried parsley
Bragg's

Wash mushrooms and remove stems. Chop stems, and set aside. Soak rose petals and mushroom caps overnight in rose water. Drain the next day, separating rose petals from the mushroom caps.

Put ground walnuts in a bowl, add rose petals, chopped mushroom stems, onion, and sunflower seeds. Mix in the ghee, add spices and Bragg's to taste. Mix into a paste. Put a spoonful of mixture into each mushroom cap.

Serve as hors d'oeuvres.

Mustard Greens

Botanical Name: Brassica juncea

Mustard belongs to a large family of plants that includes cabbages, broccoli, cauliflower, rutabaga, turnips, and kale. It is a native of Asia and China, and today is widely cultivated in the southern U.S. It is also found in abundance in the wild, and often referred to as a weed. The leaves of wild mustard can be eaten raw in salads, or cooked as a vegetable for 5 to 10 minutes. This leafy green vegetable has many medicinal properties, in the seeds and flowers as well as in the leaves. Mustard greens are extremely high in vitamin A and vitamin K. Used as a poultice, the greens can break down tumors.

Energy: Warming

Taste: Pungent, Bitter

Post Digestive: Pungent

Indications: Lung congestion, fat reducing, tumor reducing, phlegm dispeller

Systems: Respiratory, Muscular

Dosha Affected:

Vata and **Pitta**: Avoid

Kapha: Excellent

Mixes Well With: All vegetables, proteins or starches

Season: Spring, Summer

Greens a la Coconut

Serves 6

1 sweet onion, chopped

1 tablespoon ghee

10 large sized leaves and stems of mustard greens, chopped – Kapha only

3 leaves of dandelions, chopped

6 large leaves of kale, chopped

5 large leaves of collard greens, chopped

2 cups coconut milk

½ teaspoon turmeric, ground

½ teaspoon fennel, ground

1 teaspoon cardamom, ground

2 teaspoons coriander, ground

1 teaspoon mustard seed – Kapha only

1 teaspoon maple syrup

½ cup millet – Pitta

½ cup quinoa – Kapha

½ cup spelt – Vata

In large wok, sauté onions in ghee until brown. On low heat, begin adding greens to wilt; stir well. Add coconut milk, then remaining ingredients. Top with breadcrumbs or crushed rice crackers, and serve.

Okra

Botanical Name: Hibisccus esculentus

Okra is native to Africa, and was introduced to the U.S. in the 18th century. It also goes by the names of "lady finger" and "gumbo." The okra plant is in the mallow family (with such species as cotton and cocoa); it is grown for its edible pods, which are harvested when immature. The taste of cooked okra is delicious, and it is now cultivated in many parts of the world. Eating okra is soothing and moisturizing to female organs.

Energy: Cooling, Moisturizing

Taste: Sweet

Post Digestive: Sweet

Indications: Urinary tract infections, diarrhea, dysentery, leukorrhea, nerves

Systems: Urinary, Excretory

Dosha Affected:

Vata: Good (well cooked)

Pitta: Excellent

Kapha: Avoid or reduce

Mixes Well With: All vegetables, proteins or starches

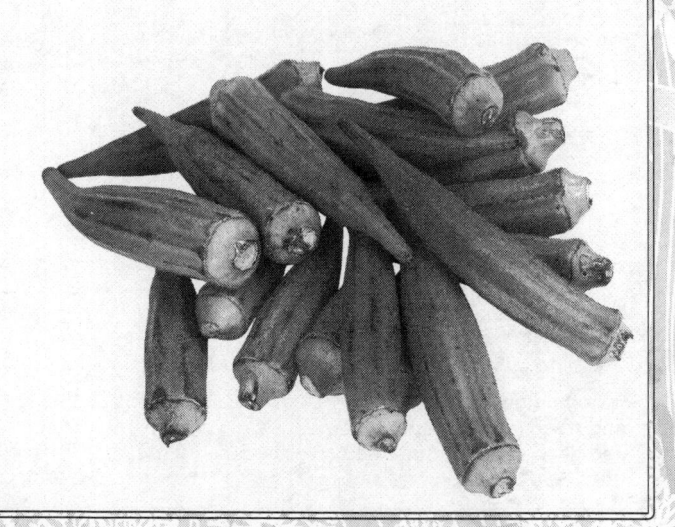

Okra Delight

Serves 4

- 2 cups okra, sliced into rings
- 2 cups broccoli flowers, leaves, and stems (peel stems), chopped
- 1 tablespoon ghee
- ½ cup of green onions, chopped
- 1 clove garlic, chopped
- 4-inch piece ginger, chopped
- ½ cup water
- ½ cup cilantro, chopped
- ½ cup parsley, chopped
- 1 teaspoon coriander, ground
- Bragg's

Steam okra and broccoli. In a wok or large skillet, met ghee and sauté the onions, garlic, and ginger. Then add okra and broccoli and ½ cup of water, and bring to a boil. Cover and steep for 10 minutes. Once tender, add cilantro, parsley, and coriander. Add Bragg's to taste.

Okra Coconut Tomato Curry

Serves 4

- 3 cups okra, cut in small circles
- 2 cups tomatoes, well chopped
- 2 mild chilies, chopped
- ¼ cup onions, chopped
- 1 tablespoons cumin
- 2 tablespoons mild curry
- 1 cup cilantro, well chopped
- 2 tablespoons ghee
- ½ cup coconut cream
- 4 cups water
- Salt to taste

In a medium pot, 4 cups of water add Okra, bring to boil lower flame cover it and steep for ten minutes strain the water out. In a skillet, roast cumin and chilli, add ghee, onions and tomatoes. Add coconut cream. Mix well. Cook for 5 minutes. Add cilantro curry and salt.

Olive

<u>Botanical Name: Oleum europaea</u>

Olives are native to the warm regions of Asia and Europe, and can be traced to the beginnings of ancient history. Egyptians grew olives 4,000 years ago. They were first introduced to California by the Franciscan monks around 1769. Approximately six to seven varieties are used commercially. The olive grows on evergreen trees or shrubs, and the wild varieties are often very spiny. For pickling, olives are gathered when they have reached full size but are still green in color. Ripe olives are also in demand and are picked from the tree when purple or black in color. Olives should not be eaten as a main food; it is best to combine them with vegetables and salads.

Energy: Warming

Taste: Sweet

Post Digestive: Sweet

Indications: Indigestion, skin rashes, bad breath, dry throat

Systems: Epithelial, Digestive, Endocrine

Dosha Affected:

Vata: Moderation

Pitta: Good

Kapha: Avoid or reduce

Mixes Well With: Vegetables, starch or protein

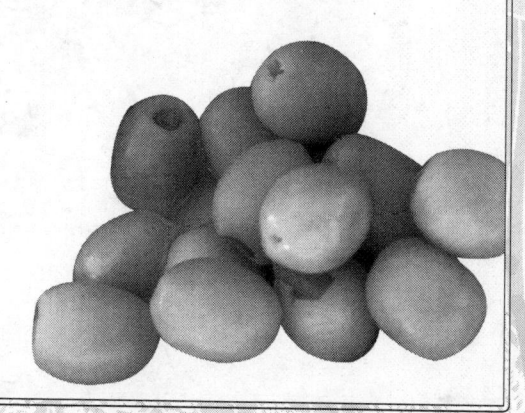

Olive Pâté

- ½ cup black olives
- 1 cup raw cashews
- 1 green onion
- 2 tablespoons olive oil
- 2 tablespoons lime juice
- 1 tablespoon Italian seasoning

Put all ingredients in blender; blend until smooth.

Serve with salad, or put on bread or crackers.

Olive Salad

Serves 4

- 1 cup green olives, large, pitted
- 1 cup black olives, large, pitted
- 2 endives, well chopped
- ½ cup radicchio, chopped
- 1 cup baby spinach, chopped
- 2 tablespoons olive oil
- 1 tablespoon lemon juice
- 1 cup parsley, chopped

Mix all ingredients together in a bowl. Add olive oil and lemon juice. Serve.

Parsnip

<u>Botanical Name: *Pastinaca sativa*</u>

Parsnips are believed to have originated in Germany where they grow along the Rhine Valley. They were known to the Romans prior to the Christian era, and also well known in England during the 16th century. The parsnip is a biennial related to carrots, grown for its long, thick, sweet, white root, and is used as a vegetable mainly from autumn to spring. It is an easy vegetable to grow, with a high nutritive value – yet not very popular. It is best steamed for 15 to 20 minutes or baked for 30 minutes (with ghee or oil added). Higher fiber than any other vegetable. Cancer fighting properties. Keeps digestive tract healthy.

Energy: Warming

Taste: Astringent, Pungent

Post Digestive: Pungent

Indications: Kidney disorders, blood purifier, colon disorders, high blood pressure, constipation, heart problems

Systems: Urinary, Circulatory

Dosha Affected:

Vata: Avoid

Pitta: Moderation

Kapha: Good

Mixes Well With: Non-starchy vegetables, greens

Season: Late Fall

Baked Parsnips with Carrots

Serves 4

- 1 tablespoon ghee
- 6 parsnips, chopped
- 3 carrots, chopped
- 1 cup dill weed, chopped
- Bragg's

Preheat the oven to 350°. Oil a baking dish with ghee, fill with chopped parsnips and carrots, and cook for 30 minutes. Mix the dill weed and Bragg's, add to vegetables, and serve.

Serve with grains.

Mashed Parsnips

Serves 4

- 6 parsnips, medium
- 1 cup chives or top of green onions
- 1 tablespoon ghee
- ½ tablespoon fennel, well chopped
- 1 tablespoon Churna
- 2 cups water

Wash parsnips and cut into pieces. Put in water & bring to boil. When tender, drain, and mash. Add remaining ingredients, except churna which is add to each individual Serving.

Peas

Botanical Name: Pisum sativum

Peas are probably native to Central Europe or Central Asia. They were known to the Aryans two thousand years before Christ, with numerous references found in Biblical history. The pea plant is an annual tendril-climbing vine grown for its edible seeds and pods. Fresh garden peas can be among the first rewards of the season. All peas should be eaten when fresh and young for the highest nutritional value. Peas have a sweet and delicate flavor and should be steamed for only 1 or 2 minutes. The pea is a legume and, in the dried state, is not as wholesome as the fresh pea. It can be used in soups or as a cooked vegetable.

Energy: Cooling

Taste: Astringent, Sweet

Post Digestive: Sweet

Indications: Kidney infections, urinary tract infections, liver and gall bladder disorders, blood purifier

Systems: Urinary Tract, Digestive, Endocrine

Dosha Affected:

Vata: Avoid or reduce

Pitta and **Kapha**: Good

Mixes Well With: Vegetables, protein or starches (when fresh).

Starchy and non-starchy vegetables (when dried and cooked).

Season: Summer

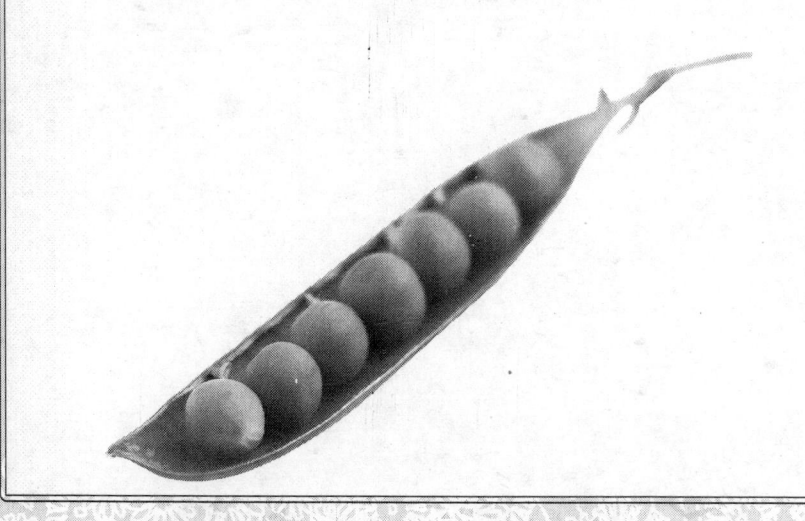

Spiced Peas

Serves 4

- 1 cup fresh or frozen peas (best if fresh)
- 4 cups water
- 1 medium onion, chopped
- 1 teaspoon ginger, well chopped
- 2 tablespoons garam masala
- 6 large leaves and stems of kale, thinly sliced
- 1 tablespoon fresh cilantro, chopped
- 4 tablespoons ghee
- 1 tablespoon dried mint leaves
- 2 teaspoon parsley
- Bragg's or salt

If using fresh peas, soak 2 hours in water; then drain. Place peas in saucepan. Add water, onion, ginger, and garam masala. Bring to a boil and simmer for 45 minutes. Add chopped kale, cilantro, mint, parsley, and ghee; cook for another 10 minutes. Add Bragg's or salt to taste. Cover and steep for 10 minutes.

Serve with grains or vegetables.

Snow Peas and Watercress

1 bunch green onions, chopped
½ bunch basil, chopped
½ tablespoon ghee
2 teaspoons cumin seeds
1 tablespoon coriander, ground
1 whole red pepper, thinly sliced
2 cups snow peas, ends removed
2 cups watercress, chopped
Bragg's or salt

In melted ghee, sauté the onions, basil, and spices. Add red pepper and snow peas, and continue cooking. Add watercress and sauté lightly. Add Bragg's to taste just before serving.

Peas & Potatoes

Serves 4

1 cup dry peas (or frozen organic peas)
1 cup potatoes, cubed small
6 cups water
1 onion, well chopped
1 tablespoon cumin
1 tablespoon ajwan
1 teaspoon turmeric
8 bay leaves
1 teaspoon mustard seeds
1 tablespoons Vata, Pitta, or Kapha churna

Soak dry peas in 1 cup of water overnight. Next day drain the water off. Add one half of the onions together with one half of the spices, except for the bay leaves, and 4-1/2 cups of the water. Cook for 40 minutes. Drain all liquids. In a large skillet, roast all remaining spices. Cook until soft. Add ghee, potatoes, and a little water. Mix in churna, salt, and peas. Serve with rice.

Ayurvedic Curative Cuisine for Everyone

Potato

Botanical Name: Solanum tuberosum

This plant was first introduced into Europe by the Spaniards and later by the English, but did not become popular in Europe until the 18th century. It is a tropical and sub-tropical perennial now extensively grown in temperate climates worldwide. The potato is a member of the nightshade family, closely related to the eggplant, tomato, and pepper. Therefore, those with allergies or a high sensitivity to foods should be careful. Potatoes are very starchy. The best ways of preparing them are either steamed or baked.

Energy: Cooling

Taste: Astringent, Sweet

Post Digestive: Sweet

Indications: Diarrhea, poor assimilation/absorption, inflamed nerves, nerves, gout, kidney disorders, intestinal cleansing

Systems: Excretory, Nervous, Urinary

Dosha Affected:

Vata: Moderation (with lots of butter)

Pitta: Good

Kapha: Moderation (baked)

Mixes Well With: Other starches and vegetables

Season: Fall

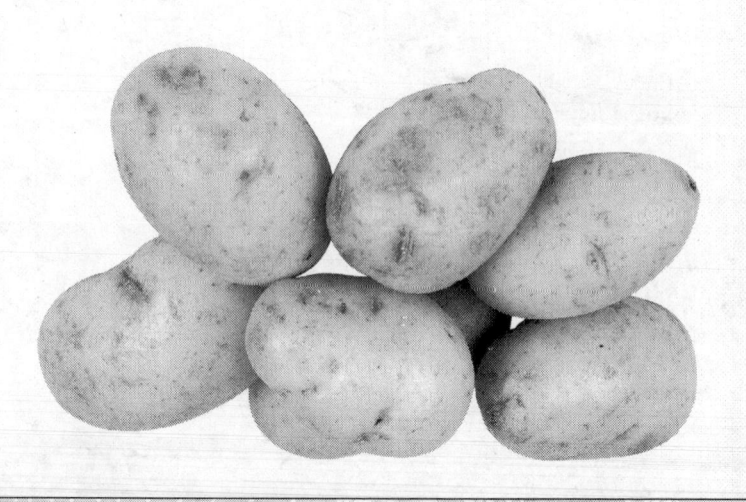

Potato Spinach Fennel Curry

Serves 6-8

- 4 medium potatoes
- 20 leaves or 2 bags of organic baby spinach
- 2 cups fennel, finely sliced
- 3 tablespoons sunflower oil
- 1 teaspoon mustard seeds
- 1/8 teaspoon hing
- 1 teaspoon turmeric
- 3 cups water
- 1 teaspoon sea salt
- 4 teaspoons coriander, ground
- 4 tablespoons lemon juice
- 1/2 green pepper, chopped

Wash spinach, potatoes, and fennel. Cut potatoes into ½-inch cubes, chop spinach and fennel. In heavy saucepan, roast mustard seeds and hing - then add oil. When seeds pop, add turmeric, potatoes, fennel and water. Stir. Cover and cook on medium heat for 7 to 10 minutes. Then add spinach and all other ingredients. Mix well. Cook covered for additional 10 to 15 minutes.

Potatoes & Kale

Serves 4

- 2 cups kale
- 2 cups water
- 2 tablespoon mustard seed
- 2 cups potatoes, cubed
- 2 tablespoons ghee
- 1 cup green onions
- Salt to taste or Bragg's

Cut potatoes into cubes. Steam for 5 minutes. In wok or skillet, roast mustard seeds at a low heat for 3-5 minutes. Add ghee, green onions, steamed potatoes

Curried Potato Patties with Carrots

Serves 8

- 6 large or 8 small red potatoes, unskinned
- 1½ tablespoons sunflower oil
- 1 tablespoon mustard seeds
- 2 cups grated carrots
- 1 tablespoon curry powder
- 1 teaspoon sea salt
- ²/₃ cup green onions, finely chopped
- 2 cups cilantro, finely chopped

In a large pot, boil for the potatoes until tender, about half an hour. Put the oil in a large skillet and add the mustard seeds. When they pop, add the grated carrot and cook just long enough to wilt them slightly. Stir in the curry powder and salt. When the potatoes are done, drain them and let them cool enough to handle them. Mash them well, with a fork or your hands, and stir or mash in the carrots, onions, and cilantro. Form the mixture into patties and cook on a skillet, browning them in ghee 1 to 2 minutes on each side. Serve hot.

German Potato Salad

Serves 6

- 6 potatoes, cubed
- 1 cup string beans, sliced
- ½ cup peas, fresh or frozen organic
- 3 tablespoons mayonnaise (see page 344)
- 1 cup carrots, grated
- 1 cup green onions, chopped
- 2 hard boiled eggs, chopped
- 2 small apples – or 1 large – chopped
- 2 teaspoons dill powder
- ½ teaspoon paprika

Remove ends from green beans. Bring potatoes and string beans to boil in water. Can also make hard boiled eggs in pot with potatoes, which adds calcium from the eggshells. Cook until potatoes are tender but not mushy – still firm. Otherwise it will turn into mashed potatoes. Drain water. Cool. Crack eggs, peel, and cut into slices – save a couple slices for garnishment. Chop apples. Add fresh or defrosted peas. Mix everything together in bowl. Slowly add the mayonnaise and mix gently without mashing the potatoes. Garnish with egg slices and paprika.

Rutabaga

Botanical Name: Brassica napus

The rutabaga, or Swedish turnip, is a hardy biennial herb cultivated as an annual vegetable. It differs from the turnip in having bloom-covered leaves, a more elongated and leafy top, and many more fibrous roots. Those with finicky or impaired digestion must avoid this vegetable, along with other root vegetables, since they easily create gas due to their mustard oil content. The rutabaga has a rajasic nature. Good for clearing mucous & congestion. Avoid when there is kidney problems. Anti-cancer properties. Very high in minerals. Avoid when there are kidney or digestive disorders

Energy: Heating

Taste: Astringent, Pungent

Post Digestive: Pungent

Indications: Blood and lymphatic cleanser, excessive bleeding, mucous, congestion, cancer

Systems: Circulatory, Lymphatic, Respiratory

Dosha Affected:

Vata: Avoid or reduce

Pitta: Moderation

Kapha: Good

Mixes Well With: Vegetables or starches

Season: Late Fall

Ayurvedic Curative Cuisine for Everyone

Sweet Rutabaga with Chard

Serves 4

- 2 rutabagas, peeled and cut into cubes
- 1 sweet potato, cut into cubes
- 1 tablespoon fresh ginger, grated
- 2 tablespoons ghee
- 1 tablespoon cinnamon
- 1 tablespoon cardamom, ground
- 1 tablespoon jaggary or sucanat
- 12 large leaves and stems of chard, well chopped
- 1 tablespoon fresh mint, well chopped
- Bragg's or salt

Preheat oven to 350°. Mix together rutabaga and sweet potato cubes. Add ginger, ghee, seasonings and sweetener. Place mixture into an oiled baking pan, and cook for 40 minutes. Mix in the chopped chard and mint, and cook for 5 minutes more.

Serve with salad or other vegetables.

Rutabaga Steamed & Mashed

Serves 4

- 3 rutabagas, peeled, chopped
- ¼ cup cream, organic
- 2 tablespoons fennel seed powder
- 2 tablespoons ghee
- 1 tablespoon coriander
- 1 quart water
- Salt to taste

Bring water to boil and add rutabagas. Cook until tender. Drain water. Mash rutabaga, using a potato masher or hand blender. Mix in remaining ingredients. Serve.

Spinach

Botanical Name: Spinacia oleracea

Spinach originated in northern Asia and was introduced into central Europe during the 16th century. It is a hardy, short-seasoned plant that may be planted in very early spring. There are two main varieties: the winter or perpetual spinach (which has small prickly leaves), and the smooth leaf variety (with thick, fleshy, and crumpled leaves). Used in salads, spinach improves flavor and variety. When cooking spinach leaves, do so for only 1 to 3 minutes. Butter, ghee, or oil dressing is all that is necessary. Spinach contains a considerable amount of oxalic acid and, for this reason, large servings should not be eaten – nor should it be eaten frequently.

Energy: Cooling

Taste: Astringent

Post Digestive: Pungent

Indications: Fevers, cough, lungs, blood toner

Systems: Respiratory, Circulatory

Dosha Affected:

Vata: Avoid or reduce

Pitta: Moderation

Kapha: Excellent

Mixes Well With: Vegetables, starch or protein

Season: Summer, Early Fall

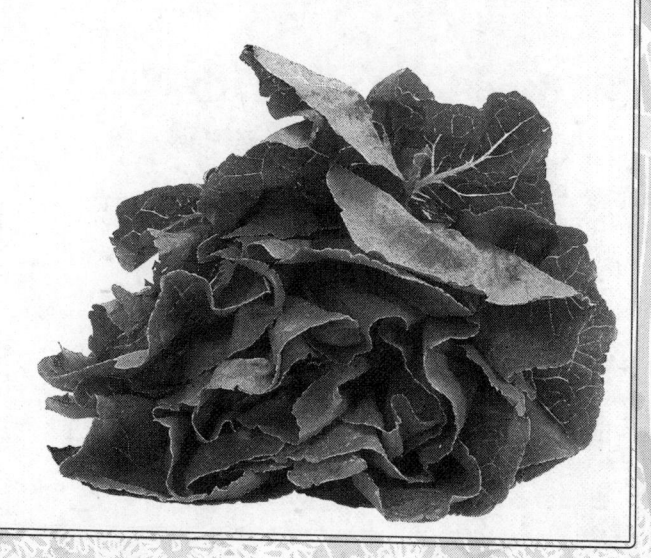

Ayurvedic Curative Cuisine for Everyone

Spinach and Goat Cheese

Serves 10

- 2 teaspoons cumin seeds
- 1 tablespoon ghee
- 1½-inch piece ginger, finely chopped
- 5 garlic cloves, finely chopped – Kapha only
- 1 large or 2 medium onions, chopped
- 1½ teaspoons red chili powder
- ½ teaspoon turmeric
- 1½ teaspoons salt
- 1 pack spinach
- 750 grams goat cheese, cut in cubes
- 1 teaspoon garam masala
- ghee or butter

Roast cumin seeds in skillet. Add ghee, ginger, garlic, and onions, and sauté until brown. Add chili powder, turmeric, and salt, and continue cooking. Add spinach and sauté lightly. You may add ½ to 1 cup of water if necessary, to make thin gravy. Pour it over cubes of goat cheese, and serve garam masala and butter on top for garnish.

Serve with rice, chapattis, etc.

Wilted Spinach With Nuts

Serves 4

- 2 bags baby spinach
- 1 cup almond slivers
- 1 cup jicama, grated
- 1 tablespoons ghee
- 1 tablespoon Vata, Pitta, or Kapha churna
- Aminos to taste

In skillet, add ghee. Slowly add the spinach, jicama and nuts. Stir well. Add aminos and chuna. Cook for 5 minutes.

Spinach Sauce #1

- 2 cups steamed spinach
- 2 tablespoons ghee
- ½ onion
- 1 tablespoon curry powder
- ½ tablespoon cumin
- Bragg's to taste

Add all ingredients in blender and blend until smooth.

Spinach Sauce #2

- 2 cups steamed spinach
- 2 tablespoons olive oil – Kapha
- 2 tablespoons ghee – Vata & Pitta
- ¼ lb. soy mozzarella cheese
- ½ onion
- 1 tablespoon curry powder
- ½ tablespoon cumin
- Bragg's to taste

Add all ingredients in blender and blend until smooth.

Spinach Sauce #3

Serves 4-6

- 2 cups steamed spinach
- ½ sweet onion, steamed
- 2 tablespoons ghee
- 1 tablespoon Bombay curry powder
- ½ tablespoon coriander
- 1 tablespoon Bragg's

After steaming vegetables, place all ingredients in blender and blend until smooth. Serve on top of steamed broccoli.

Saag Paneer

Serves 8

- 2 packages frozen chopped spinach, thawed
- 1 green chili (serrano, Thai or jalapeño), split lengthwise
- 2 tablespoons cardamom pods
- 2 teaspoons salt (divided)
- 1 cup thinly sliced onion
- 3 tablespoons olive oil
- 1 teaspoon ginger, minced
- 1 cup tomatoes, chopped
- 1¼ cup water (divided)
- 1 teaspoon coriander, ground
- 1 teaspoon cumin, ground
- ¼ teaspoon turmeric, ground
- 1/8 teaspoon cayenne pepper
- 1 recipe paneer (see page 430)
- 1 teaspoon garam masala

In 2-quart saucepan over medium heat, cook spinach with green chili, cardamom pods and 1 teaspoon salt for about 5 minutes, or until spinach is soft. Remove from heat and set aside. In large skillet over medium-high heat, sauté onion in oil until edges are nicely browned. Add ginger and stir for another minute. Add tomatoes and 1 more teaspoon salt; sauté until tomato pieces begin to break up. Add coriander, cumin, coriander, cayenne, and ¼ cup of water; continue cooking. Stir in cooked spinach, 1 cup of water, and paneer; simmer until water is absorbed. Stir in garam masala and remove from heat.

Squash

Botanical Name: Cucurbita species

The name "squash" is the corrupted, short, Indian name for the fruits and plants of several members of the gourd family. There are many, many varieties grown, all with a similar chemical composition. For practical purposes, squash can be divided into two groups: one group being the so-called bush or running variety, the other group contains the summer and winter varieties. The bush and summer squash are comprised of relatively small plants that are eaten before maturity. The other group occupies large spaces because the squash are large, maturing during autumn and winter. All squash is tender to frost; therefore, do not plant too early nor too late, in order to avoid the autumn frost. The most popular summer varieties are the Zucchini, Yellow Crookneck, Fordhook, Early Yellow Bush, Pineapple, Turban, Pattypan, and Grant Summer. The chief winter varieties include the Acorn, Spaghetti, Gregory Delicious, Hubbard, Boston Marrow, and the Canada Crookneck. Pumpkins are also winter squashes. Summer squash should be steamed and given a ghee or olive oil dressing. Winter squash lends itself very favorably to baking.

Energy: Warming

Taste: Sweet

Post Digestive: Sweet

Indications: Blood stagnation, diarrhea, kidney disorders, expectorant

Systems: Circulatory, Digestive, Urinary, Respiratory

Dosha Affected:

Vata: Moderation

Pitta: Good

Kapha: Avoid

Mixes Well With: Vegetables, starches. Squash should not be combined with protein.

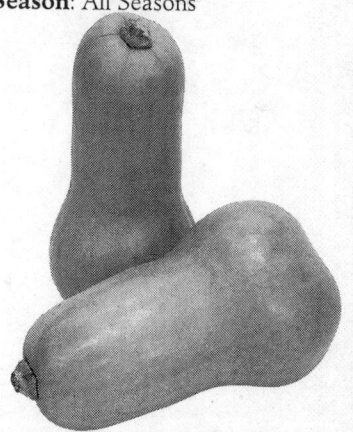

Season: All Seasons

Zucchini Ratatouille

Serves 2

- 1 sweet onion
- 3 cups zucchini, chopped
- 1 cup yellow squash, chopped
- 1 cup basil, chopped (or 2 teaspoons dry)
- ¼ cup fresh oregano, chopped (or 1 teaspoon dry)
- 1 cup water
- 1 teaspoon salt
- 2 large tomatoes, chopped

Sauté onion until soft. Add squash, then basil, oregano, water, and salt. Cover pan and cook for 20 minutes, then add tomatoes, and cook for 5 to 10 minutes more.

Raw Tip: This recipe can also be served raw with a few changes. You will need to grate the zucchini & squash. Add other ingredients as listed, add 1 tablespoon olive oil and 1 tablespoon Balsamic vinegar. Sit overnight & serve.

Stuffed Acorn Squash

Serves 4

- 2 acorn squash
- 4 tablespoons ghee (divided)
- 1 tablespoon cardamom (divided)
- ½ teaspoon cinnamon
- ½ teaspoon coriander
- ½ teaspoon fennel, ground
- 1 teaspoon ajwan seeds – Kapha only
- 2 green onions, chopped
- ½ bulb fennel, finely chopped
- 6 stalks celery, finely chopped
- 1 cup basil, chopped
- 1 cup water
- 2 sheets nori, crushed
- 1 cup cashew butter or 1 cup ground cashews, unsalted

Cut each squash in half, and clean out center. Thinly slice off bottom so they are flat and stable on pan. Prick with fork all around and generously rub ghee (about 2 tablespoons), cinnamon and half the cardamom inside each squash. Bake at 350° for 25 minutes or until very soft; remove from oven. Sauté in 2 tablespoons ghee: coriander, ground fennel, and ajwan, then add onions, fresh fennel, celery and basil. Add water, crushed nori, and cashew butter, **stir well** and let simmer until vegetables are well cooked (about 20 minutes). Put scoop of vegetable stuffing in center of each squash. Garnish with fresh basil leaves.

Baked Spaghetti Squash

Serves 2

- 1 large spaghetti squash
- 2 tablespoons ghee
- ¼ teaspoon dried rosemary
- ¼ teaspoon sage, ground

Cut squash in half and remove seeds. Pierce squash with a fork all around, and place in baking pan. Bake for 45 minutes at 275°. Remove from oven. Scoop out pulp and place in bowl with remaining ingredients. Serve with salad or vegetables.

Use removed seeds - roast them in oven - then blend with 1 tablespoon of ghee, 1/3 cup cilantro, 2 tablespoons lemon juice, 1/2 cup chopped onions, and 1/4 teaspoon jaggery. Blend until smooth. Makes an excellent sauce or chutney - to be used on squash or any other vegetable.

Pumpkin Soup

- 1 medium pumpkin, chopped
- 1 large onion, well chopped
- 2 tablespoons ghee or olive oil
- 2 tablespoons coriander, ground
- 1 teaspoon cinnamon
- 1 teaspoon cardamom
- 1 teaspoon nutmeg
- 1 cup rice (or soy) milk
- Bragg's

Steam pumpkin until soft. In another pan, sauté the onions well in ghee or oil. Put pumpkin in blender, add all spices and onions, and blend well into a creamy texture. Add rice milk, and Bragg's to taste. Serve with garnish of cilantro or parsley in center of bowl.

Sweet Potato

Botanical Name: Ipomoea batatas

Sweet potatoes are native to the Americas, and considered to be the oldest cultivated vegetable in America. In the tropics, the sweet potato is perhaps the most popular food plant. It belongs to the morning glory family, having an abundance of the many branched trailing vines and white, funnel-shaped flowers. The fleshy, rooted tubers are highly nutritious and delicious. Unless carefully stored, they are hard to keep. After removal from the ground, they should be left to dry for several hours, then stored in a dry warm place. For storing, they can be arranged in barrels or boxes in layers of sand and potatoes.

The edible tuberous root is long and tapered, with a smooth skin ranging in color between red, purple, brown and white. Its flesh can be white, yellow, orange, or purple. The moister, usually orange-colored, sweet potato is sometimes referred to as a "yam" in the U.S., but it is not related at all to the true yam (Dioscorea) – see Yam, page 226. The USDA requires the word "yam" to be accompanied by the words "sweet potato" when referring to these sweet potatoes, but that rule is ignored in most stores and markets.

Energy: Cooling

Taste: Sweet

Post Digestive: Sweet

Indications: Constipation, immune builder, hemorrhoids

Systems: Immune, Digestive

Dosha Affected:

Vata: Good

Pitta: Moderation

Kapha: Avoid or reduce

Mixes Well With: Vegetables

Season: Late Fall

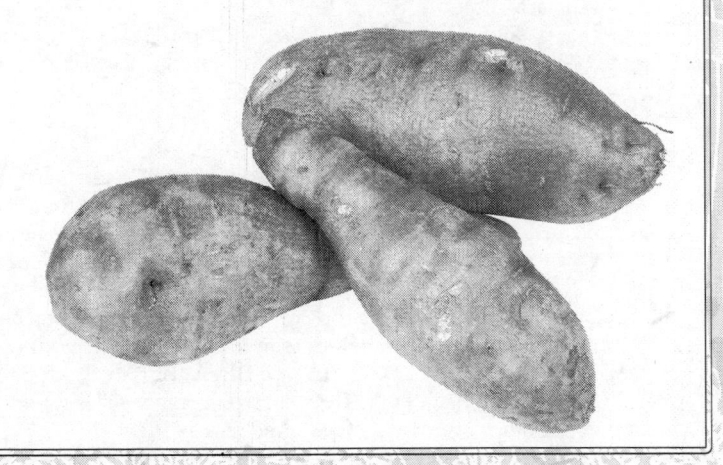

Sweet Potato Subzi

Serves 2

- 1 cup sweet onions, chopped
- 2 tablespoons ghee
- 2 large sweet potatos
- 2 carrots, sliced
- ½ cup water
- 1 head broccoli, chopped
- 3 stalks celery, chopped
- ½ cup cilantro, chopped
- 2 teaspoons coriander, ground
- 2 teaspoons cumin, ground
- 1 teaspoon fennel, ground
- Bragg's

Sauté onions in ghee. Add potatoes, carrots, and water, and simmer for 10 minutes. Add broccoli, celery, cilantro, and spices; simmer for more 10 minutes. Add Bragg's to taste; serve over rice.

Sweet Potato Lasagna

Serves 4-6

- 4 large sweet potatoes
- 1 bunch red chard, chopped
- 2 cups spinach, sliced
- 2 ounces soy mozzarella cheese, grated
- 1 cup olive oil
- 2 cups basil, fresh
- 2 tablespoons Bragg's

Peel sweet potatoes, and slice them lengthwise as thin as you can make them. Then blanch. **Prepare sauce:** In blender, mix olive oil with basil leaves and Bragg's; blend well. **Assemble lasagna:** Place a third of the sweet potato slices in baking pan (like lasagna noodles). Layer a third of the chopped chard on sweet potatoes, then sprinkle on a quarter of the cheese, and add a third of the sauce. Continue layering; on the top layer, sprinkle the remaining cheese. Bake at 350° for 45 minutes. (The potatoes tend to get a little crispy – if desired, add a little ghee on top, or cover while baking.) **Blanching Method:** Bring 2 quarts water to boil with a pinch of salt. Throw in sweet potato slices for approximately 5-6 minutes. Do not overcook. They should remain firm.

Tapioca (from Cassava)

Botanical Name: Manihot esculenta

Tapioca is made from the root of the cassava (also called manioc and yuca) plant, native to South America and an important staple in Africa as well. The root is processed into flour, and the flour into small white "pearls" that must be soaked before cooking. Tapioca is high in carbohydrates, and should be eaten in small quantities. It is considered to be highly non-allergenic. In today's markets, it is also available as a wonderful flour. This starchy flour can be used as a thickener for sauces or baking. This food is high in carbohydrates and excellent for soups and desserts.

Energy: Warming

Taste: Sweet

Post Digestive: Sweet

Indications: Colitis, infection, low immunity

Systems: Digestive, Immune, Excretory, Muscular

Dosha Affected:

Vata: Excellent

Pitta: Good

Kapha: Avoid

Mixes Well With: Starchy vegetables

Season: Tropical, Winter

Tapioca Soup

Serves 8

- 2 cups pearl tapioca
- 12 cups water (divided)
- 1 cup rice milk
- 2 tablespoons olive oil
- 1 onion, well chopped
- ½ cup grated carrots
- 1 cup yuca root, grated (available in Latin grocery stores)
- 2 tablespoons basil, well chopped
- 2 tablespoons cilantro, chopped
- 1 tablespoon mild curry powder

Soak the tapioca overnight in 8 cups of water; drain the next day. Add tapioca to 4 cups of fresh water, and bring to a boil. Add rice milk and cook until the tapioca becomes translucent (another 10 minutes). Sauté the onion in oil, then add grated carrots and yuca. Add to tapioca with basil, cilantro, and curry powder. Take off the heat and let it steep for 10 minutes. Serve with salad.

Tapioca Pudding

Serves 6

- 1 cup pearl tapioca
- 2 cups water
- 2 cups coconut milk
- 2 teaspoons cinnamon
- 2 teaspoons cardamom
- 1 teaspoon nutmeg
- 1 teaspoon ginger, ground
- 2 teaspoons sucanat or jaggary
- 1 teaspoon vanilla

Soak tapioca overnight; drain in the morning. Put in double boiler and add 2 cups fresh water; bring to boil and cook for 15 minutes. Lower heat and slowly add coconut milk; cook on low for 20 minutes. Add spices, sucanat and vanilla; stir well.

Tapioca Sauce

Makes 1 ½ cup sauce

½ cup tapioca flour

1 tablespoon ghee

1 cup cream

½ cup water

1 teaspoon curry powder

Coconut aminos to taste or Bragg's aminos

In a saucepan, briskly mix tapioca and water together on medium heat. When it begins to boil, turn heat to low, slowly add cream, curry, and aminos, while continuing to stir with whisk until consistency is of a sauce.

Curry Sabudana (Tapioca)

Serves 4

1 cup tapioca

1 cup corn kernels, fresh, organic

1 cup carrots, grated

1 teaspoon mustard seeds

1 teaspoon cumin seeds

1 teaspoon ajwan

1 green chili, well chopped

2 tablespoons ghee

1 cup green onions, chopped

1 cup cilantro, chopped

1 cup water

3 tablespoons water

Salt to taste

Soak tapioca for 8 hours. In skillet, roast cumin seeds, mustard seeds, & ajwan seeds in ghee. Add green onions and green chili. Cook for 5-10 minutes on low heat. Drain tapioca well. Add tapioca to mixture. Add 3 tablespoons water. Cover. Cook for another 10 minutes. Add cilantro, curry, & salt to taste. In Hindi, the word for tapioca is "sabudana."

Taro Root

Botanical Name: Colocasia esculenta

Taro is a plant believed to be native to Southeast Asia; it grows in tropical as well as warmer temperate regions, having its natural habitat in virgin forests. Cultivation dates back some 4,000 to 7,000 years, but it was probably introduced to Japan and China at a later period. Taro belongs to a family of ornamental plants that include philodendron and dieffenbachia. The taro root is a staple food in several tropical countries of Asia, the Pacific Islands, and the West Indies, where it is also known as dasheen. Over 100 different varieties exist, with some resembling a sweet potato, while others resemble celeriac. The tubers have a thick, brownish, ringed skin that is rather rugged and hairy. The flesh can be white, cream-colored, or purple-gray, and sometimes veined with pink or brown color. Taro roots contain a high starch content with a sweet flavor. The Hawaiians make a fermented mixture called "poi" resembling yogurt, which they feed to their small children or anyone convalescing. This mixture has a sour taste.

Energy: Warming

Taste: Sweet

Post Digestive: Sweet

Indications: Digestive aid, to gain weight, general weakness, chronic illnesses

Systems: Digestion

Dosha Affected:

Vata: Good (well cooked)

Pitta: Moderation

Kapha: Avoid or reduce

Mixes Well With: Vegetables (especially green), starches

Mashed Taro

Serves 4

- 8 taro roots, skinned and chopped
- 4 cups water
- 1 tablespoon ghee
- 1 cup Chinese chives, chopped
- 2 tablespoons parsley, chopped
- 1 tablespoon coriander, ground
- salt

Put taro roots and water in saucepan; bring to a boil and cook for 20 minutes. When the roots are soft, drain, then mash the roots with a potato masher. Add ghee and mix in chives, parsley, and coriander. Salt to taste.
Serve with vegetables or protein.

Taro Sauce

- 2 cups tarot, skinned, chopped
- 1 tablespoon oregano
- 4 cups water
- 2 tablespoons ghee
- 2 carrots, medium, chopped
- ½ cup green onion
- 1 tablespoon of Vata, Pitta, Kapha Churna
- Bragg's or salt to taste

Place carrots & tarot into saucepan with water. Boil until tender or soft. Drain. Place carrots & tarot into blender with remaining ingredients. Add left over water slowly until desired consistency. Add Vata, Pitta, or Kapha churna for body type.

Turnip

Botanical Name: Brassica rapa

This semi-hardy vegetable originated in Europe or Asia. It differs from the Swedish turnip, or "rutabaga", by its closer cropping of leaf stems, its hairy leaves, the flatter swollen root, almost naked taproot, and light colored flesh. Innumerable varieties are grown throughout the temperate zone, of which the most common are the white and yellow. The white varieties are preferred in the summer, while during the winter, the yellow turnips are more frequently consumed. The pungent odor and flavor is due to the large amount of sulphur. Shape is important in selecting turnips; smoothness, regularity, and firmness indicate quality. Wrinkled or spongy roots have been kept too long and may be pithy. Large, coarse, overgrown turnips, that are light in weight for their size, may be tough, woody, pithy, hollow, and strong in flavor. When cooking, the best method is to steam approximately 15 to 20 minutes and serve with ghee or olive oil dressing. Turnip leaves, when fresh, also make a delicious wholesome salad. Turnips are good for pregnant women and for children under fifteen years of age, as they contain phytoestrogens.

Energy: Cooling
Taste: Astringent, Pungent
Post Digestive: Pungent
Indications: Hemorrhoids, acid conditions
Systems: Excretory, Digestive

Dosha Affected:
Vata: Avoid
Pitta: Moderation
Kapha: Excellent
Mixes Well With: Vegetables, starches
Season: Fall

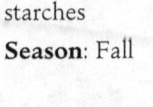

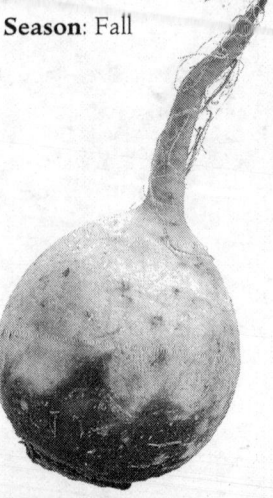

Turnip Combo

Serves 6

- 3 cups turnips, cut into small cubes
- 1 large fennel bulb, thinly sliced
- 1 cup carrots, well chopped
- 1 tablespoon coriander, ground
- 2 tablespoons fennel, ground
- 1½ teaspoon cinnamon
- 1 tablespoon ghee
- 3 tablespoons fresh mint, chopped

Preheat oven to 350°.

Combine chopped turnips, fennel and carrots in oiled baking dish; mix in spices. Pour ghee over all; bake for 30 minutes. When vegetables are soft, stir in the mint.

Serve with rice or protein.

Raw tip: Ingredients can also be pulsed in a food processor until they are well-blended but chunky.

Turnip Soup

Serves 4

- 6 turnips, cut into cubes
- 3 carrots, cut into rings
- 1 potato, cut into cubes
- 1 large leek, cut into rings
- 1 cup tomato sauce
- 2 tablespoons ginger, fresh, grated
- 2 tablespoons celery
- 1 tablespoon marjoram
- 2 tablespoons miso paste
- Salt to taste

Bring water to boil in a large soup pot. Add all ingredients except the miso and tomato sauce. Cook for 25 minutes. Add tomato and miso just before serving. Salt to taste.

Yam

Botanical Name: Dioscorea

The origin of yams is unknown. Archeological excavations provide some evidence that indicates that they were cultivated over 10,000 years ago in Asia and Africa. The yam is one of the most widely consumed foods in the world, and a staple food in South America and the West Indies. True yams are not to be confused with the sweet potatoes that are often mislabeled as "yams" in U.S. stores (see Sweet Potato, page 217). They are not easy to find outside of Latin, Asian, and African specialty food markets. These tubers can grow up to 6 or 7 feet in length, and weigh up to 150 pounds (and are, therefore, often sold by the "chunk," cut and wrapped in plastic wrap). The yam family includes over 600 varieties. Dioscorea opposita, the Chinese yam, is somewhat smaller than African yams, and was the yam that was introduced to Europe in the 1800's when the potato crops were failing. Some species of African yams must be cooked very carefully, as they contain toxins when raw. The flesh of the yam can be white, yellow, orange, or purple. It is great in soups, baked breads, cakes, and purees. If stored in plastic bags, yams will spoil quickly; store in a cool, dry place instead.

Yucca is in the same botanical family as Yams and has similar constituents. Yucca is a tropical tuber found in Spanish stores and some supermarkets. Highly nutritional. High in potassium.

Energy: Cooling
Taste: Sweet
Post Digestive: Sweet
Indications: Constipation, immune builder, hemorrhoids
Systems: Immune, Digestive

Dosha Affected:
Vata: Good
Pitta: Moderation
Kapha: Avoid or reduce
Mixes Well With: Vegetables
Season: Fall

Roasted Yams

Serves 6

4 yams, cut into cubes
1 large onion, cut into rings
2 zucchini, sliced into rounds
2 carrots, cut into rounds
1 tablespoon sucanat or jaggary
2 tablespoons balsamic vinegar
3 tablespoons ghee
1½ tablespoon Italian seasoning
Bragg's to taste

Preheat oven to 350°. Mix all ingredients together, and spread on oiled baking pan. Bake for 45 minutes to an hour, stirring occasionally, then broil for a few minutes until crisp.

Serve with salad.

Yucca Patties

Serves 4

2 cups yucca, peeled, cut small
1 cup carrots, grated
4 cups water
½ cup flour
1 teaspoon baking powder
2 tablespoons ghee
½ teaspoon nutmeg
2 teaspoons coriander

Peel yucca well. Cut into small pieces. Bring water to boil. Add yucca. When soft, blend in food processor until creamy.

Add spices, baking powder, and grated carrots. Make into patties. Cook on baking sheet, turning on each side.

Bake at 325 for 30 minutes.

Ayurvedic Curative Cuisine for Everyone

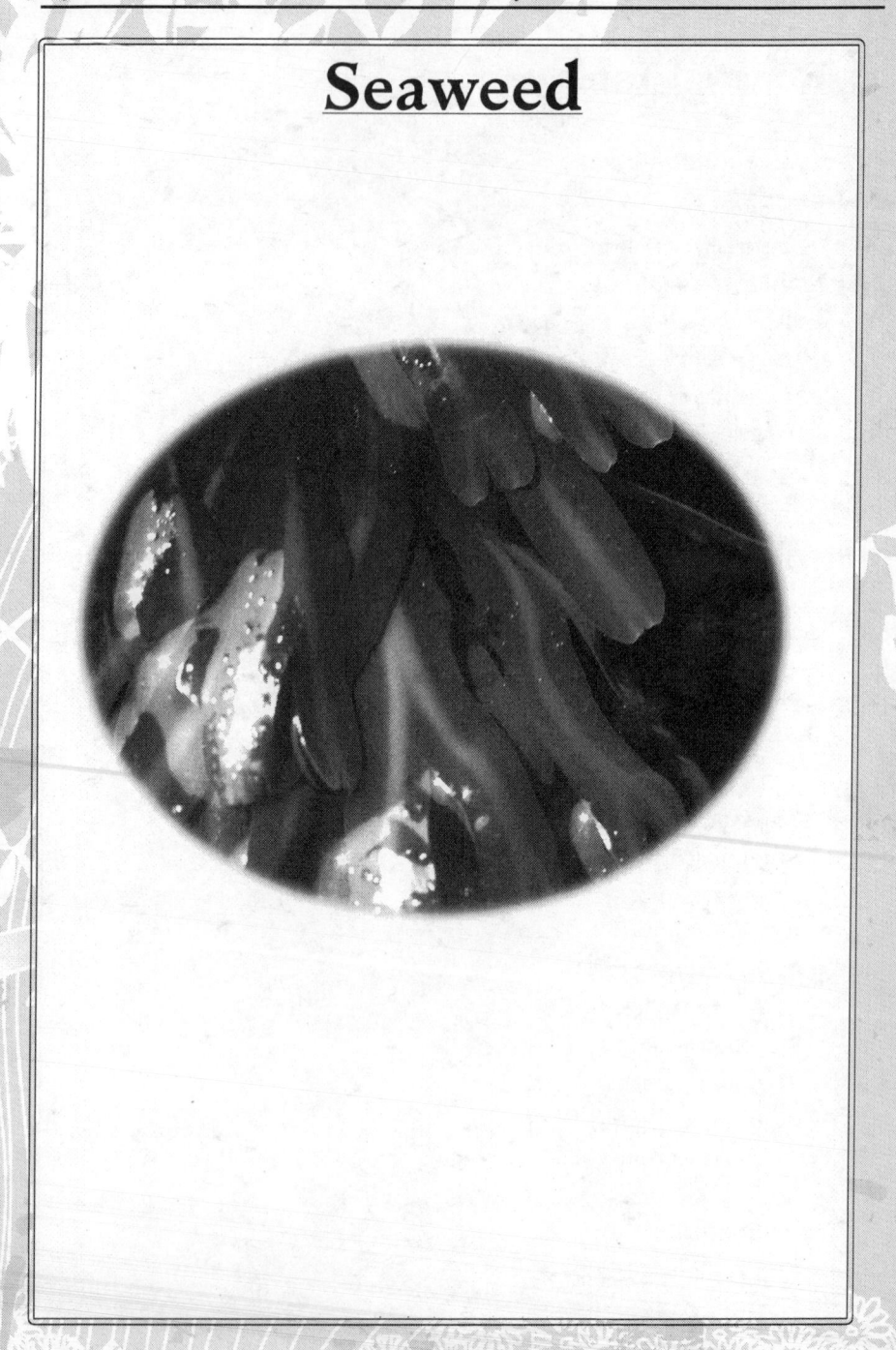

Seaweed

Seaweed

All marine plants are called seaweeds. Most varieties that are available come from Scandinavia and Ireland and are once again being harvested off the coasts of North America in Maine, Nova Scotia, Oregon, and California. Seaweeds are not traditionally part of Ayurveda lore, but it is good to be knowledgeable of them because many Europeans and Asians use them. Today, even Americans are now consuming large quantities of seaweeds. They are exceptionally high in protein and may contain 17 to 20 grams of protein per 100 grams of algae. The dark black and purple seaweeds have a unique, rich taste and flavor which are used to strengthen the kidneys, intestines, digestive system, and sexual organs, as well as to improve the power of the will and provide clear judgment. Seaweeds are also taken medicinally to dissolve excess fat and cholesterol deposits which assist in reversing hardening of the arteries and high blood pressure. These sea vegetables are also good for the maintenance of a healthy thyroid and the regression of tumors. It has been scientifically documented that common seaweeds helped eliminate nuclear radiation and fallout, enabling the Japanese survival of Hiroshima.

It is recommended to add seaweed to your daily diet whether you are a meat-eater or a vegetarian. As a general food group, seaweeds rank second in the amount of calcium and phosphorous and first in the amount of magnesium, iron, iodine, and sodium. They contain up to 25% more protein than milk and are naturally free of calories since they are low in fat. They also contain vitamins A, B, C, D-3, E, and K as well as digestible carbohydrates called fructose.

Due to their mineral and alkaline content, seaweeds purify the blood by eliminating the acidic effects of a modern diet. Most importantly, sea vegetables are rich in vitamin B-12, which is required for the functioning of the neuromuscular system, a deficiency of which results in pernicious anemia.

Seaweeds are known to protect endocrine organs – such as the pituitary, thyroid, gall bladder, liver, and other vital organs. According to many health experts (including Brigitte Mars in her book Beauty by Nature), seaweed added to one's bathwater can help to draw environmental pollutants from the body, including radiation and other chemicals. Any edible seaweed can be used for this purpose.

If eating seaweeds is new to you, begin with the milder tasting ones such as Dulse, Kombu, Arame, and Nori. Others, such as Kelp, Wakame, and Hiziki, have a stronger flavor. You may also want to introduce only one kind at a time into your diet. It is best to use them in soups and casseroles, or try sprinkling seaweed flakes (dulse, for example) on your salads.

Always store sea vegetables in airtight jars after their package has been opened. If they become damp, simply dry briefly in the oven on low heat, or in the sun. White spots that may form on the surface are crystals of salt that have been brought to the surface by a change in temperature.

The following recipe uses five different kinds of seaweed:

Seaweed Soup

Serves 8

- 1 cup sesame seeds
- 1 tablespoon cumin seed
- 1 tablespoon ajwan
- 8 cups water
- 12 inches of wakame, cut into small pieces
- 6 inches of kombu, cut in small pieces
- 2 ounces hiziki
- 2 ounces dulse flakes
- 2 tablespoons grated ginger
- 1 bunch green onions, chopped
- 1 cup carrots, sliced
- 1 cup snow peas
- 1 cup celery, finely chopped
- 1 cup baby corn
- 6 sheets of nori
- 2 ounces cellophane rice noodles
- ¼ cup miso of choice
- ¼ cup parsley
- ¼ cup cilantro

In a large pot, roast sesame, cumin, and ajwan seeds for 5 minutes, stirring constantly. Add water, wakame, kombu, hiziki, dulse, and ginger, and cook for 20 minutes, until soft. Add vegetables, and bring to a boil; cook for 15 minutes.

Crush the nori sheets into the soup; add noodles, miso, parsley, and cilantro. Let steep for 10 minutes. Daily consumption of this soup is an effective way to get your minerals.

Agar Agar (Kanten)

<u>Botanical Name: *Gelidiella acerosa*</u>

Agar Agar is a transparent substance that is used like gelatin as a food thickener. It is made from many kinds of seaweed in the genus gelidium. Chopped dried seaweeds are boiled in water with acetic acid or sulphuric acid. The hot liquid is strained, removing any remaining pieces of seaweed, and then neutralized with bicarbonate (baking soda). A jelly is formed at a temperature of 104°. To eliminate the seaweed taste, the jelly is formed and dehydrated. This sea gel produces great snacks or desserts when made into jello with added nutritional fruits or juices, such as cherry, pineapple, carrot, lemon, grape, or pomegranate. Your loved ones will not even know that you are not using the commercial jello. When you purchase agar agar in bulk, it comes in a bar about 12 inches long. When used as a thickener, it must be cut into about 4" pieces and soaked in 2 cups warm water. Keep in mind, that it thickens when it cools down.

Energy: Warming, Moisturizing

Taste: Sweet, salty

Post Digestive: Sweet

Indications: Arteriosclerosis, arthritis, osteoporosis, cramps, spasms, high blood pressure, tumors, radiation, exposure, constipation

Systems: Circulatory, Muscular, Urinary, Digestive, Reproductive, Skeletal

<u>**Dosha Affected:**</u>

Vata: Excellent

Pitta: Good in small amounts

Kapha: Avoid or reduce

Mixes Well With: Salads, vegetables, starches or proteins

Healthy Jello

2 cups apple juice
½ cup fruit of your choice, well chopped
2 teaspoon agar agar

Bring apple juice to a boil. Add fruit and agar agar, and continue stirring until thickened. Let it cool. Place in refrigerator until it gels (for at least 2 hours).

Optional: 2 cups chopped fruits of your choice.

Arame

Botanical Name: Eisenia bicyclis

This firm sea vegetable grows on both coasts of the Pacific as well as regions of Japan and Peru. It is also known as "sea oak", and its fronds resemble big, very tough, oak leaves. After harvesting, shredding, and drying, arame becomes like wiry black threads. In cooking, it turns dark brown with a sweet, delicate taste, and is commonly sautéed with root vegetables, tofu, or soybeans. Arame is high in complex carbohydrates, fiber, niacin, calcium, iron, and iodine. This seaweed is stringy. Can be cooked for 15 minutes, or when eaten raw, must be soaked overnight. Drain water next day and add seaweed to your favorite vegetable dish.

Energy: Warming, Moisturizing

Taste: Sweet, salty

Post Digestive: Sweet

Indications: Arteriosclerosis, arthritis, osteoporosis, cramps, spasms, lowers high blood pressure, tumors, radiation exposure, female disorders

Systems: Circulatory, Muscular, Urinary, Digestive, Reproductive, Skeletal

Dosha Affected:

Vata: Excellent

Pitta: Good in small amounts

Kapha: Avoid or reduce

Mixes Well With: Salads, vegetables, starches or proteins

Arame Salad

- ½ cup raisins
- 1 cup arame seaweed, cut into small pieces
- 1 cup grated jicama
- 1 cup grated carrots
- 1 tablespoon grated ginger
- 1 cup ground almonds
- ½ cup chives, chopped
- 1 cup baby greens
- 1 cup baby spinach
- ¼ cup olives

Soak arame and raisins for 4-5 hours in warm water. Drain water, mix all ingredients in a salad bowl, toss, and add your favorite dressing.

Dulse

Botanical Name: Palmaria palmata

This tufted, purplish-red seaweed is abundant on the rocky coast of the Atlantic Ocean and has been eaten in Europe for thousands of years. It is also a traditional staple in Scotland, Wales, Ireland, Japan, Canada, and New England. In Japan, it is called, "darusu." It is very high in iron and, although moderate in flavor compared to some other seaweeds, it adds zest to food. Dulse can be eaten as a snack, by chewing a small piece at a time. In powdered or flaked form, it can be sprinkled in soups or on salads. It is the most user-friendly seaweed, as it need not be cooked. Dulse can also be found in flakes that can be used as a seasoning when used in a salt shaker. It is rich in vitamins and has a very distinct flavor. When soaked it becomes soft and is easy to incorporate into a salad chopped into small pieces. Another name for it is "Sea Lettuce." Dried dulse can be eaten as a snack, especially for Vata imbalance, can also be added to sandwiches, as well as soups and grains. Of all the seaweeds, it is the highest in protein. Dulse can be purchased in individual packages or in bulk in health food stores. Normally, seaweeds can be found in Asian stores at a lower price.

Energy: Warming, Moisturizing

Taste: Sweet, salty

Post Digestive: Sweet

Indications: Arteriosclerosis, arthritis, osteoporosis, cramps, spasms, high blood pressure, tumors, radiation exposure

Systems: Circulatory, Muscular, Urinary, Digestive, Reproductive, Skeletal

Dosha Affected:

Vata: Excellent

Pitta: Good in small amounts

Kapha: Avoid or reduce

Mixes Well With: Salads, vegetables, starches or proteins

Dulse Salad

Serves 2

2 ounces dulse – cut into small pieces
1 head romaine lettuce, torn in bite-size pieces
1 cup celery, well chopped
1 tomato, well chopped

Soak dulse for 15 minutes, then drain. Mix all ingredients in a bowl; toss well. Serve with your favorite dressing.

Hiziki

Botanical Name: Hizikia fusiforme

Hiziki (also spelled Hijiki) can be found in the East Asian waters stretching from Japan along the China coast to Hong Kong. Hiziki is a pine needle shaped seaweed that is harvested at low tide in the spring, and sun-dried. Its course, black, crispy strands become very tender when properly cooked, and have a strong ocean flavor with a nutty aroma. To prepare hiziki, it can be boiled, steamed, or baked. It is high in minerals, iron, protein, vitamins A, B-1, and B-12, and contains ten times more calcium than a comparable amount of milk, cheese, or other dairy food. When you first begin using this seaweed, start with small amounts until you get used to it. Best soaked before adding to soups because it is quite salty and fishy. Hiziki is black in color and expands 5-6 times original size after cooking. Great in casseroles or stews.

Energy: Warming, Moisturizing

Taste: Sweet, salty

Post Digestive: Sweet

Indications: Arteriosclerosis, arthritis, osteoporosis, cramps, spasms, high blood pressure, tumors, radiation exposure, strengthens the intestines, beautiful shining hair, blood purifier

Systems: Circulatory, Muscular, Urinary, Digestive, Reproductive, Skeletal

Dosha Affected:

Vata: Excellent

Pitta: Good in small amounts

Kapha: Avoid or reduce

Mixes Well With: Salads, vegetables, starches or proteins

Hiziki Bok Choy Combo

Serves 4

- 1 cup hiziki, dry and crushed
- 1 teaspoon cumin seed
- 1 tablespoon sesame oil
- 1 bunch green onions, chopped
- 1 tablespoon ginger, grated
- 1 red pepper slice
- 2 small (or 1 large) Chinese bok choy
- ¼ cup water
- 2 cups soybean or mung sprouts
- soy sauce to taste
- 1 teaspoon agave syrup
- 1 tablespoon mild curry

Soak hiziki for 3 hours. In a large pot, roast the cumin seed for 5 minutes; add oil, onions, ginger, and pepper, and cook for 5 minutes or until soft. Add bok choy and water; cook for another 5 minutes. Drain seaweed, and add to pot with sprouts, soy sauce, agave, and curry powder. Stir all ingredients, and serve over rice or meat.

Kombu

<u>Botanical Name: Laminaria, various species</u>

This sea vegetable grows in abundance in Japan and off the Pacific coast between British Columbia and San Francisco. After harvesting, it is dried on the ground by the sun and wind, then stored in a dark place. The Japanese city of Osaka is known for its superior kombu. It is used extensively in Japanese diets with grains, beans, and root vegetables, as well as being made into teas, pickles, condiments, snacks, and candy. When purchasing kombu, do not scrub the tiny white flecks off its outer surface as these are mineral salts and complex sugars which contribute to its delicious taste and energy. Kombu is high in vitamins A, B-2, and C, as well as calcium and iodine. There are many varities of kombu, the Japanese variety is called "Atlantic Kelp" and is sweeter tasting. Kombu provides mega minerals. It is also very high in glumatic acid. It often has the white powder of glumatic acid on it – do not confuse this with mold. It is best used in rice, beans, and soups.

Energy: Warming, Moisturizing

Taste: Sweet, salty

Post Digestive: Sweet

Indications: Arteriosclerosis, arthritis, osteoporosis, cramps, spasms, high blood pressure, tumors, radiation exposure, protects against degenerative diseases, flatulence

Systems: Circulatory, Muscular, Urinary, Digestive, Reproductive, Skeletal

Dosha Affected:

Vata: Excellent

Pitta: Good in small amounts

Kapha: Avoid or reduce

Mixes Well With: Salads, vegetables, starches or proteins

Kombu Dill Salad

Serves 2

2 ounces kombu "crumbles"

1 small head lettuce, Bibb or Boston

1 cup fresh dillweed, well chopped

½ cup pine nuts

1 cup fresh bean sprouts

Soak kombu crumbles in warm water for 15 minutes; drain. Cut lettuce into bowl and mix in dillweed. Add nuts and sprouts. Dress with your favorite dressing.

Kombu Soup

Serves 10-12

2 tablespoons sesame seeds

2 tablespoons olive oil

1 bunch green onions or scallions, well chopped

1 tablespoon lemon juice

2 quarts water

4 carrots, sliced

1 head broccoli (including peeled stalk), chopped

1 cup green beans, cut up

½ head cabbage, chopped

1 fennel, greens and bulb, well chopped

1 package kombu, cut up in small pieces

1 package cellophane rice noodles

1 tablespoon white barley miso

1 tablespoon coriander, ground

In a pan, roast sesame seeds. When toasted, add olive oil, onion and lemon juice. Bring 2 quarts of water to boil, add chopped vegetables and kombu pieces. Stir all ingredients together. Boil until almost tender. Add rice noodles and cook until tender. Add barley miso and coriander; mix all together. (Do not boil again as it will kill the enzymes in the miso.)

Nori

<u>Botanical Name:</u> *Porphyra, various species*

This seaweed is processed almost exclusively in Japan where the name was given, although it grows throughout the world. Nori is primarily cultivated in Japanese islets rather than being harvested wild, as are other seaweeds. After harvesting, nori is washed and dried into thin sheets, which are then folded in half. Nori is related to red algae. In Scotland it is known as "laver" while in Ireland it is known as "sloke." The highest grades of nori are expensive and are used only for very special occasions. The cheaper grades will be purple, limp, uneven, and may also be dyed green and chemically lacquered. Nori is used in sushi. This industry employs over 300,000 people in Japan. Unlike other seaweeds, nori does not need to be washed or soaked before using. It is an exceptionally nutritious sea vegetable, high in carotene (vitamin A) – from 2 to 4 times the amount of an equal volume of carrots. It is also high in protein (twice as high as beefsteak), and contains high amounts of vitamins B-12 and C, calcium, and iron. Nori can be found roasted and toasted and eaten as chips. It can also be found as 8 x 11 sheets that are used for making sushi. **Note:** When using mineral supplements, cut down their intake if eating a lot of seaweed.

Energy: Warming, Moisturizing

Taste: Sweet, salty

Post Digestive: Sweet

Indications: Arteriosclerosis, arthritis, osteoporosis, cramps, spasms, high blood pressure, tumors, radiation exposure, reduces serum cholesterol, relieves beriberi

Systems: Circulatory, Muscular, Urinary, Digestive, Reproductive, Skeletal

<u>**Dosha Affected:**</u>

Vata: Excellent

Pitta: Good in small amounts

Kapha: Avoid or reduce

Mixes Well With: Salads, vegetables, starches or proteins

Nori Ginger Sauce

- ¼ cup water
- 2 ½ teaspoons sesame oil
- 1 teaspoon agave syrup
- 1 tablespoon fresh ginger, grated or chopped
- ¼ teaspoon kelp
- 1 tablespoon, radish, chopped
- ½ teaspoon alfalfa powder
- 3 sheets of nori

Put all ingredients in blender; blend until smooth. Serve over vegetables, salad, or protein. This recipe can be used to support thyroid function, hair and nail growth. Helps with mental imbalances, anxiety, confusion, etc.

Spirulina and Blue-Green Algae

Botanical Name: Arthrospira platensis Arthrospira maximus

There are many varieties of algae, and one of the most well known is blue-green algae. Grown in fresh alkaline water, it is said to have been in existence for one to three billion years. It reproduces very rapidly into two plants every 24 hours. Many native people, the Aztecs included, ate this weed on the lake shores of Mexico and the lakes of Chad in Central Africa. It was returned to the marketplace in 1960. Spirulina is a micro-algae that thrives in hot, humid climates. This algae is 20 times higher in protein than soybeans – it is extremely high in gamma linoic acid and flax seed. A great food for vegetarians.

Energy: Cooling

Taste: Sweet, Bitter

Post Digestive: Sweet

Indications: Allergies, Obesity, Immune problems

Systems: Immune, Endocrine, Muscular, Circulatory

Dosha Affected:

Vata: Avoid or reduce

Pitta: Excellent

Kapha: Moderation

Mixes Well With: Fruits, green leafy vegetables, juice

Green Shake

- 1 cup blueberries
- 1 cup soy milk or almond milk
- 1 tablespoon spirulina
- 1 teaspoon vanilla
- fruit of your choice

Put all ingredients in blender; blend until smooth.

Longevity Shake

Serves 2

- 2 cups milk of your choice – or fruit or Vegetable juice
- 1 teaspoon Ashwagandha
- ½ tablespoon spirulina
- ½ tablespoon bhrami
- ¼ teaspoon cinnamon
- ¼ thumb size, fresh ginger, chopped
- ¼ teaspoon cardamom

Place all ingredients in blender until smooth. Drink.

Wakame

Botanical Name: Undaria pinnatifida

This sea vegetable is harvested in Japan, as well as along the coasts of Korea and China. In appearance, texture, and taste, it is similar to another seaweed, Alaria (Alaria esculenta), which is traditionally used in Scotland, Ireland, and northern Europe. It is extremely high in calcium, with large amounts of iron, vitamins A and C, niacin, and protein. Wakame is a long, dark, green seaweed and is often confused with kombu. Always cut and soak before using.

Energy: Warming, Moisturizing

Taste: Sweet, salty

Post Digestive: Sweet

Indications: Arteriosclerosis, arthritis, osteoporosis, cramps, spasms, high blood pressure, tumors, radiation exposure, anti-bacterial properties, blood cleanser after childbirth

Systems: Circulatory, Muscular, Urinary, Digestive, Reproductive, Skeletal

Dosha Affected:

Vata: Excellent

Pitta: Good in small amounts

Kapha: Avoid or reduce

Mixes Well With: Salads, vegetables, starches or proteins

Ayurvedic Curative Cuisine for Everyone

Wakame Salad

Serves 4

- 2 cups wakame, cut into small pieces
- 2 cups water
- 1 large head Bibb lettuce, torn into bite-size pieces
- 1 cup grated carrots
- 1 tomato, sliced
- 1 bunch cilantro, well chopped
- ¼ cup sesame seeds
- 2 tablespoons olive oil
- ½ tablespoon rice vinegar
- 1 tablespoon soy sauce

Cook wakame for 15 minutes or until soft; then drain. Mix vegetables together, add wakame, oil, rice vinegar, and soy sauce. Toss well.

Beans

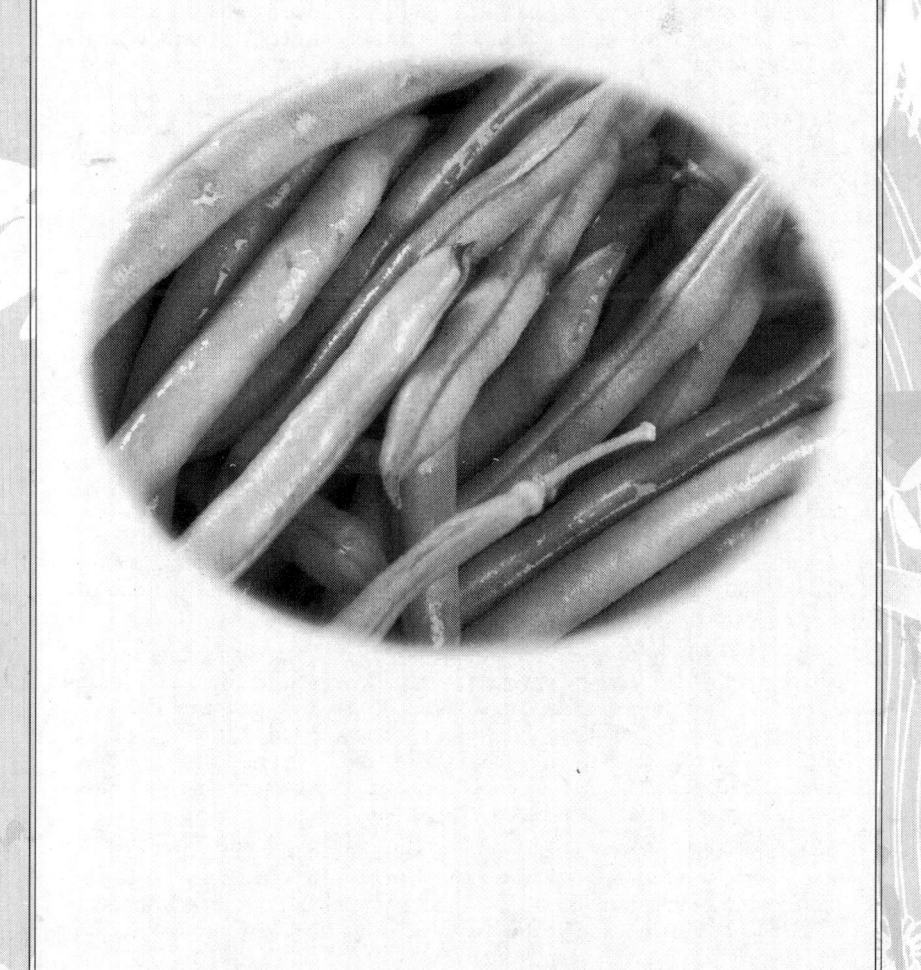

Beans

General Considerations

Beans have been around for thousands of years, and are perhaps the most common and widely used vegetable throughout the world. The plants range in habit of growth from low and bushy forms to tall and climbing "pole" beans, with many gradations in between. Different beans are edible at different stages of maturity. Some are eaten green, when the whole pod is edible – such as string beans and snow peas. "Shell" beans are those large seeded varieties whose immature, but fully formed, seeds are edible – such as green peas and edamame (immature soybeans). Those beans allowed to fully mature are called "dried" beans. The seed characteristics of beans vary in that they may be large or small, "eyed," mottled, and a variety of colors – white, brown, red, black, yellow, and green.

When used in the immature form, about one-half fully ripened, beans are still alkaline in reaction since they contain more lime and less phosphoric acid than they do when dry. All legumes in their dry, mature state contain a very high 20% protein and about 50% carbohydrate. Much of the protein, however, is not easy assimilated by the human digestive system. As a result, fermentation, flatulence, and irritation occur in the digestive tract. Beans are decidedly acid-forming. The red bean of the tropics that is commonly used in Latin America is less prone to cause gastro-intestinal disturbances.

Beans all belong to the legume family, but there are hundreds of varieties. Some of the beans most well- known in the U.S. include adzuki beans, black-eyed peas, chickpeas, lentils, lima beans, mung beans, soybeans, and split peas. The "common bean" species (Phaseolus vulgaris) includes pinto beans, red kidney beans, white navy beans, and black turtle beans, among others. The fava or broad bean (Vicia faba) is a native of southwestern Asia and northern Africa, where it has been cultivated from prehistoric times and from whence it has spread throughout the world to be grown in cold climates and seasons. This plant differs from other beans in that it is hardy. It grows well in Canada and the states of Washington and Oregon, as well as in California as a winter vegetable.

Used in salads, beans add nutrition, quality, and flavor. All legumes should be eaten with salads and green vegetables and are excellent either alone or in soups. The best procedure for preparation is to soak overnight in an ample quantity of pure water. Experiments have demonstrated that soft water or distilled water greatly facilitates the digestion of all legumes. After soaking, drain, add fresh water, and then cook long enough to make them soft. Other herbs and vegetables may be added.

When soaking is not possible, bring them to a boil in water for 10 to 15 minutes, pour water out, add fresh water, and then cook for 1 to 2 hours. Legumes should not be eaten more than 2 to 4 times per week due to the large amount of nitrogenous matter and acid-forming elements therein, which may cause digestive disturbances if eaten frequently.

Bean Sprouts

Almost all beans can be sprouted. Today, the most common sprouts found in the marketplace are mung and alfalfa. Sprouted beans have an increased nutritional value of ten times that of dry or cooked beans. They contain high contents of vitamins and minerals and are an easily assimilated vegetable protein.

Energy: Cooling

Taste: Sweet, Sour, Astringent

Post Digestive: Sweet

Indications: Liver disorders, fevers, alcoholism, stomach acidity

Systems: Circulatory, Immune

Dosha Affected:

Vata: Avoid (unless well cooked)

Pitta: Good

Kapha: Excellent

Mixes Well With: All proteins, vegetables, starches

How to Sprout Dried Beans

The following simple method is recommended:

1. Select a stock of clean bright new beans.

2. Hand pick thoroughly and discard everything except clean, whole beans.

3. Wash beans and place in a suitable container for sprouting, such as a one-quart or two-quart glass canning jar. The bean sprouts will increase to about six times the original volume.

4. Cover the seeds with at least four times their volume of lukewarm water and let stand for a few hours until they are swollen, or at most overnight.

5. Pour off the water, rinse the swollen beans thoroughly, then drain well.

6. Cover the top of the jar with a piece of cheesecloth or other thin cloth, and tie it on securely. Quarter-inch mesh screening also makes a good cover. (Sprouting lids can be found in most health food stores.)

7. Invert the jar and place in a cupboard or dark place, in a slightly tilted position so that the excess water can drain away.

8. At least three times per day (every four hours is better), place the jar under the water tap or pour on plenty of cool water, thoroughly and carefully washing the swelling and sprouting seeds so that bacteria or molds which may have developed are carried away. The better the washing, the better the sprouts. After washing, place the jar back in its inverted, slanted position.

The sprouts will be fully grown in 4 to 6 days, when they are approximately 1½ to 2 inches long. After the sprouts are washed to free them from loose hulls or seed coats, they are ready to be used in cooking, stored in the refrigerator, or to be used raw in salad.

Note: For those who might encounter difficulty in their first experiments with sprouting and become discouraged, the following suggestions are offered:

• Beans will become moldy or even rot during the sprouting if they are too old and lack germination. The only remedy for this is to use new seeds with high germination values.

• The spoilage may be caused by soaking the beans for too long initially. If this is the case, soaking should be omitted. The dry beans, after being thoroughly washed, are placed in the container and watered three or four times per day. Any defective beans noted after each watering must be picked out and discarded.

- In case the decay of the beans is due to bacterial action, frequent changing of soaking water is of greatest necessity.

- It might be well to gain some experience from sprouting mung beans before attempting to sprout soybeans. Mung beans are the tiny green beans out of which the bean sprouts used in chop suey dishes are prepared. They are excellent as an addition to salad, though their food value cannot compare with that of soybean sprouts.

Sprouted beans can be cooked by gently sautéing in small amount of olive oil or ghee. Cooking time should be about 1-5 minutes, depending upon amount used. This helps to get rid of the raw taste when added to soups or stir fry, always add last.

Alfalfa is the most popular of the sprouts. Always watch for mold when purchasing store bought sprouts. It is best to sprout your own.

Sprouts may be cooked gently by sautéing in small amount of oil or ghee. To get rid of the raw taste, cooking time should be about 5 minutes, depending upon the amount. When adding to soup or stir fry, always add last.

Raw tip: Most raw fooders would only eat sprouted lentils, mung, garbanzo or adzuki. Other bean spouts can be difficult to digest.

Sprouted Lentil Sauté

Serves 2

- 1 tablespoon sesame oil
- 1 green onion, chopped
- 1 cup celery, chopped
- 1 red pepper, chopped
- 8 ounces baby corn
- 1 tablespoon fresh ginger, grated
- 1 tablespoon ajwan
- 2 cups sprouted lentils
- 1 teaspoon agave or ¼ teaspoon Stevia

Sauté chopped onion, celery, and peppers in sesame oil at a low heat for 10 minutes, or until soft. Add baby corn, ginger, and ajwan seeds; cook for another 10 minutes. Add the lentil sprouts and agave last, and cook only long enough to heat sprouts. Lentils are high in iron and protein. 1 cup of lentils yields 2 cups of sprouts.

Serve with protein or starches.

Adzuki Beans

<u>Botanical Name: Vigna angularis</u>

Adzuki (also spelled aduki and azuki) beans are the small, red "mung" type beans used in Japan and China. They are good for strengthening the kidneys. They are rajasic in nature (stimulating; causing excessive energy and agitation, creating a distracting, restless state of mind).

Energy: Cooling

Taste: Sweet, Astringent

Post Digestive: Sweet

Indications: Kidney stones, blood tonic, circulation, chronic illness, weight loss, inflammation

Systems: Circulatory, Immune

Dosha Affected:

  Vata: Moderation

  Pitta: Excellent

  Kapha: Moderation

  Mixes Well With: All vegetables, starches

Ayurvedic Curative Cuisine for Everyone

Adzuki Moon Cakes

Serves 6

1 ½ cups dried adzuki beans

8 cups water

¼ teaspoon baking powder

1 cup flour

1 egg - optional

1 onion, well chopped

12 inches kombu, cut into small pieces

6 bay leaves

½ cup fresh ginger, grated

2 tablespoons soy sauce or Bragg's

Soak beans overnight. The next day, drain beans and add to 8 cups fresh water, chopped onion, kombu, and bay leaves. Bring to a boil, then lower to medium heat and cook about 30 minutes, until soft. Drain most of the water, but not all (keep just enough to keep beans moist). Put beans into food processor, or mash by hand. Add the ginger, flour, baking powder, eggs (optional), and soy or Bragg's. Make into patties (small cakes), place on baking sheet, and bake at 250° for 10 minutes.

Serve with salad. When sprouted, ½ cup aduki beans yields 2 cups of sprouts.

Black-Eyed Peas

Botanical Name: Vigna unguiculata

Black-eyed peas are native to Africa, but now grow in Asia and the Americas. In the Southern US, they are a popular ingredient in soul food. A traditional New Year's meal features these beans with collard greens, and is supposed to bring one good luck and financial enrichment. Black-eyed peas are an excellent source of calcium, folate, and vitamin A. In the U.S., this food has traditionally been used in the south with collard greens, tomatoes, and animal fat.

Energy: Warming

Taste: Astringent, Sweet

Post digestive: Sweet

Indications: Excellent for weak conditions, strengthening kidneys, immune builder, gives stamina when overworking, helps all muscle tissues, to gain weight, good source of minerals – particularly iron and calcium

Systems: Muscular, Circulatory

Dosha Affected:

Vata: Good (when well cooked, made into a paste)

Pitta: Excellent

Kapha: Moderation

Mixes Well With: Starches, greens, other beans

Black-Eyed Peas and Collard Greens

Serves 8

- 1½ cups black-eyed peas
- 2 tablespoons olive oil or ghee
- 1 onion, chopped
- 1 clove garlic, chopped (Kapha only)
- 8 cups water
- 6 bay leaves
- ½ tablespoon turmeric, ground
- 6 large leaves and stems of collard greens, well chopped
- ½ cup cilantro, chopped
- 2 tablespoons coriander, ground
- 2 tablespoons dried basil
- 1½ cups tomatoes, chopped (optional)
- salt to taste

Soak beans overnight; drain the next day. In a large pot, sauté onions and garlic in oil. Add beans and 8 cups of fresh water, bay leaves, and turmeric; cook for 35 minutes on medium heat. When beans are boiling, add collard greens, cilantro, coriander, and basil. Steep for 15 minutes. If tomatoes are allowed in the diet, add with collard greens. Add salt to taste.

Chickpeas
(Garbanzo Beans)

<u>Botanical Name: *Cicer arietinum*</u>

Chickpeas, also known as Garbanzo Beans, are native to India and the Mediterranean area. They are used to make hummus, a popular East Indian food. This bean is hardy, very high in minerals, and often prepared by salting and roasting. It can be found in packages of Chinese trail mix. In India, it is called Chana. Traditionally, this flour is used in many Ayurvedic practices. It is excellent for skin treatments, face masks, beauty and creams. It is also good for removing excel oil after an abyangha self-massage.

Energy: Cooling

Taste: Sweet, Astringent

Post Digestive: Sweet

Indications: PMS, urinary tract infection, immune builder, gall stones

Systems: Reproductive, Urinary, Immune

Dosha Affected:

Vata: Moderation (best in hummus)

Pitta: Excellent

Kapha: Moderation

Mixes Well With: All vegetables, starches

Chana Marsala

Serves 4

- 1 cup dried chickpeas
- 6 cups water
- 1 small sweet onion, chopped
- 6 bay leaves
- 6 inches kombu, cut into small pieces
- ¼ teaspoon hing (asafoetida)
- 1 tablespoon yellow mustard seeds
- 2 tablespoons ajwan
- 1 tablespoons ghee
- 2 stalks celery, chopped
- 1 red or green pepper, chopped
- 1 tablespoon garam masala
- 1 cup baby spinach, chopped
- 2 teaspoon dried cilantro
- Bragg's or salt

Soak chickpeas overnight; drain the next day. Put beans in saucepan with 6 cups of fresh water, onions, bay leaves, kombu, and hing; bring to a boil. Cook gently for 45 minutes, or until beans are soft. In a large pan, roast mustard seeds and ajwan. Add ghee, celery, and peppers, and sauté until soft. When beans are cooked, drain well and add to the celery-pepper mixture. Stir in garam masala, spinach, and cilantro; add Bragg's or salt to taste.

Serve with vegetables or grains.

Homemade Falafel

- 1 cup dried chickpeas
- 4 cups water
- 1 onion, chopped
- 6 bay leaves
- ¼ teaspoon hing (asafoetida)
- 1 cup oat flour
- 1 cup breadcrumbs
- ½ cup parsley, well chopped
- 2 tablespoons cumin, ground
- 2 tablespoons coriander, ground
- 1½ teaspoons turmeric, ground
- 2 tablespoons Bragg's
- sesame oil

Soak chickpeas overnight; drain the next day. Cook for 45 to 60 minutes in 4 cups fresh water with onion, bay leaves, and hing; drain. Grind the cooked beans in a food processor or blender; set aside. Mix oat flour, breadcrumbs, parsley, cumin, coriander, turmeric, and Bragg's. Add chickpea mixture, stirring to make a soft dough (add a little water if necessary). Roll into 1-inch balls; sauté in sesame oil. (For crispier falafel balls, roll in extra breadcrumbs before frying.)

Serve with cucumber salad.

Ayurvedic Curative Cuisine for Everyone

Basil Hummus

- 2 cups dried chickpeas
- 12 inches kombu, cut into small pieces
- 1 medium or 2 small onions, chopped
- 1 teaspoon cumin seeds
- 6 bay leaves
- ¼ teaspoon hing (asafoetida)
- 1 cup lemon or lime juice
- ½ cup olive oil
- 15 ounces tahini (sesame butter)
- 2½ cup basil, fresh (well chopped)
- 1 tablespoon coriander, ground
- 1½ tablespoon Bragg's

Soak chickpeas overnight; drain and rinse well the next day. Put in large pot with 8 cups of fresh water, kombu, onions, cumin, bay leaves, and hing. Bring to a boil, turn to simmer and cook for 45 minutes, until beans are soft. Drain water off, reserving 1½ cups of the "bean broth." Put beans in blender, and blend with lemon juice, olive oil, tahini, basil, coriander, and Bragg's until smooth. Add some of the reserved "bean broth" if mixture is too thick to blend easily. Serve as a spread or dip with crackers or vegetables.

Variations: Add roasted red peppers or sun-dried tomatoes.

Fava Beans

<u>Botanical Name:</u> *Vicia faba*

Fava (or broad) beans are native to Africa, and one of the oldest types of bean available. They can be toxic; therefore, avoid when cancer or any auto-immune disorder is present. They are difficult to digest. When cooking, add three times the amount of water.

Energy: Warming

Taste: Sweet, Astringent

Post Digestive: Sweet

Indications: Ulcer, liver disorders, urinary tract infection

Systems: Digestive, Urinary, Immune, Circulatory

<u>Dosha Affected:</u>

Vata: Avoid

Pitta: Good

Kapha: Moderation

Mixes Well With: All vegetables, starches

Fava Loaf

- 1 lb. dried fava beans
- 10 cups water
- 1 onion, chopped
- 8 bay leaves
- 12 inches of kombu, cut in small pieces
- ½ cups rice
- ½ bunch cilantro, chopped
- ½ bunch parsley, chopped
- 2 tablespoons tomato sauce
- 2 tablespoons flour
- 2 tablespoons mild curry powder
- 1 tablespoon Bragg's

Soak beans overnight. Drain the next day, add 10 cups of fresh water, and cook with onions, bay leaves, and kombu for 45 minutes; add rice and cook for another 15 minutes. When rice is done, add cilantro, parsley, and tomato sauce; cover pot, let steep for another 10 minutes. Strain off all liquid. Mash well; add flour, curry powder, and Bragg's, and place mixture into an oiled loaf pan. Bake at 350° for 10 minutes.

Fava Stew

Serves 4

- 1 cup fava beans
- ¼ cup tomato sauce
- 3 tablespoons potato, cooked, sliced
- 1 red onion, chopped
- 1 red pepper, chopped
- 5 bay leaves
- 1 teaspoon oregano, well chopped
- 2" piece of kombu, well chopped
- ¼ cup leeks, sliced thin
- 3 cups water
- 1 teaspoon salt

Soak beans overnight in 1 cup water. Next day, drain & discard water. Put remaining water & other ingredients together with the beans in pot, except the peppers. Bring to boil. Lower heat to simmer, add peppers & cover. This recipe can also be made with various types of beans.

Kidney Beans

<u>Botanical Name:</u> *Phaseolus vulgaris*

Kidney beans are the large, red beans favored in Latin America, and commonly used in soups and chili. They contain a toxin that can only be removed by soaking the beans, discarding the water, then boiling in fresh water for at least 10 minutes. One of the richest in fiber.

Energy: Cooling

Taste: Sweet, Astringent

Post Digestive: Sweet

Indications: Protein deficiency, muscle builder, weak constitution, edema, kidney disorders

Systems: Muscular, Urinary

Dosha Affected:

Vata: Avoid

Pitta: Excellent

Kapha: Moderation

Mixes Well With: All vegetables, starches

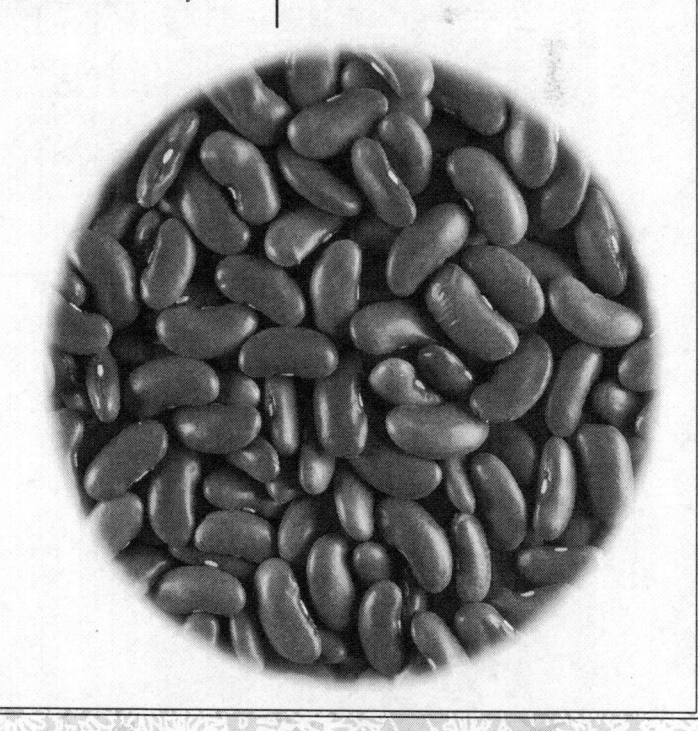

Kidney Bean Stew

Serves 6

- 1 cup dried kidney beans
- 4 cups water
- 1 large onion, chopped
- 4 inches of wakame, cut into small pieces
- 4 bay leaves
- ¼ teaspoon hing (asafoetida)
- 2 tomatoes, chopped
- ½ bunch of cilantro, chopped
- ¼ cups ghee or olive oil
- Bragg's or salt

Soak beans overnight; drain the next day and rinse well. Bring 4 cups of fresh water to a boil, add the soaked kidney beans, onions, wakame, bay leaves, and hing, and cook over medium heat for 45 to 60 minutes. When beans are soft, add tomatoes, cilantro, and ghee; cook for another 10 to 15 minutes on low heat. Add Bragg's or salt to taste.

Serve with cornbread, crackers, or grains.

Kidney Bean Salad

- 2 cups dried red kidney beans
- 5 cups water
- ½ lb. fresh string beans
- 8-10 asparagus
- 1 cup green onions, chopped
- ½ cup cilantro or parsley, chopped
- 2 tablespoons cumin, ground
- 1 tablespoon fennel, ground
- ½ cup lemon juice
- 1 large or 2 medium carrots, grated
- 2 tablespoons olive oil
- Bragg's

Soak beans overnight; drain the next day. Place in pot with 5 cups of fresh water and cook for 30 minutes on medium (do not overcook). Drain. Cut string beans & asparagus into 1½-inch pieces, remove hard end pieces of asparagus and discard. Then blanch by placing in a bowl and pouring boiling water over them; let steep for 5 minutes. Drain, then add beans, onions, cilantro, cumin and fennel, lemon juice, and grated carrots. Cover and let steep for about 1 hour in bowl. Add olive oil and Bragg's to taste, and serve.

Lentils

<u>Botanical Name: Lens esculenta</u>

Lentils are one of the most ancient foods known. A large, purplish green lentil is widely used in Europe, while the red lentil comes from Egypt. In New Mexico, Arizona, and Mexico, a small variety is grown, the seed of which was first brought to America by the Spanish missionaries. Lentils are 26% protein, making it the bean with the second highest level of protein (after the soybean).

Energy: Warming

Taste: Sweet

Post Digestive: Sweet

Indications: Anemia, debility, urinary tract infection, blood builder

Systems: Circulatory, Urinary

Dosha Affected:

Vata: Avoid

Pitta: Excellent

Kapha: Moderation

Mixes Well With: All vegetables, starches

Lentil Patties

Makes 12 patties

2 cups dried lentils

4 cups water

6 bay leaves

1 tablespoon ajwan seeds

1 tablespoon cumin seeds

1 medium onion, well chopped

10 inches of kombu, cut into small pieces

½ cup tomato sauce

1 egg, beaten (or egg substitute)

1 green pepper, chopped

¼ bunch cilantro, chopped

1 tablespoon sesame oil

1 tablespoon Bragg's or salt

Soak lentils overnight; drain. Put lentils in pot with 4 cups of fresh water, bay leaves, ajwan and cumin seeds, onion, and kombu. Bring to a boil; cook 30 to 40 minutes or until soft. Drain off water, and mash lentils. Add tomato sauce, egg, peppers, cilantro, sesame oil, and Bragg's or salt. Form into patties, place on baking sheet, and bake at 300° for 10 minutes. Serve with vegetables or salad.

Lima Beans

Botanical Name: Phaseolus limensis

Lima (also called Butter) beans are natives of Central America, and are higher in fat and starch than any other bean. In South America, they are often eaten with potatoes, olive oil, or butter. In many parts of Asia, they are roasted with sugar or salt added, and are eaten as a snack.

Energy: Slightly cooling

Taste: Sweet, Astringent

Post Digestive: Sweet

Indications: Blood builder, urinary tract infection, edema, inflammations, to gain weight

Systems: Circulatory, Urinary, Immune

Dosha Affected:

Vata: Avoid

Pitta: Excellent

Kapha: Moderation

Mixes Well With: All vegetables, starches

Lima Bean Patties

- 1 cup dried lima beans
- 2 eggs well beaten
- 4 cups water
- 1 onion, chopped
- 1 bunch parsley, chopped
- 1 cup breadcrumbs
- 2 tablespoons mild salsa
- 2 tablespoons Italian seasoning

Soak beans overnight; drain water the next day. Put in pot with 4 cups of fresh water and onions, and bring to a boil. Cook for 45 minutes, until beans are soft; drain water off, and mash beans well. Add parsley, breadcrumbs, salsa, and Italian seasoning, and well beaten eggs. Form into patties, place on baking sheet, and bake at 350° for 15 minutes, or until crisp.

Lima Beans and Rice

Serves 6

- 1 cup lima beans
- 1 cup basmati rice
- 4 ¼ cups water
- 1 teaspoon cilantro, fresh, chopped
- 1 green pepper, chopped
- ¼ cup green onions, chopped
- ½ cup pumpkin or butternut squash, chopped small
- 1 cup tomato sauce
- 1 tablespoon nutritional yeast

Soak beans overnight in 1 cup water. Next day, drain. Cook beans and squash in 2½ cups water until tender. Then add remaining ingredients, except cilantro, green peppers, and rice. When it comes to a boil, then add rice, cilantro, peppers, and 1 ¼ water.

Mung Beans

<u>Botanical Name: Vigna radiata</u>

Mung beans are small, bright green beans that are highly nutritious, and one of the most digestible of the legumes. They are a good meat substitute, as they are high in protein. Mixed with rice, they are an essential ingredient in the Indian dish called Khichari. They are also the bean used to make bean sprouts in Asian cooking.

Energy: Neutral

Taste: Sweet

Post Digestive: Sweet

Indications: Building tissue, convalescence, chronic illnesses, anemia, blood disorders, kidney stones, detoxification

Systems: All systems

<u>**Dosha Affected:**</u>

Vata: Good (if in khichari)

Pitta and **Kapha**: Excellent

Mixes Well With: All vegetables, starches, proteins

Khichari

(Also known as Khichadee and many other spellings)

Serves 8-10

- 2 cups dried mung beans – or Moon Dahl
- 1 teaspoon cumin seeds
- 1 teaspoon ajwan
- 2 tablespoons ghee
- 2 tablespoons fresh ginger, grated
- ½ sweet onion, well chopped
- 12 inches kombu, cut into small pieces
- 8 cups water
- $1/16$ teaspoon hing (asafoetida)
- 2 cups basmati rice or quinoa
- 1 teaspoon coriander, ground
- 1 teaspoon turmeric, ground
- 1½ teaspoon Bombay curry
- $1/16$ teaspoon saffron
- ½ bunch cilantro, well chopped
- ½ bunch basil, well chopped

Soak mung beans overnight; drain the next day. Roast cumin and ajwan seeds in pan, then add ghee and sauté ginger, onion, and kombu for 15 minutes. Add 8 cups of fresh water, hing, and beans. Bring to a boil and cook for 30 minutes, then add rice while water is boiling. Continue cooking for about 10 minutes, then add coriander, turmeric, curry, and saffron. Lower heat, and continue to cook for about 1 hour – or until water has been absorbed. Do not stir at all while cooking on low heat. Remove form heat, and stir in cilantro and basil; serve.

Note: If using moon dahl instead of mung beans, cook for only 15 minutes.

Peanuts

Botanical Name: Arachis hypogaea

Peanuts (also called Ground nuts and Goober Peas), are thought to be native to Brazil, and were later introduced into all tropical countries. Two well-known varieties are the Spanish and Virginia peanuts grown in this country. In Costa Rica, a variety grows which has pod-like beans containing 4 to 6 peanuts. The plant is a tender, annual, herbaceous vine, and is grown in the southern United States for forage and hay, to improve soil, and for its pods. Even though the composition closely resembles that of a nut, and most people consider peanuts to be nuts, they are actually members of the legume family. Ordinary peanut butter is far from being a wholesome food, because the peanuts are made indigestible by long roasting and abundant salting. Nuts should only be very slightly roasted for making butter, and the addition of salt is unnecessary and harmful. The hydrogenated oils in which nuts are boiled are especially harmful to the digestive system, as well as the saturated fats that contribute so much to diseases of the circulatory system. Learn to eat peanuts raw and unadulterated, and they will prove a valuable addition to the natural diet.

Energy: Warming

Taste: Astringent, Sweet

Post Digestive: Sweet

Indications: To gain weight, muscle spasm, nerves, constipation

Systems: Muscular, Nervous

Dosha Affected:

Vata: Good (best cooked or boiled – not roasted)

Pitta and **Kapha**: Best sprouted

Mixes Well With: All vegetables, starches

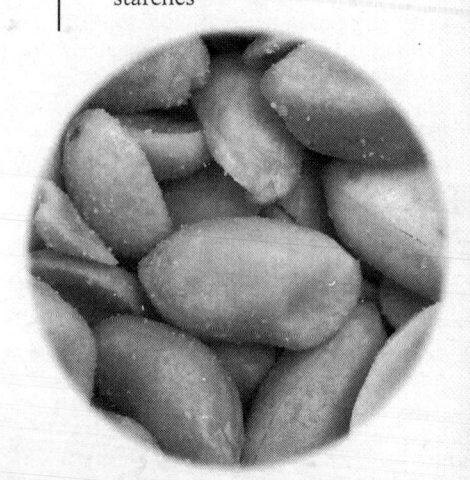

Peanut Sauce

- 1 cup raw peanuts
- 1 tablespoon sunflower oil
- ¼ cup lemon juice
- 1 cup water
- 1 tablespoon Bragg's

In blender, blend all ingredients until smooth.

Serve with salad or vegetables.

Peanuts, Greens, Tofu

Serves 4

- 2 cups peanuts, halved
- 1 (8 oz.) cake of tofu, firm
- 1 cup tomatoes, chopped
- 1 cup kale, well chopped
- 2 cups onions, chopped
- 1 ½ cup celery, chopped
- 4 cups zucchini, sliced
- 2 tablespoons ginger, fresh, grated
- 1/3 cup cilantro, fresh, chopped
- 2 cups water

In a large skillet on medium heat, boil onions & zucchini until soft. Add grated ginger. Cook for 10 minutes. Add tomato sauce and celery. Cover. Simmer for about 5 minutes. Add peanuts and remaining ingredients. Serve with grains.

Soybeans

Botanical Name: Glycine max

The soybean is a native of Japan and China. It is a bushy annual, growing from 2 to 6 feet in height, with little pendant pods that contain small yellow, brown, green, or black seeds. In Asia, the ripe seeds are primarily used for making oil, as well as being made into fermented forms, such as tempeh, miso, tamari, and soy sauce. In America, soy products have grown in popularity as soy is an excellent food and can be used advantageously in the diet. During the long winter months, in regions where the availability of fresh green vegetables is scarce, soybeans are a welcome and extremely valuable adjunct to salads and cooked as a vegetable. When three-fourths grown, soybeans make a very palatable and wholesome green vegetable similar to the green pea and lima bean. They contain a rich amount of potassium and phosphorus and small amount of calcium, magnesium, and sulphur.

Note: It is important to buy only organically-grown soybeans and soybean products, as the majority of soybeans now grown in the US and several other countries are genetically modified. Look for "non-GMO" labeling.

Energy: Warming

Taste: Sweet

Post Digestive: Sweet

Indications: Phlegm expeller, colds, flu, urinary tract infection, inflammation, fever

Systems: Respiratory, Urinary, Immune

Dosha Affected:

Vata: Avoid

Pitta: Excellent

Kapha: Moderation

Mixes Well With: All vegetables, starches

Creamy Soybean Soup

Serves 4

- 2 cups dried soybeans
- 6 cups water
- ¼ cup chopped sweet onion
- 6 bay leaves
- ¼ teaspoon hing (asafoetida)
- 2 cups tomatoes, chopped
- 1 cup soy milk (for a sweeter taste use vanilla soy milk)
- 1 clove garlic, chopped
- 1 tablespoon Italian seasoning
- 1 tablespoon cumin, ground
- 2 tablespoons fresh basil, chopped
- soy sauce

Soak the soybeans in ample water overnight; drain and rinse the next day. Place the soaked beans in a pot with 6 cups of fresh water, onion, bay leaves, and hing; bring to a boil. Lower to medium heat and add tomatoes, soy milk, garlic, Italian seasoning, and cumin. Cook 45 to 60 minutes, until beans are soft. Add basil, then place soup in blender and blend until smooth. Add soy sauce to taste.

Serve with salad and vegetables.

Tofu

Tofu is made from soy milk, and has a milk flavor and cheese-like qualities. Tofu is to soy milk what cheese is to dairy milk. Tofu is versatile in food preparation as it absorbs the flavors of other foods. It can be made into sauces, and with a high protein content, tofu makes a good meat substitute. It is a traditional staple of the East. Tofu can be made at home, or purchased in various forms, including soft ("silken"), firm, and baked with flavoring.

Energy: Cooling. Moisturizing
Taste: Sweet, Astringent
Post Digestive: Sweet
Indications: Heart disorders, lowers cholesterol
Systems: Circulatory, Endocrine

Dosha Affected:
Vata & **Pitta**: Good
Kapha: Moderation
Mixes Well With: Green vegetables

Baked Tofu

- 2 blocks of firm tofu
- 2 tablespoons ghee
- 2 tablespoons grated ginger
- 1 teaspoon coriander, ground
- ¼ cup cilantro, chopped
- ¼ cup lemon juice
- 1 tablespoon soy sauce

Slice tofu in half and place in a wide baking dish. In blender, mix ghee, ginger, coriander, cilantro, lemon juice and soy sauce. Pour the mixture over the tofu. Marinate tofu for ½ hour. Bake for 20 to 30 minutes at 250°. While baking, occasionally drizzle the sauce over the tofu.

Serve with salad or vegetables.

Tofu Bean Soup

Serves 6

- 2 cups dried adzuki beans
- 2 tablespoons olive oil
- 2 sweet onions, chopped
- 2 cloves garlic, chopped – Kapha only
- 2 teaspoons cumin, ground
- 6 cups water
- 4 bay leaves
- 2 pieces kombu or wakami seaweed, cut into small pieces
- 1 lb. firm tofu – OR – ½ lb. chicken meat, organic
- 1 bunch cilantro, chopped
- 2 teaspoons coriander, ground
- Bragg's

Soak beans overnight; the next day, drain beans and rinse well. Sauté onions and garlic in olive oil. Add cumin, water, and drained beans. Add bay leaves (crushed up with hand), and seaweed. Bring to a boil, lower heat, and cook 25 minutes. Add tofu or chicken, cilantro, and coriander. Add Bragg's to taste.

Split Peas

Botanical Name: Pisum sativum

The pea is a legume and, in the dried state, is not as wholesome as when fresh. However, if used sparingly and in combination with an ample amount of fresh raw vegetables, it may be used either in soups or as a cooked vegetable. The split pea is a pea cut in half to make it easier to cook and to digest.

Energy: Cooling

Taste: Sweet, Astringent

Post Digestive: Sweet

Indications: Ulcers, stomach disorders (high acidity), infections, increases endurance

Systems: Digestive, Immune

Dosha Affected:

Vata: Moderation (best as a dahl)

Pitta and **Kapha**: Good

Mixes Well With: Non-starchy vegetables

Split Pea Soup

Serves 4

- 2 cups split peas
- 6 cups water
- 1 large onion, chopped
- 3 stalks celery, chopped
- 2 carrots, grated
- ¼ cup cilantro, chopped
- 2 cloves of garlic, chopped
- ½ teaspoon hing (asafoetida)
- ¼ cup ghee
- 1 teaspoon black pepper
- 1 tablespoon mild curry or churna
- Bragg's or salt

Soak split peas for 2 to 3 hours; drain. Add peas to pot with 6 cups boiling water and onion, celery, carrots, cilantro, garlic, and hing. Cook for 30 to 45 minutes on medium heat. Add ghee, pepper, curry powder, and Bragg's to taste.

Serve with garlic bread.

Dhal with Coconut

Serves 8

- ¼ teaspoon mustard seeds
- 2 tablespoons olive oil
- ¼ cup chopped onion
- 1 teaspoon minced garlic
- ½ teaspoon cumin, ground
- ⅛ teaspoon red pepper, ground
- ⅛ teaspoon turmeric, ground
- 1 cup yellow split peas
- 2½ cups water
- ¼ cup grated coconut (unsweetened)
- 1 teaspoon salt
- 2 teaspoons lemon juice
- 2 teaspoons ghee

In covered skillet, heat mustard seeds over medium-high heat in oil until seeds begin to pop. Uncover, add onion, and sauté until edges are nicely browned. Add garlic, cumin, red pepper, and turmeric, and sauté for 20 seconds, stirring constantly. Remove from heat and set aside. In saucepan, bring split peas and water to a boil. Turn heat down and add onion mixture to simmering dhal. Cover and continue simmering for 45 minutes. The peas will hold their shape even as water level drops, but will break under the slightest pressure when cooked. Mash dhal with potato masher or back of spoon 6 to 8 times to break up roughly. Stir in coconut and salt. Partially cover and simmer for 5 to 10 minutes, adding a small amount of water if mixture gets too thick. Check often to make sure peas are not sticking to bottom. Mixture should be consistency of thick soup. Stir in lemon juice. Remove from heat and stir in ghee.

Spicy Dhal

<u>Serves 6-8</u>

1 cup yellow split peas

2½ cups water

¼ teaspoon turmeric, ground

¼ teaspoon cumin seeds

¼ teaspoon mustard seeds

¼ teaspoon crushed red pepper

2 tablespoons olive oil

1 cup sweet onion, chopped

2-3 green chilis (serrano, Thai or jalapeno), split lengthwise

1 cup tomatoes, chopped

2 tablespoons mild curry powder

1 teaspoon salt or Bragg's

2 tablespoons cilantro, chopped

In saucepan bring split peas, water, and turmeric to a boil. Turn heat down, cover, and let simmer 45 minutes, watching for spilling. While dhal cooks over medium-high heat, in heavy covered saucepan, heat cumin seeds, mustard seeds, and crushed red pepper in oil until mustard seeds begin to pop. Turn heat down to medium, add onion and green chilis and sauté for about 5 minutes until onion is soft. Add tomatoes and cook, stirring until they are soft. Do not overcook – tomato pieces should hold their shape. When dhal is cooked and completely tender, mash with potato masher or back of spoon 6 to 8 times to break up roughly. Add curry powder; simmer for 2 minutes, adding more water if necessary for pourable consistency. Remove from heat, add Bragg's to taste, and garnish with chopped cilantro.

Indian Dahl

- 2 cups yellow or green peas (or lentils)
- 2 teaspoons ajwan (Kapha only)
- 1 teaspoon cumin seeds
- 2 tablespoons ghee
- 1 sweet onion, chopped
- 2 cloves garlic, chopped (Kapha only)
- ¼ teaspoon hing (asafoetida)
- 12 inches kombu, cut into small pieces
- 8 cups water
- ¼ cup basil, chopped
- 1 teaspoon coriander, ground
- 1 teaspoon mild curry powder
- Bragg's to taste

Soak beans overnight; drain the next day. Roast ajwan and cumin seeds in a pan, then add ghee, and sauté onion and garlic. Add beans, hing, kombu, and 8 cups fresh water; bring to a boil, then lower heat to medium for 45 minutes. Add basil, coriander, and curry powder, and cook on low for 10 more minutes. Add Bragg's to taste.

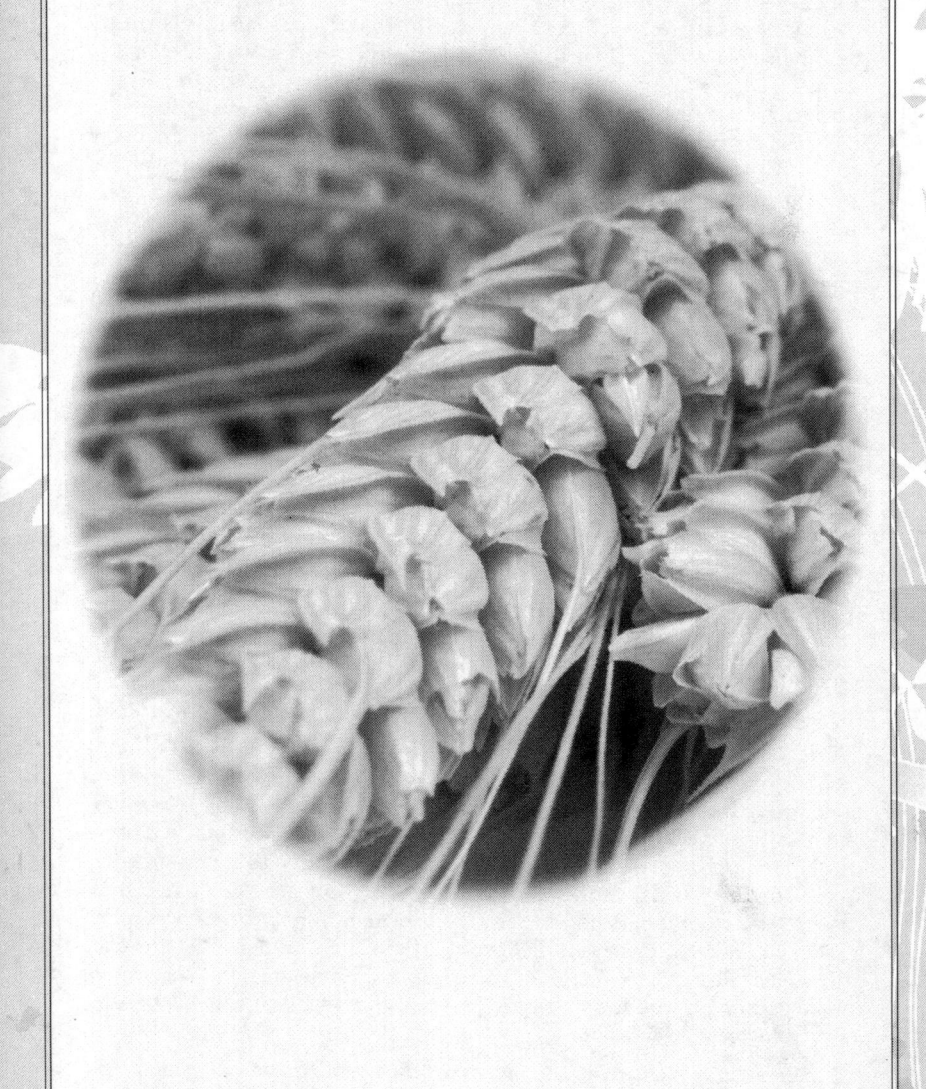

Grains

Grains

General Considerations

Grains – or cereal crops – are the edible seeds of the grass family. (There are two grains that do not belong to the grass family; buckwheat, which belongs to the polygonacea family, and quinoa, which is a species of goosefoot.) Grains have been an essential part of the human diet since the beginning of agriculture. The Egyptians and Syrians had mastered the techniques of irrigation by 3000 B.C. Grain has played a vital role in world history. Each continent has a dominant grain that is part of their culture: rice is the grain of Asia; wheat and barley were from Southern Europe; rye and oats have dominated most of northern Europe; corn was the original staple of the Americas; and millet and sorghum were predominantly used in Africa. Grains are the most important crop in the third world, where it is the major source of food – in many countries up to 90%. This compares to a 25% portion of the diet in industrialized countries. Whole grain consumption has been declining over the last century with the polishing and bleaching of grains, and its replacement with other food groups.

Grain consists of three main parts; an outer layer (the bran), the kernel, and the germ. The seed is enclosed in an outer shell, or hull, that cannot be assimilated by the human digestive system. For this reason, grains need to be hulled to make them edible. The kernel is the largest part of the grain, composed mainly of starch, a complex carbohydrate, that is absorbed slowly by the body, producing a long-lasting feeling of satiety. The bran, which is made of several fibrous layers, is rich in minerals and vitamins and plays a most important function within the G.I. tract, providing fiber (assisting with constipation). The germ, located in the lower grain, contains the seed of a new plant and has the highest concentration of nutrition, vitamins, and minerals. It also has the highest level of oil.

Grains play a central role in the human diet. They can be cooked, crushed, dried, made into flour, pastas, puffed, or flaked. They can be cooked in soups and fruit dishes. Many alcoholic beverages are made from grains, such as beer, whiskey, bourbon, and sake. Grains are usually cooked with water, milk, or stock; cooking transforms the flavor of the grain. Most grains require 2 to 3 times the volume with liquid. It is best to soak grains for 12 to 24 hours prior to cooking in order to shorten the cooking time and to reduce the effect of phytic acid. Phytic acid interferes with digestion, producing gas. Much of it can be poured off with the soak water. Always store grains in tight containers away from heat and moisture.

A vegetarian diet must include foods that are complementary in amino acids, such as beans and grains. Amino acids are the building blocks of proteins. There are 20 amino acids, 8 of which are essential because they cannot be synthesized by the human body. These essential amino acids must come from the foods that we eat. Some of the essential amino acids are found in grains, but not legumes. Some are found in legumes but not in grains. Almost every culture was based on a grain–legume diet that provided ingredients for complete protein.

Sprouting grains increases food value and makes it more digestible. Raw sprouted grains are up to 10 times more nutritionally potent.

Many grains have diuretic properties; especially barley, corn, rye and buckwheat. Because they are sweet in nature, most grains are particularly good for Vata due to their strengthening properties, particularly during chronic illness. All humours benefit from grains, with some too cool for Vatas (barley), too wet/mucous producing for Kaphas (oats), or too heating for Pittas (corn). Fortunately, there is enough variety for all doshic types to have several grains.

Cooking Grains

1 Cup	Liquid (cups)	Cooking Time
Oats (whole)	2-3	1 Hour
Rolled Oats	1	5 Minutes
Whole Wheat Grain	2	60-90 Minutes
Cracked Wheat	2-3	30-40 Minutes
Bulgur	2	25-35 Cover & Simmer
Millet	2	30-40 Minutes
Barley (Whole Grain)	2	45 Minutes
Basmati Rice (white)	1½	30-45 Minutes
Brown Rice	2	45-60 Minutes
Wild Rice	3	45-60 Minutes
Buckwheat	2	15-20 Minutes
Corn Meal	4	25-30 Minutes
Spelt	2	30-40 Minutes
Amaranth	2	12-15 Minutes
Quinoa	2	30 Minutes

Amaranth

Botanical Name: Amaranthus, several species

Amaranth played an important part of the history of the Aztec Indians in Mexico, with 60 individual species now growing all over the world. The Spanish prohibited its cultivation, thinking it was worshiped as a God. Amaranth is to grains what the soybean is to its fellow legumes. Amaranth is higher in oils than any other grain. This super grain is high in protein and is unusually high in lysine, mellenonine, and other amino acids, which are often in short supply in grains. The seeds are very small, about the size of a poppy seed. In India, amaranth is a major ingredient in the sweets (laddus) prepared for Hindu festivities.

Energy: Warming

Taste: Sweet

Post Digestive: Sweet

Indications: Improves urinary flow, constipation, helps balance large intestines, blood tonic, liver disorder, enlarged spleen, eye disease, fevers

Systems: All systems

Dosha Affected:

Vata: Good

Pitta: Excellent

Kapha: Moderation (best toasted)

Mixes Well With: All vegetables and starches

Coconut Amaranth

Serves 2

- 1 cup amaranth
- ¼ cup raisins
- 2 cups coconut milk (or almond milk)
- 2 teaspoons cardamom
- 1 teaspoon vanilla
- 1 teaspoon cinnamon

Soak amaranth and raisins for 4 hours (or overnight); drain. Add coconut milk, bring to a boil, and cook for 10 to 15 minutes on low heat. Add spices at end of cooking time.

Amaranth a la Saffron

Serves 2

- 1 cup amaranth
- ¼ teaspoon saffron threads
- 3 cups water
- ½ cup rice (or soy) milk
- ½ cup raisins
- ¼ teaspoon cinnamon
- ¼ teaspoon cardamom
- ¼ teaspoon coriander
- 1 tablespoon ghee
- 1 teaspoon vanilla
- 1 tablespoon agave syrup or stevia

Place amaranth, saffron, and water in saucepan; bring to a boil and cook for 30 minutes. Add milk, raisins, cinnamon, cardamom, and coriander; stir well. Turn off heat, add ghee and vanilla. Cover pan, and let stand for 10 minutes. Sweeten to taste with agave or stevia.

Barley

Botanical Name: Hordeum vulgare

Barley is extremely hardy, one of the most ancient cultivated plants, and has been found in the earliest Egyptian monuments. It grows at great altitudes (15,000 feet in Tibet) and in Timbuktu, near the Equator. In countries such as Tunisia, Algeria, and Morocco, barley is used chiefly for making bread. In Scotland, barley "porridge" is very popular. In the U. S., the grain is first demineralized, producing an acceptable taste; "pearled" barley is the result. A wholesome flour can be made with the plain hulled barley in combination with whole wheat and whole rye flours.

Energy: Cooling

Taste: Sweet

Post Digestive: Sweet

Indications: Edema, kidney stones, rheumatic and arthritic joints, diarrhea, assimilation, chronic illnesses

Systems: Urinary, Auto-immune system

Dosha Affected:

Vata: Moderation (well-spiced)

Pitta & **Kapha**: Good

Mixes Well With: Vegetables, oils, legumes

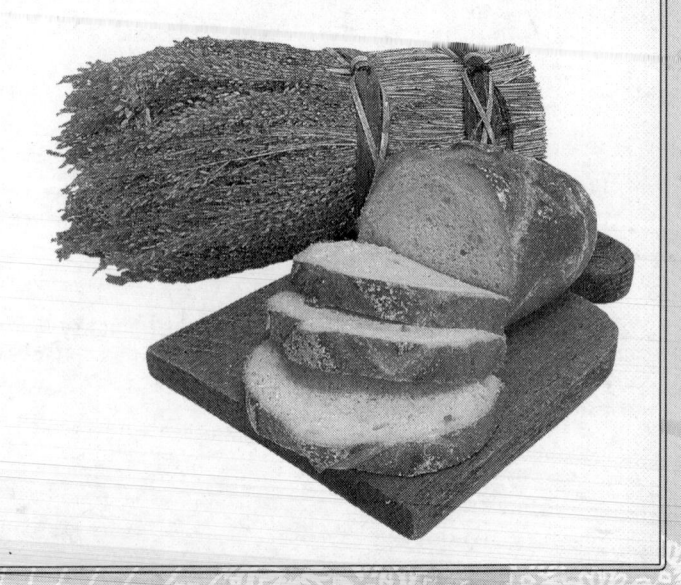

Miso Barley Soup

Serves 8-10

- 2 cups barley
- 1 onion, chopped (Kapha)- or -1 bunch green onions or scallions, chopped (Pitta)
- 2 cloves garlic, chopped (Kapha only)
- 2 tablespoons olive oil
- 8 cups water
- 5 large stalks of celery, chopped
- 12 large leaves and stems of chard, thinly sliced
- ¼ lb. green string beans, chopped
- 2 sheets nori, cut into small pieces
- ½ cup parsley, chopped
- 2 teaspoons coriander, ground
- 1 tablespoon fennel, ground
- ¼ cup barley or rice miso (no wheat)

Soak barley overnight. The next day, drain and rinse barley grains. Sauté onion and garlic in olive oil, then add barley and 8 cups of fresh water. Bring water to a boil, lower heat to medium and cook for 30 minutes. Add celery, chard, and string beans, bring to a boil again. Lower heat and cook for 10 to 15 minutes. Add nori, parsley, and spices; turn off heat and add miso. Do not boil miso – it will lose nutritive value and enzymes. Serve and eat with rice crackers and ghee.

Buckwheat

Botanical Name: Fagopyrum esculentum

Buckwheat is the seed of an annual herb native to Siberia. Its name is derived from the German Buchweizen, "beech wheat", because its shape resembles that of the beechnut. It is known in France as Ble Sarrasin, because it was reported to have been brought to Europe by the Crusaders. The "kasha" popularly eaten in Russia, is a cereal made up of buckwheat, millet, and other crushed grains. Buckwheat is grown chiefly in the eastern portions of the United States, the northwest of Europe, and in the mountains of Japan where it is used instead of rice. It will grow on poor thin soil and hilly lands where most other grains cannot be grown. There is no other flour subjected to as much adulteration as buckwheat flour. A large percentage of wheat is usually added because pure buckwheat flour produces mucous when water is added.

Energy: Warming

Taste: Sweet

Post Digestive: Sweet

Indications: Varicose veins, bleeding disorders, nosebleed, muscle building, to gain weight, fluid retention

Systems: Circulatory, Muscular, Endocrine, Urinary

Dosha Affected:

Vata: Good (best made into kasha)

Pitta: Moderation

Kapha: Moderation

Mixes Well With: Non-starchy vegetables, oils

Buckwheat Seaweed

Serves 6

1½ cups roasted buckwheat

2 cups water, divided

4 inches of kombu, cut in small pieces

½ cup sweet onion, chopped

1 teaspoon cumin, ground

1 tablespoon coriander

¼ cup cilantro, chopped

Bragg's

Toast buckwheat for 10 minutes in wok. Add ½ cup of the water, kombu, and onions; cover pan and cook on low heat. Stir occasionally, slowly adding the rest of the water, until buckwheat is fluffy and the seaweed is soft. Then add cumin, coriander, cilantro, and Bragg's to taste.

Serve with salad or vegetables.

Bulgur (wheat)

<u>Botanical Name:</u> *Triticum durum*

Bulgur is made from wheat (usually durum) – the wheat grains are parboiled, dried, and then ground into particles. It has more nutritional value than rice or couscous, and because it is pre-cooked, needs only to be soaked or cooked for a short time. It is different than "cracked wheat," which is not pre-cooked.

Tabouli

- 2 cups bulgar
- 3 cups water
- ½ cup olive oil
- ¼ cup lemon juice
- 1 teaspoon fennel, ground
- ½ onion, finely chopped
- 1 red pepper, finely chopped
- ¼ cup parsley, finely chopped
- ½ cup black olives, chopped
- soy sauce

Soak bulgar in water for 15 minutes. Make sure all the water has been absorbed. Mix olive oil, lemon juice, and fennel powder together, and add to bulgar. Add chopped onion, pepper, parsley, and olives, and mix well. Let the tabouli flavors mix together for 20 minutes, then add soy sauce to taste.

Serve with vegetables.

Corn (Dried)

<u>Botanical Name: Zea mays</u>

While young (immature) corn is considered a vegetable (see page 161), it is really a grain as well, when the seeds are used in the dried (mature) state. Cornmeal, grits, hominy, and posole are all processed from the mature kernels of corn. Popcorn is another variety of this grain.

Energy: Warming
Taste: Sweet
Post Digestive: Sweet
Indications: Liver tonic, gallbladder disorders, edema
Systems: Endocrine, Urinary

<u>**Dosha Affected:**</u>
Vata: Moderation (avoid corn chips)
Pitta: Moderation (blue corn is best)
Kapha: Good
Mixes Well With: Vegetables, starches

Corn Tortilla Soup

Serves 4

- 1 onion, well chopped
- 3 tomatoes, chopped
- 3 carrots, chopped
- 1 tablespoon coriander, ground
- 2 tablespoons ghee (divided)
- 10 corn tortillas
- 6 cups vegetable broth
- 1 piece epazote, chopped
- ½ bunch parsley
- 1 tablespoon cumin, ground
- 1 teaspoon chili powder
- 1 bunch cilantro, chopped
- 1 tablespoon lemon juice
- salt

Preheat oven to 350°. Sauté onions, tomatoes, carrots, and coriander over medium heat in 1 tablespoon. ghee. Brush 1 tablespoon. ghee over the tortillas; bake for 10 minutes or until golden brown. After the tortillas are done baking, crush them up. Bring the vegetable broth to a boil; add the epazote and parsley. Add sautéed vegetables and crushed tortillas, and reduce to low heat. Add cumin, chili powder, cilantro, lemon juice, and salt to taste.

Millet

Botanical Names: Panicum miliaceum,

Millet is the common name for several groups of small-seeded grasses. Millet, or grain sorghum, produces small round seeds resembling corn in chemical composition. Many varieties have been grown for ages in the eastern hemisphere. In Russia and China, it is a common staple food, while in Africa, its consumption is greater than that of wheat.

Energy: Cooling
Taste: Sweet
Post Digestive: Sweet
Indications: Indigestion, acidity, high agni, blood purifier, long term illnesses
Systems: Digestive, Circulatory

Dosha Affected:
Vata: Avoid
Pitta: Good (the only alkaline grain)
Kapha: Moderation (well spiced)
Mixes Well With: All vegetables

Millet Loaf

- 2 cups millet
- 3½ cups water
- 1 cup mushrooms, chopped
- 1 cup cooked green beans, chopped
- 2 onions, well chopped
- ¼ cup parsley
- ½ tablespoon Italian seasoning
- 1 tablespoon lecithin
- ¼ cup pastry flour
- 1 tablespoon Bragg's or salt

Put millet and water in a pot, bring to a boil, and cook on low heat for 30 minutes. In a bowl, mix together the chopped mushrooms, green beans, onions, parsley, Italian seasoning, lecithin, flour, and Bragg's. Add cooked millet, mix well, and pour into a well-oiled loaf pan. Bake at 350° for 10 minutes.

Optional: Sprinkle cheese on top before baking.

Oats

<u>Botanical Name: *Avena sativa, Avena fatua*</u>

Oats grow well in high altitudes such as China and Tibet, and readily grows in poor quality soil where other grains will not thrive. Oats have always assumed a role of importance as a staple item in Scotland. "Steel Cut Oats" are made from whole oats which have been passed through a steel blade, thereby cutting them into slices. "Old Fashioned Oats" are made by rolling steamed whole oats to produce flat flakes. "Quick Oats" are steamed oats which have been finely cut. Oats are very rich in minerals, perhaps more so than any other grain. An important British nutritionist proved, however, that due to the presence of phytic acid, oats have a tendency, if not compensated for by other foods rich in calcium and vitamin D, to rob the body of calcium and produce rickets. They should be used in the form of "old fashioned" rolled oats and soaked a couple of hours, or even overnight, before cooking. The soaking water is then discarded and replaced with fresh water before cooking.

Energy: Cool

Taste: Sweet

Post Digestive: Sweet

Indications: Chronic constipation, nerves, insomnia, muscle weakness, immune builder, mental clarity, excellent for children

Systems: All systems

Dosha Affected:

Vata: Excellent (best used with lots of spices)

Pitta: Moderation

Kapha: Avoid

Mixes Well With: All vegetables, starches, ghee, oil or butter

Oatmeal à la Bryan

- 1½ cups rolled oats
- ½ cup raisins
- 3 cups water
- 2 apples, diced
- 1 pear, diced
- 2 tablespoons cinnamon
- 2 tablespoons cardamom
- 1 tablespoon grated ginger
- ¼ teaspoon cloves, ground
- agave syrup to taste

Soak oatmeal and raisins overnight. The next morning, drain off water. Heat in pan with water, diced fruits, spices, and agave to taste.

Oatmeal Cookies

- 1 cup apple juice
- ½ cup dates, well chopped
- 1 cup rolled oats
- ¼ cup barley flour
- 1 large egg, beaten
- ½ teaspoon baking powder (aluminum-free)
- ¼ cup walnuts, chopped
- 2 tablespoons sucanat or jaggary
- ½ teaspoon nutmeg
- 1 teaspoon cinnamon
- ½ teaspoon fennel, ground
- ¼ teaspoon salt
- 1½ teaspoons vanilla extract
- ½ cup ghee

Soak dates in apple juice overnight (in refrigerator). Preheat oven to 375°. Drain apple juice off the dates and simmer until warm. In a bowl, mix dates, rolled oats, flour, egg, and baking powder. Add the warmed apple juice to this mixture, then add walnuts, sucanat, spices, salt, and vanilla. After oiling a large cookie sheet with ghee, add remaining ghee to the mixture. Roll dough into small balls, place on cookie sheet, and flatten slightly. Bake at 375° for 35 minutes.

Quinoa

Botanical Name: Chenopodium quinoa

This ancient food is pronounced keen-wah, and is the historic companion to the grain, amaranth. Quinoa is not actually a cereal grain, although it is treated as such – it is the seed of an herb in the goosefoot family (and related to chard, spinach, and lamb's quarters). Quinoa traditionally grows in South America and was the staple of the Inca Indians. Its cultivation was forbidden by the Spanish, because it was such an important part of Inca festivities. Today, this plant is grown in the high mountains of Colorado. The plant is harvested by hand, has seed clusters at the end of the stalk, does not need good soil, yet it thrives at high altitudes and with low rainfall. In today's natural food stores, quinoa is a great hit as a substitute for wheat. It is high in essential amino acids and very rich in minerals, particularly calcium. It has a distinctly nutty flavor with a light and fluffy texture. The Indians of Bolivia use the entire plant to make a fermented drink, called chichi, and eat the greens as a vegetable. The plant contains a natural insect repellent called saponin. This substance makes the seeds taste bitter and needs to be washed off before cooking. (Quinoa sold in boxes, however, has already been washed.)

Energy: Cooling

Taste: Bitter, Sweet

Post Digestive: Sweet

Indications: Good substitute for wheat allergies, osteoporosis, bone injuries, blood cleanser, arthritic joints and rheumatism

Systems: All systems

Dosha Affected:

Vata: Avoid

Pitta: Excellent

Kapha: Excellent

Mixes Well With: All fruits, all vegetables and legumes.

Quinoa Pasta with Broccoli and Seaweed

<u>Serves 6</u>

- 1 box quinoa pasta
- 1 bunch green onions, chopped
- 1-2 tablespoons ghee or olive oil
- 1 head broccoli, cut into small pieces
- 1 tablespoon dulse flakes
- ¼ cup cilantro
- ¼ cup parmesan, grated

Follow instructions on box to cook pasta; drain. Sauté onions in ghee or olive oil. Steam the broccoli. Pour onions over spaghetti. Add broccoli, dulse, cilantro, and grated cheese.

Saffron Quinoa

- 1 cup quinoa
- 2 cups water
- 1 tablespoon ghee
- 4-5 threads of saffron
- 1 teaspoon cardamom
- Bragg's

Wash quinoa well (best if soaked overnight). Put quinoa in pot with water and ghee, and bring to a boil. Add saffron and cardamom; lower heat and simmer until done, approximately 15 minutes. Add Bragg's to taste.

Rice

Botanical Name: Oryza sativa, Oryza glaberrima

Dependable information regarding the origin of rice is scarce. The earliest rice cultivation recorded is from China, around 2800 B.C. Every part of the plant is used. Rice straw is used for making paper, matting, sandals, brooms, hats, and numerous other useful articles. Hulls can be used for pillow stuffing. Rice is the most extensively cultivated of grains and the principal food of a significant portion of the world's population. In the commonly cultivated types, it must be kept flooded during the growing season and is, therefore, more easily raised on level lowlands. It can also be grown at higher elevations on terraces and mountainsides. Cultivation in the U. S. began in 1694 in Charleston, S. C. The industry developed steadily with significant production in Georgia and South Carolina prior to the Civil War.

The first process to which the rice is subjected produces the unpolished or "brown" rice, which is the best form. When modern methods refined this grain, however, nutritional diseases, such as beriberi, resulted wherever polished rice was introduced. The removal of the outer layers robs the rice of nutritious value as well as much of its flavor. This is a matter for serious consideration, particularly when the diet is also lacking in nutritional elements. Basmati rice is native of India, very flavorful, nutritious, and easy to digest. It is naturally white and has not been milled.

Energy: Neutral

Taste: Sweet

Post Digestive: Sweet

Indications: Vomiting, anorexia, aids digestion, blood tonic, builds all tissues, convalescence, assists all body functions, depression, thirst quenching, balances emotions, improves circulation

Systems: All systems

Dosha Affected:

Vata: Excellent – both brown and basmati

Pitta: Good – basmati; avoid short grain brown rice

Kapha: Good – basmati; reduce brown rice

Mixes Well With: All vegetables, legumes

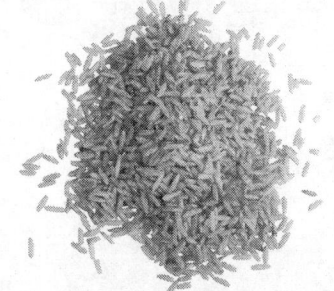

Saffron Rice

- 2 cups basmati rice
- ½ teaspoon saffron threads
- 2 tablespoons warm milk
- 1-inch piece cinnamon stick
- 4 whole cloves
- 4 cardamom pods, crushed lightly to break pods
- 1 tablespoon vegetable oil
- 3¼ cups water
- 1½ teaspoons salt
- 1/3 cup cashews (raw pieces) or almonds (blanched, slivered)
- 1/3 cup raisins (dark or golden)
- 1 tablespoon ghee

Rinse basmati by placing it in a large bowl, then fill bowl with water and drain it off repeatedly until water is no longer cloudy. Drain rice completely and set aside. In a small bowl soak saffron in warm milk for 10 minutes. In a 5- to 6-quart saucepan over medium-high heat, sauté cinnamon, cloves, and cardamom pods in oil for 1 to 2 minutes, until they release their fragrance. Add rice, soaked saffron (with milk), water, and salt, and bring to a full boil. Stir briefly to break up clumps. Turn heat down to low, cover tightly (weighing down lid if necessary), and simmer without removing lid for 20 minutes. Turn off heat and allow rice to sit with cover on for 10 minutes. Fluff up rice with a fork. In a small frying pan over medium heat, sauté nuts and raisins in ghee until nuts turn reddish brown. Stir thoroughly into rice and serve.

Rice Biriyani

- 1 recipe Saffron Rice (page 302)
- 1 head cauliflower, cut into small pieces
- 7 tablespoons ghee (divided)
- 2 large onions, sliced

Preheat oven to 350°. Prepare rice up to the point of preparing the nuts and raisins (golden raisins are prettiest for this dish). While rice is cooking, steam the cauliflower. In a large skillet over medium heat, melt 6 tablespoons of the ghee. Add onion and sauté until edges are golden brown; set aside. Brush bottom of Dutch oven or casserole with remaining 1 tablespoon of ghee, then layer these ingredients in the following order:

- cauliflower pieces
- half of cooked Saffron Rice
- cooking water from cauliflower spooned evenly over rice
- remaining rice
- sautéed onions spread in an even layer, plus 2 tablespoons of the ghee that onions were cooked in, sprinkled over the top.

Tightly seal top of Dutch oven or casserole with aluminum foil, then place lid over foil. Bake in preheated oven for 30 minutes. Meanwhile, sauté nuts and raisins as for Saffron Rice. When rice and cauliflower have baked for 30 minutes, carefully transfer to large serving platter, trying not to stir mixture too much. Garnish with sautéed nuts and raisins.

Ayurvedic Curative Cuisine for Everyone

Rice Pudding #1

- 2 cups water
- 1 cup basmati rice
- 5 cups coconut milk
- 2 cups agave or jaggary
- 1 teaspoon cardamom
- pinch of salt
- 1 teaspoon vanilla

Bring water to boil in medium saucepan. Add rice, cover and reduce heat to low and simmer until liquid is absorbed, about 18 minutes. Add coconut milk, sweetener, cardamom, and salt. Simmer uncovered over medium heat, stirring frequently until thickened, for about 20 minutes. Remove from heat and stir in vanilla. Serve warm or chilled.

Rice Pudding #2

- 1 cup rice
- ¼ cup date pieces
- ¼ cup raisins
- 3 cups coconut milk (divided)
- 3 cups water (divided)
- 2 tablespoons ghee
- ½ teaspoon grated ginger
- ¼ teaspoon saffron
- 2 teaspoons cardamom
- ½ teaspoon cinnamon
- 1 tablespoon agave (or maple syrup or honey)

Soak rice, dates, and raisins overnight in 2 cups of coconut milk plus 2 cups of water. Next day cook all ingredients by bringing to a boil. Add 1 more cup each of water and coconut milk. Add ghee, turn burner to low, and cook for another hour. Add spices, and let steep for 15 minutes. Add sweetener; serve.

Semolina

(made from durum wheat)

Semolina is made by coarsely grinding hard (durum) wheat. It is made from the endosperm left on the bottom of the sifting machine after the finer particles have passed through into a flour. It is the protein matter of wheat and makes excellent flour. This by-product is easier to digest than wheat or corn, and is the preferred flour for making pasta. It is also used to make couscous granules.

Energy: Cooling

Taste: Sweet

Post Digestive: Sweet

Indications: Wheat allergies, substitute for wheat, kidney tonic, convalescence (also refer to wheat)

Systems: Same as Wheat

Dosha Affected:
Good for all doshas

Mixes Well With: Starches, vegetables

Pasta Primavera

Serves 4

- 2 heads of broccoli flowers and leaves, cut into small pieces
- 1 box semolina spaghetti
- 4 cups water
- 2 tablespoons olive oil (divided)
- ½ cup green onions, well chopped
- 1 cup grated carrots
- 1 tablespoon Italian seasoning
- 1 cup spaghetti sauce
- ½ cup cilantro, chopped
- ½ cup parsley

Steam broccoli. In a large pot, boil spaghetti noodles in water with 1 tablespoon of the oil. Sauté onions and carrots in the remaining tablespoon of oil. Add Italian seasoning and broccoli. Drain noodles, and add to vegetables with spaghetti sauce. Add cilantro and remove from heat.

Couscous

- 1 tablespoon cumin seeds
- 2 tablespoons ghee
- 1 bunch green onions, well chopped
- 5 stalks celery, well chopped
- ½ green pepper, well chopped
- 1 cup peas, cooked
- 1 cup carrots, grated
- 1 teaspoon curry powder
- 1 teaspoon coriander
- ½ cup almonds, sliced (optional)
- 2½ cups boiling water
- 2 cups couscous
- ½ cup cilantro, well chopped
- ½ cup parsley, well chopped

Roast cumin seeds in skillet; add ghee, and sauté onions, celery, and peppers. When soft, add peas, carrots, curry, coriander, and almonds. Cover and simmer for 10 minutes; then add cilantro and parsley. Add boiling water to couscous, and let stand for 10 minutes. Mix couscous into vegetable mixture until evenly blended.

Spelt

<u>Botanical Name: *Triticum spelta*</u>

Spelt is a variety of wheat native to the Mediterranean Sea. Spelt wheat was the staff of life for Ancient Europe. The Roman Legionnaires marched with a pouch of spelt on their sides and conquered most of the known world. It is a high gluten wheat, ancestor to the modern wheat. Spelt is used as an alternative for those who are allergic to wheat. This grain is not suited to people who are sensitive to gluten.

Energy: Warming
Taste: Sweet
Post Digestive: Sweet
Indications: Same as wheat
Systems: All systems

<u>**Dosha Affected:**</u>
Vata: Good
Pitta: Moderation
Kapha: Good
Mixes Well With: All vegetables

Macaroni à la Seaweed

- 1 box spelt macaroni
- 3 cups water
- 1 tablespoon olive oil (divided)
- 1 cup dulse flakes
- ½ cup parsley, well chopped
- ½ cup parmesan cheese, grated

In a medium saucepan, put macaroni, water, and ½ tablespoon of olive oil; bring to a boil. Cook until macaroni is soft, then drain water. Add the remaining ½ tablespoon. of olive oil, mix in dulse and parsley. Sprinkle cheese over all.

Spelt Berry Muffins

- 1½ cups spelt flour
- 1 egg
- 1 cup blueberries or raspberries
- ½ cup almond milk
- 2 tablespoons baking soda
- 1 teaspoon cinnamon
- ½ cup raw sugar
- 1 teaspoon vanilla
- ¼ cup ghee

Mix eggs, milk, ghee, and sugar. Add the flour, baking soda and mix. Slowly fold in blueberries or raspberries. Mix together and add cinnamon and vanilla. Oil cup cake pan and using cup cake papers, fill each with batter. Preheat at 400. Bake for approximately 40 minutes – or until toothpick comes out clean.

Wheat

Botanical Name: Triticum aestivum

There is much uncertainty as to the origin of wheat, but the final conclusion seems to be that, at the dawn of history, it was indigenous to western Asia. The most ancient names for wheat are: summana and hodhuma (Sanskrit); mai (Chinese); chittah (Hebrew). It is grown in all regions where the average yearly rainfall is no more than thirty inches. In the U.S., it is perhaps the best known and most widely used grain. Unfortunately, white flour is highly processed with many nutrients destroyed. Diabetics have been advised that gluten flour is beneficial for them because of the elimination of carbohydrate elements. Contrary to this belief, it is detrimental to diabetics, because most of the alkaline elements are removed in the manufacturing process. Wheat is the most acid-forming of the grains and should be used in its whole grain form.

Energy: Warming

Taste: Sweet

Post Digestive: Sweet

Indications: Anorexia, heart tonic, insomnia, ulcer, colitis, diarrhea, bleeding disorders, nerve disorders, increases muscle mass

Systems: Circulatory, Nervous, Digestive, Excretory, Muscular

Dosha Affected:

Vata: Good

Pitta: Moderation

Kapha: Avoid (mucous forming)

Mixes Well With: Non-starchy vegetables

Sooji Halva
Serves 8

- 1/3 cup dark raisins, soaked overnight
- 1/3 cup cashews (raw pieces)
- 1 teaspoon ghee
- 1½ cups water
- 1 cup cream of wheat cereal
- ¼ cup ghee
- 1 cup sucanat or jaggary
- 1/8 teaspoon cardamom

Lightly butter an 8-inch square cake pan with ghee. In skillet over medium heat, sauté raisins and cashews in 1 teaspoon of ghee until lightly golden; set aside. Bring water to a boil; set aside. In wok or skillet, combine cream of wheat and ¼ cup of ghee. Stir constantly over medium-high heat until light brown spots start to appear. Add hot water and stir, preferably with a wire whisk. When water is mostly absorbed, add sucanat, cardamom, raisins and cashews. Continue stirring over medium heat for 1 minute or until mixture becomes semi-solid. Transfer mixture to buttered pan, pressing lightly to a thickness of 1 inch. Cut into 25 squares or diamond shapes. Serve warm or at room temperature.

Pancakes à la Bryan
Serves 2

- 1 cup whole wheat flour
- 1¼ teaspoons baking powder
- ½ teaspoon coriander
- ½ teaspoon cinnamon
- 1 teaspoon ginger, ground
- 2 eggs
- 1 tablespoon ghee, butter, or oil
- 1 teaspoon honey, agave, maple or rice syrup
- 1 teaspoon vanilla extract
- fruit or berries, diced (mango, apple, pineapple, kiwi, papaya, raisins)
- water or milk as needed

Mix dry ingredients together in a bowl. Beat eggs, add ghee, sweetener, and vanilla, then pour into dry ingredients and mix well. Add diced fruit, then add enough water or milk to thin batter to desired consistency. Ladle onto hot skillet or griddle to form pancakes.

Wild Rice

Botanical Name: Zizania palustris, Zizania aquatica

Though belonging to a different botanical group than regular rice, wild rice is similar in appearance. It contains twice as much protein as white polished rice, four times as much phosphorous, eight times as much thiamin, and twenty times as much riboflavin. This grain has a long slender hull, which greatly resembles that of oats except that it is longer and darker. It is a tall, tubular, reedy, and aquatic plant which springs up from six or seven feet in depth and rises to nearly the same distance above the water.

Called by the Ojibway Indians, mahnomen, wild rice is found in the greatest abundance on the marshy margins of the northern lakes and waters of the upper branches of the Mississippi.

Energy: Cooling

Taste: Sweet

Post Digestive: Sweet

Indications: Malnutrition, vomiting, debility, brings harmony to stomach and lungs

Systems: All systems

Dosha Affected:
Good for all Doshas

Mixes Well With: Non-starchy vegetables

Ayurvedic Curative Cuisine for Everyone

Poultry

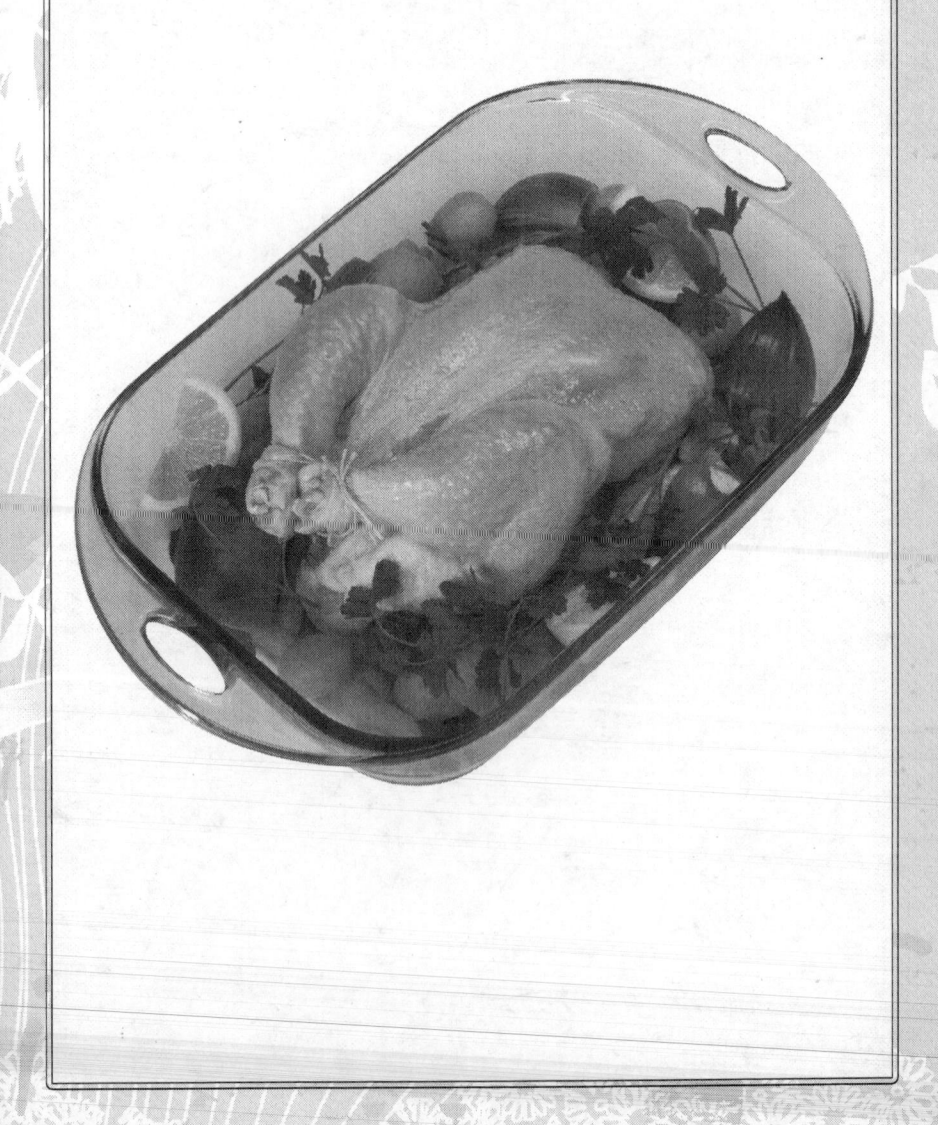

Poultry

General Considerations

The term "poultry" comes from the Latin word pulla, meaning a young female animal, and refers to all domestic fowl (duck, turkey, hens, chickens, pigeons, goose, guinea hens, and fowl). In cooking, the term refers generally to the flesh of the chicken hen. It is important to consider the risk of salmonella poisoning when preparing poultry, as it is a bacteria that annually produces illness in many people. When purchasing poultry, make sure that it is fresh and then refrigerate it immediately. Do not keep more than a day without freezing or cooking it. Testing indicates that as much as 60% of all chicken is contaminated due to processing methods using recycled water and mechanical processes that spread fecal bacteria.

Chicken

Energy: Warming

Taste: Sweet

Post Digestive: Sweet

Indications: Cold, flu, long term illnesses (in soup), immune builder

Systems: Respiratory

Dosha Affected:

Vata: Good

Pitta: Moderation (white meat best)

Kapha: Moderation (dark meat best)

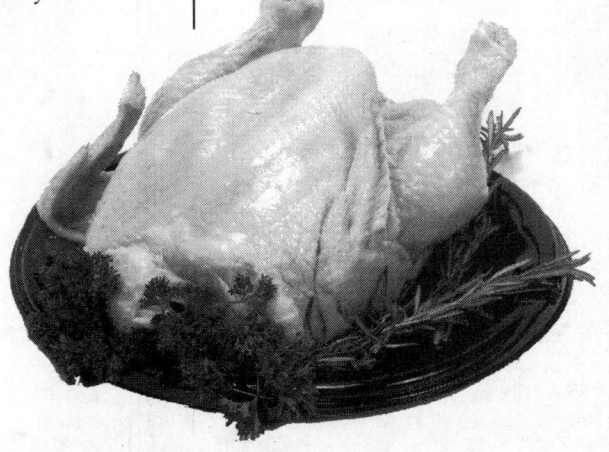

Ayurvedic Curative Cuisine for Everyone

Lemon Curry Chicken

Serves 4

- 2 chicken breasts, cut into cubes
- 2 tablespoons lemon juice
- 1 sweet onion, sliced into rings
- 1 tablespoon ghee
- ¼ cup water
- 2 tablespoons mild curry or pita churna
- 1 tablespoon Bragg's or salt
- ¼ cup cilantro, chopped

Marinate chicken cubes in lemon juice for one hour. Sauté onion rings in ghee until caramelized, on low to medium heat. Strain chicken cubes and set lemon juice aside. Add chicken and water to onions; cover and cook for 15 minutes, stirring occasionally. Then add curry, lemon juice marinade, and Bragg's; continue cooking uncovered for 5 minutes. Mix in chopped cilantro just before serving.

Serve with vegetables or salad.

Curry Chicken Salad

Serves 6

- 2 chicken breasts, organic best
- 1 cup celery, chopped
- ½ cup carrots, grated
- 1 cup green onions, chopped
- ½ cup fennel stalk, well chopped
- 4 tablespoons mayonnaise
- 2 tablespoons mild curry or Vata, Pitta, or Kapha churna
- 1 tablespoons vegetable oil
- ¼ cup water

Cut chicken into small cubes. Place in skillet with olive oil and water. Cover. Cook until tender at low heat. Remove chicken from heat and let cool. In a large bowl mix remaining ingredients together with mayonnaise. Stir well. Serve on lettuce leaves and roll up like a burrito or as a side dish.

Turkey

Native to North America, turkeys were introduced to Europe by the Spanish. During a certain period in Europe, it was only served at royal tables. This meat is high in tryptophan, a natural amino acid.

Energy: Warming

Taste: Sweet

Post Digestive: Sweet

Indications: Nervous disorders, headache, convalescence, cold, flu, antidepressant, promotes sleep

Systems: Nervous

Dosha Affected:
 Vata: Good
 Pitta: Moderation (white meat)
 Kapha: Moderation (dark meat)

Mixes Well With: Green leafy vegetables.

Turkey Loaf

<u>Serves 6</u>

- 1 lb. ground turkey
- ½ bunch green onions, chopped
- 2½ tablespoons breadcrumbs
- 2 eggs, well beaten
- 2 tablespoons Italian seasoning
- 1½ tablespoons Bragg's or salt

Preheat oven to 350°. In a bowl, mix ground turkey with chopped onion, then mix in breadcrumbs, eggs, Italian seasoning, and Bragg's. Shape the mixture into a loaf (or place in loaf pan). Bake for 30 minutes, drizzling the liquid from the pan over the meat several times. Cook for 20 more minutes (or until done).

Serve with salad.

Turkey Wraps

- 24 wraps of spelt or wheat
- 8 oz spinach leaves, fresh
- 8 oz turkey slices
- 8 oz cream cheese
- 1 cup cilantro, well chopped
- 3 tablespoons mayonnaise

Soften cream cheese. Mix cilantro & cream cheese together. Apply mayonnaise on each wrap to cover with thin layer. Then spread cream cheese on each wrap. Place turkey slices on top of cream cheese. Place spinach Leaves on top of turkey. Roll tightly and place on platter. Cut wrap in sections. Serve with salads or as an appetizer.

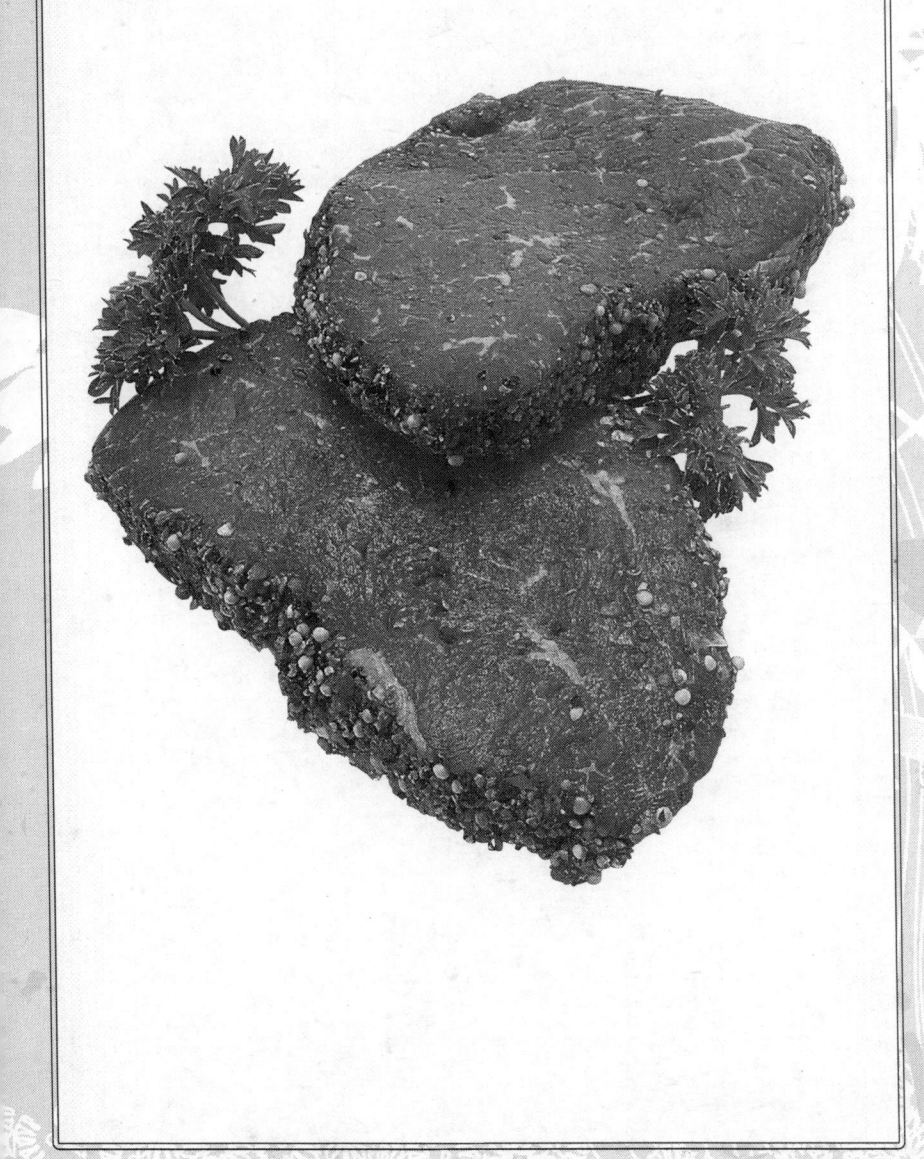

Meat

Meat

General Considerations

In the Ayurvedic system, meat is found to be Tamasic due to the fact that it comes from a dead animal, which creates a dulling effect on the mind and can reduce all Sattvic awareness. Many avoid meat because of the karmic implications and for religious reasons. Also, pesticides and herbicides in the food chain are concentrated many times higher in flesh than in natural plant sources. It is best to buy organic meat from health food stores when there is a need or desire to eat meat. Additionally, commercial animal practices utilize hormones to speed growth and antibiotics to offset crowding and unsanitary conditions.

Yet, meat is the highest source of nourishment or strengthening, especially in a broth form. It can be used as a medicine when needed. Unfortunately, meat has many disadvantages associated with it, such as feeding fevers, infections, and tumors. In large amounts, meat creates Ama. If eating meat becomes a regular habit, then it is best to raise animals and kill them yourself.

Meats are also harder to digest than other foods and must be cooked well with lots of spices in order to assist the breakdown and assimilation process. Always cook meat well – never eat it raw. Broiled, steamed, or cooked in broth is best.

Meat is best for Eskimos and for people who live in northern and/or mountainous climates, or those who have a genetic background for a high meat diet.

Ayurveda does not historically recommend meat except for medicinal purposes. Meats are one of the highest forms of protein, increasing Pitta and Kapha. When cooking, it should be charcoal-broiled. steamed, or in soup. Meat should be well cooked with the use of spices beneficial for digestion. It can be strong medicine for rebuilding a weakened individual. An older principle of healing believes that people who have heart problems should eat the heart, etc. The animal's organs contain nutrients that our organs also need.

Beef

The word beef refers to meat from heifers, cows, bulls, calves, and steers. Beef was one of the first animals domesticated. Approximately 4,000 years ago, it was used in Macedonia, Crete, and Australia. In India and parts of Africa, the cow is considered sacred. In many countries, beef is a symbol of prosperity. Today, there are several hundred species of cattle. Do not eat with starches or milk products. When beef is needed in a diet, make sure the meat is organic.

Energy: Warming

Taste: Sweet

Post Digestive: Sweet

Indications: Strengthens muscle tissue and bones

Systems: Muscular, Skeletal

Dosha Affected:

Vata: Good

Pitta and **Kapha**: Avoid or reduce

Mixes Well With: Green leafy vegetables

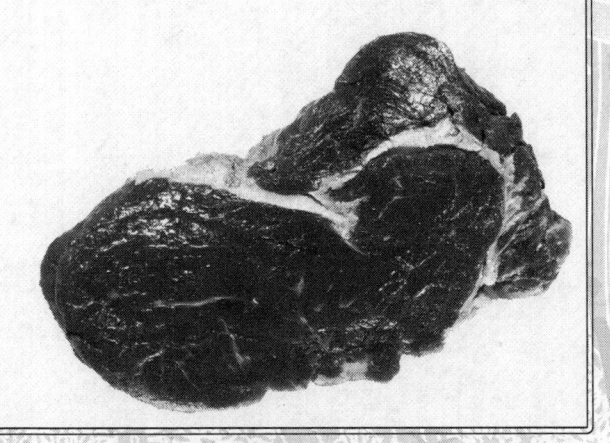

Ayurvedic Curative Cuisine for Everyone

Beef Stew

Serves 6

- 2 onions, well chopped
- 2 cloves garlic, well chopped
- 2 tablespoons ghee
- 2 lbs. beef chunks
- 2 tomatoes, well chopped
- 6 large leaves and stems of kale, well chopped
- 1 teaspoon sage
- 1 teaspoon thyme

Sauté onions and garlic in ghee for 5 minutes. Add the beef, cover pan, cook for 10 minutes. Add tomatoes, kale, and herbs. Serve with salad.

Bodhie's Beef Scallopini with Madeira Wine Demi-glace

- 1 lb. beef
- ½ cup flour
- salt and pepper
- 1 tablespoon ghee

Select desired cut of beef, then pound out thin. Take flour (all-purpose) and season with salt and pepper. Pan-sear in ghee until desired temperature. Make sauce:

Sauce:

- 1 cup madeira wine
- 2 shallots, diced
- 1 clove garlic, chopped
- any fresh herb added for flavor

Into saucepan put wine, shallots, and garlic, simmer and reduce, then add to demi-glace (see page 328).

Pour sauce over beef.

Lamb and Goat

Sheep were first domesticated in Iran 13,000 years ago and have long played an important economic role in many societies. The young lambs are slaughtered up to 12 months of age, and the meat is usually tender. The fat solidifies in cold air and, for this reason, should be served right away. Meat from lambs has a religious symbolism; the flesh was offered in favor to the deities of certain religions. In Ayurveda, this is the only meat which is considered Sattvic. Goat meat is similar to lamb, but less fatty. Goats are tree and bush feeders, like deer.

Energy: Heating

Taste: Sweet

Post Digestive: Sweet

Indications: Energy builder, strengthens all tissues

Systems: All systems

Dosha Affected:

Vata: Best

Pitta and **Kapha**: Small amounts

Mixes Well With: Mints, ginger and all green vegetables

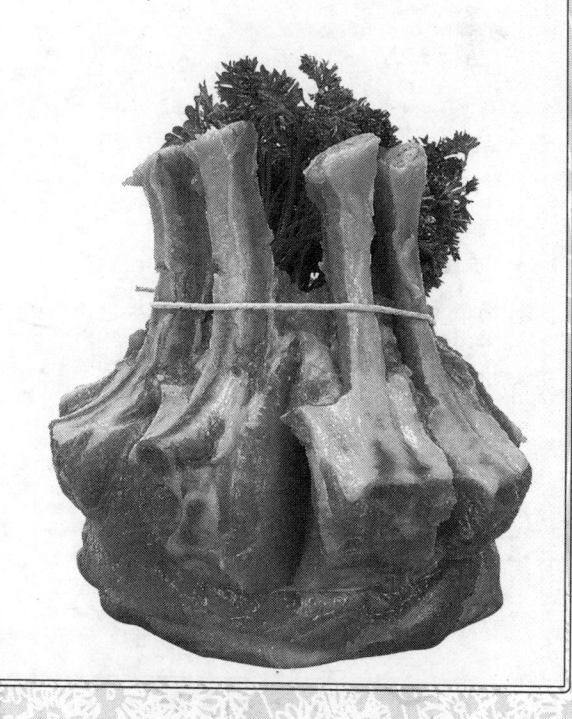

Bodhie's Tuscan Lamb Chops

- 2 cups organic fig balsamic vinegar
- 1 cup red wine (merlot)
- 1 sprig rosemary
- fresh-ground black pepper to taste
- 4 lamb chops

Combine vinegar, wine, rosemary, and pepper. Marinate chops in this mixture for up to 4 hours. Grill or pan-sear. Serve with merlot lamb demi-glace (see page 320). Plate and serve.

Lamb Marsala

Serves 4

- 1 pound lamb, cubes
- 2 tablespoons ghee or vegetable oil
- 1 onion, chopped
- 1 green chili, chopped
- 1 tablespoon cumin seeds
- ½ tablespoon turmeric
- 1 tablespoon coriander powder
- 1 tablespoon ajwan seeds
- 1 cup curry leaves or cilantro, fresh
- 1 cup water

Roast cumin seeds, ajwan seeds, coriander and turmeric in skillet for 3-4 minutes. Add the oil and onions and sauté until soft. Add meat, lower heat, add water, and cover. Cook for 10-15 minutes and mix together. When meat is tender, add chopped curry leaves or cilantro. Serve with salad.

Pork

Historians once thought that the pig was directly descended from the boar, which had more prominent teeth. Male pigs today are referred to as boars. Pigs are easier to breed than other animals, because they eat anything. Pigs are valued because of their fat. The Jewish and Muslim have dietary restrictions regarding pork that are thought to have been adopted because of the pig's feeding habits. The ancients believed that eating pork speeded up leprosy and many illnesses of those times. Pork is higher in the B-complex nutrients than other meats and is also rich in zinc and potassium. Pork is very high in fat. In Ayurveda, pork is considered to be highly Tamasic creating dullness and heaviness.

Energy: Cooling

Taste: Sweet

Post Digestive: Sweet

Indications: Liver nourishment, to gain weight

Systems: Endocrine

Dosha Affected:

Vata and **Pitta**: Moderation

Kapha: Avoid

Mixes Well With: Green leafy vegetables

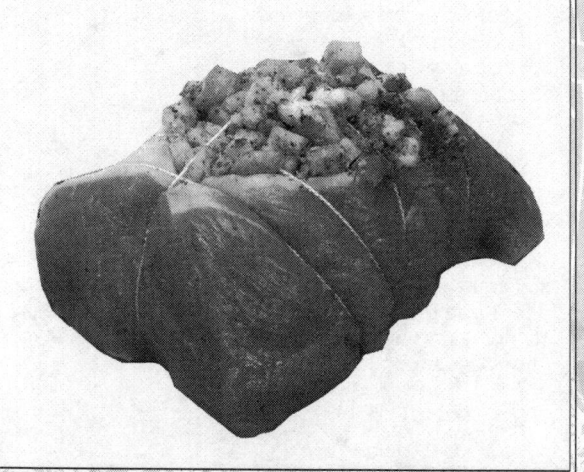

Bodhie's Prosciutto-wrapped Apricot-stuffed Pork Tenderloin

served with a sherry demi-glace – see page 328

6 ounces dried apricots, chopped
4 ounces pecans, chopped
2 ounces breadcrumbs
1 egg
2 lb. pork loin
1 teaspoon ground Schezwan peppercorns
1 teaspoon black pepper
1 teaspoon cumin, ground
1 egg
¼ lb. prosciutto

Combine apricots, pecans, bread-crumbs and egg until moist enough to form. Set this stuffing aside.

Prepare pork tenderloin: Slice pork loin vertically, and fan open. Then pound thin – the thinner the pork, the faster the cooking time. Season loin with dry spice mixture of ground peppers and cumin. Place stuffing on flattened meat, and roll from top to bottom; chill. Tie prosciutto around the loin with string. Sear until desired color, then finish in 350° oven until desired temperature.

Mint Cilantro Pork Chops

Serves 6

6 pork shops
1 cup mint, fresh, chopped
1 cup cilantro, fresh, chopped
1 clove garlic, crushed
3 tablespoons lemon or lime juice
2 teaspoons coriander powder
1 teaspoon turmeric powder
1 tablespoon coconut aminos
1 teaspoon cumin powder
1 tablespoon ghee

Mix lemon, turmeric, coriander, and garlic together with coconut aminos (non soy aminos) and ghee. Then marinate pork chops for 3 hours. Preheat oven at 325. Place marinated pork chops in baking dish. Bake for 30 minutes – or until tender – do not overcook. Sprinkle green onions, mint, and cilantro on each chop. Cook for another 10 to 15 minutes.

Rabbit

This animal is thought to have originated in southern Europe and North Africa. In Australia, where the rabbit was introduced as a domestic animal during the 19th century, there are now approximately 300 million wild rabbits. The female rabbit begins reproducing at the age of 4 or 5 months and gives birth to an average of 8 to 9 offspring at a time. Domestic doe rabbits can give birth to over 100 offspring. Rabbits are so prolific that they have become a symbol of fertility. This animal is related to the hare, a wild species regarded as game, which has darker, stronger tasting flesh. The wild rabbit, which is probably the ancestor of the domestic rabbit, has lean, dark flesh with a gamy flavor. Meat from domestic rabbits resembles chicken.

Energy: Warming
Taste: Sweet
Post Digestive: Sweet

Dosha Affected:
Vata: Plus
Pitta: Minus
Kapha: Minus
Mixes Well With: Green, non-starchy vegetables

Rabbit ala Fricassee – (Stew)

Serves 4

1 full rabbit, cut into 6 pieces (best to buy at Halal Meat Market because meat is blessed with prayers)
2 tablespoons olive oil
2 tablespoons crushed garlic
1 onion, well chopped
1 red pepper, chopped
1 cup tomato sauce
1 tablespoon marjoram
1 tablespoon rosemary
6 bay leaves, whole (remove when serving)
1 tablespoon thyme
2 tablespoons liquid aminos

Veal

This is meat from a calf less than one year old, although they are generally killed when between 4 and 6 months old. These young animals are kept in cages to keep the meat tender and away from the sun. This appears to be the cruelest form of animal treatment, making it karmically darkened. Most animals used for veal are males as they keep the females for dairy cows. The origin of veal came from the Romans and is still a very popular food in Italy. Eating veal is considered a symbol of wealth.

Veal Parmesan

Serves 4

- 1 ½ pounds veal cutlets, about six cutlets
- 2 eggs, well beaten
- 1 cup spaghetti sauce
- 1 tablespoon Italian seasoning
- 1 tablespoon fresh basil, chopped
- 1 cup green onions, chopped
- 1 cup bread crumbs
- 1 tablespoon olive oil
- ½ pound parmesan cheese in thin slices

In a bowl, mix eggs adding one teaspoon Italian seasoning. In another bowl, add bread crumbs and the other teaspoon of Italian seasoning. Then dip one cutlet at a time into the egg mixture, then dip into the breadcrumbs. Do both sides. Oil a baking pan and place cutlets in pan. Cook for 20 minutes at 350. Then blend the basil into the spaghetti sauce and pour over the cutlets. Add sliced Parmesan cheese. Cook until cheese is melted.

Venison

This meat is the flesh from any kind of deer. The Greeks first introduced deer hunting. The Romans and Gauls took pleasure in the sport as well, while the French kings and noblemen reserved hunting privileges for themselves. Today, hunting is subject to various state regulations designed to promote a measure of protection for animal populations. The flavor of venison depends on the animal's diet. Meat from a young deer is better than that of an older animal. If one eats meat, this is a better meat to consume. Deer have not been domesticated, therefore, there are no chemical additives in their diet. In areas where there is an over population, they need to be hunted to prevent them from dying of starvation.

Energy: Warming

Taste: Sweet

Post Digestive: Sweet

Indications: Hormonal stimulant, kidney tonic, fertility, child retardation

Systems: Endocrine, Urinary, Reproductive

Dosha Affected:

Vata: Good

Pitta and **Kapha**: Moderation

Mixes Well With: Green vegetables, non-starchy vegetables

Marinated Venison

- ½ cup lemon juice
- 2 cloves garlic, finely chopped
- 1 onion, well chopped
- 1 tablespoon Bragg's
- ¼ cup grated ginger
- 1 teaspoon turmeric
- 1 tablespoon mild curry powder
- 2 lbs venison, cut in chunks
- 1 bunch parsley, chopped

Mix lemon juice, garlic, onion, Bragg's, and all spices in a large bowl. Add meat, and marinate overnight. The next day, put meat and marinade in baking dish, and bake, covered, at 350° for 1 hour. Add parsley and serve.

Bohdi's Demi-Glace

Roast veal, lamb, or venison bones with mirepoix (onions, carrots, and celery), bay leaf, black pepper, and 6 cups water. Reduce by simmering for 48 hours.

Fish

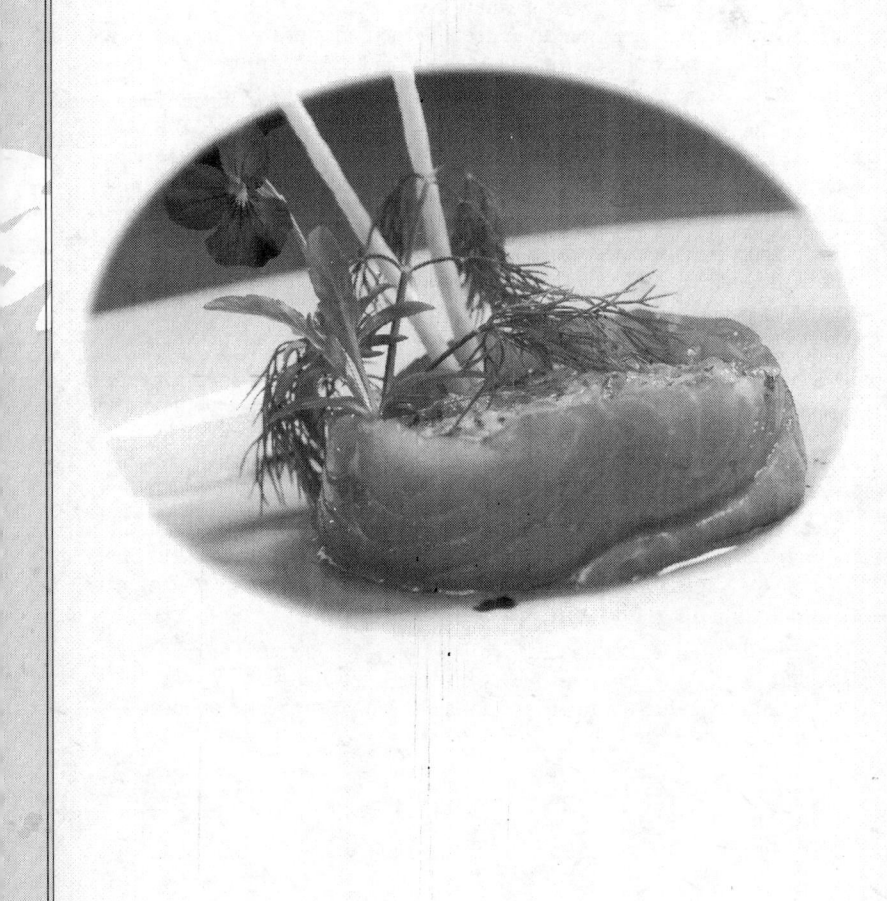

Fish

General Considerations

Fish are vertebrate animals that live in water. They have always been a staple of the human diet, especially among people of the coastal regions. At one time, fish were an abundant resource. The various species are slowly disappearing, however, due to polluted waters and over-fishing precipitated by the development of industrial fishing techniques.

Fish farming is expanding rapidly, and it has compensated for the decline of fish in nature. Although fish farming has existed for over 4,000 years, it initially involved nothing more than keeping them in captivity. They were not bred until 1733 when the Germans succeeded in breeding trout.

White meat fish are less fatty than either red meat or blue skinned varieties and may be used more frequently. The fat in fish is mainly omega-3 polyunsaturated fatty acid. Numerous studies show that polyunsaturated fatty acids have a beneficial impact on health. In Ayurveda, fish is considered less Tamasic than meat and not as dulling or as grounding as other flesh products.

Today, contaminated or toxic fish is abundant, so one must be careful when purchasing fish or even when fishing. Generally, deep ocean fish are preferable to fresh water fish that absorb more pollutants in the food chain. Many tropical fish contain a poison called ciguatera, which could cause liver damage and death.

When cooking fish, they are best when baked, broiled, or steamed, as well as slightly cooking them in ghee. Avoid canned fish; whenever possible, eat it fresh. Always cook with spices such as ginger, garlic, onions, mustard, mints, tarragon, coriander, cilantro, chives, and horseradish.

Ocean fish is better for Vata because of the salty taste, minerals, high iodine content, and warming nature. Fresh water fish is best for Pitta and has less minerals for Kapha. Pitta should avoid sour sauces. Appropriate spicing can assist digestion (i.e. pungent for Kapha; cooling for Pitta).

In general, fish does not go with dairy or fruit (except lemon juice). Treated as a pure protein, it combines best with green and non-starchy vegetables. Many cultures eat fish with rice, and for those with a strong metabolism, this combination is tolerated.

Tips for Buying Fish

(This criteria will vary depending on whether the fish is whole fresh, fresh pieces, frozen, salted, or smoked.)

- Gills should be moist and bright red.
- Eyes should be full, shiny, and slightly protruding.
- Skin should be shiny, iridescent, tight, and firmly attached to the flesh.
- The elastic, unmarked flesh should spring back when pressed and should not fall away easily from the bones.
- The shiny, intact scales should adhere firmly to the skin.
- Belly should not be swollen or faded, and the fish should have a mild, pleasant smell (a strong, fishy odor indicates that it is less than fresh).
- A muddy odor does not indicate that the fish is no longer fresh, but rather that the fish was caught in muddy waters.

Fresh Fish (fillets, steaks, or pieces)

- It should have firm, shiny, elastic flesh that has a pleasant odor and is firmly attached to the bones. It should not be brownish, yellowish, or dry.

Frozen Fish

- The fresh, firm, and shiny flesh should not show any traces of dryness or freezer burn; it should also be thoroughly frozen and wrapped in airtight, intact packaging that contains no frost or ice crystals.

Salted Fish

(Good for Vata; bad for Kapha & Pitta)

- The flesh should be an attractive color, have a pleasant odor, and should not be dried out.

Smoked Fish

(Good for Vata)

* The flesh should have a pleasant odor and should retain its juices.

* Note: U.S. regulations require that defrosted fish be clearly labeled as such. Freezing slightly alters the taste and texture. Fish should be eaten as soon as possible after it is defrosted and should never be refrozen until after it has been cooked.

Ayurvedic Curative Cuisine for Everyone

Cooking with Fish

Breaded Fish

- 1 cup breadcrumbs
- 1 teaspoon cumin, ground
- 1 teaspoon paprika
- ½ teaspoon coriander
- 1 teaspoon salt
- 1 teaspoon black pepper
- oil
- 2 fillets of fish (¼ inch thick)

Mix all spices with breadcrumbs. Dip fish into mixture, covering both sides by pressing into the mixture firmly. Sauté in oil of your choice, for 2 minutes per side. Do not overcook – fish is done when a fork goes all the way to the bottom of the pan.

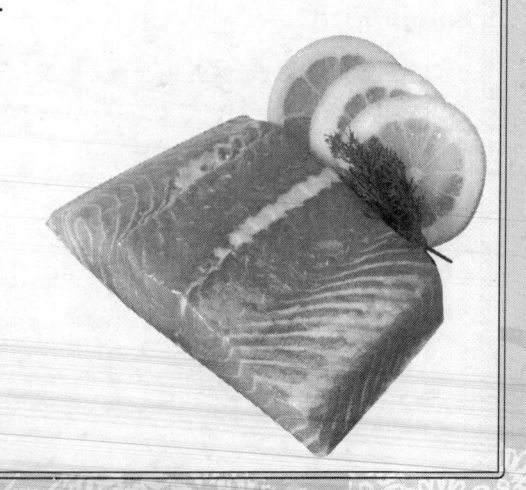

Curry Fish

Serves 4

- 1 cup breadcrumbs
- 2 tablespoons curry powder
- 1 teaspoon coriander
- 1-2 tablespoons ghee
- ¼ teaspoon salt

Mix curry powder, coriander, and bread crumbs in a plate. Press each fish filet into mixture, turning to coat both sides. Cook in ghee. When the fish turns white, cook on the other side. Pierce the fish with a fork and when it goes all the way to the bottom the fish is done.

Baked Salmon

- 4 fillets of salmon
- 1 tablespoon ghee
- ½ bunch dill weed, chopped – or ginger
- ¼ teaspoon black pepper, freshly ground
- ¼ teaspoon salt

Baste salmon with ghee, top with dill. Bake in oven at 250° for 15 minutes.

Fish Caldo (Broth)

Serves 4

- 2 fish heads
- 8 cups water
- 2 onions, large, sliced
- 2 cups carrots, sliced
- 2 cloves garlic
- 6 bay leaves
- ¼ cup ginger
- 1 tablespoons coriander
- 1 tablespoons cumin seeds
- 1 tablespoons ajwan seeds
- 2 tablespoons aminos

In a large covered pot add all ingredients and cook for 30 minutes on medium heat. Then simmer on low for another 15 minutes. Strain the vegetable and fish head out. Serve. Garnish with well chopped parsley.

Shellfish

Ayurveda does not recommend the use of crabs, oysters and shrimp, because they are scavengers. They are very Tamasic in nature. Clams, abalone, and scallops are okay.

Energy: Warming

Taste: Sweet

Post Digestive: Sweet

Indications: Production of semen, kidney tonic, impotence

Systems: Reproductive, Urinary

<u>Dosha Affected:</u>

Vata: Good

Pitta and **Kapha**: Moderation

Mixes Well With: Vegetables

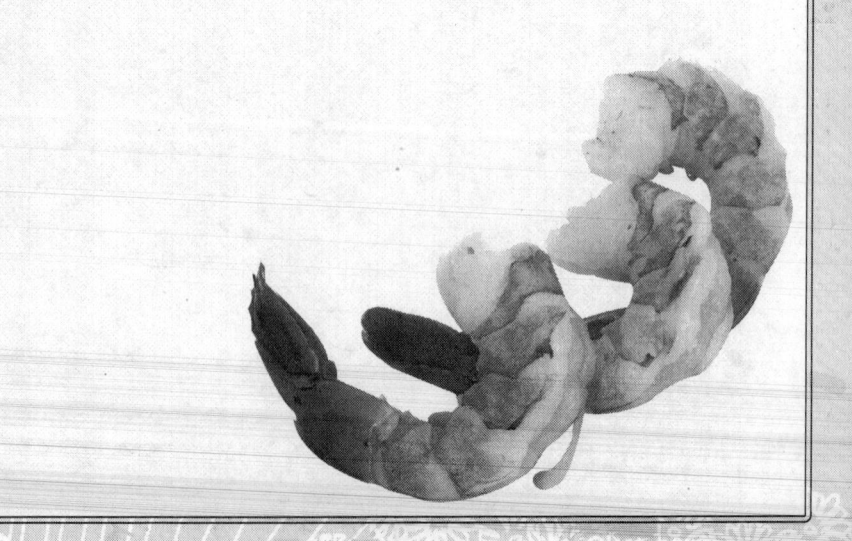

Shrimp Salad

- 1 lb. shelled shrimp, cut in half
- 4 celery stalks, well chopped
- 2 tablespoons eggless mayonnaise (see page 345)
- ½ teaspoon sage
- ½ teaspoon bay leaves, ground
- ½ teaspoon coriander
- ½ green onion, well chopped
- ½ teaspoon garam masala

Cook shrimp by putting in boiling water for 2 minutes; drain and chop. Put all ingredients in a bowl, mix well. Serve with green salad or vegetables.

Shrimp Salad & Peppers

Serves 4

- 1 pound shrimp, cooked
- 2 tablespoons vegan mayonnaise (page 345)
- ½ cup green onions, chopped
- 1 cup yellow or red peppers, chopped
- 1 cup cilantro, well chopped
- 1 tablespoon Vata, Pitta, or Kapha churna

Place all ingredients in bowl. Mix. Serve with sandwiches, crackers, or as a side dish.

Ayurvedic Curative Cuisine for Everyone

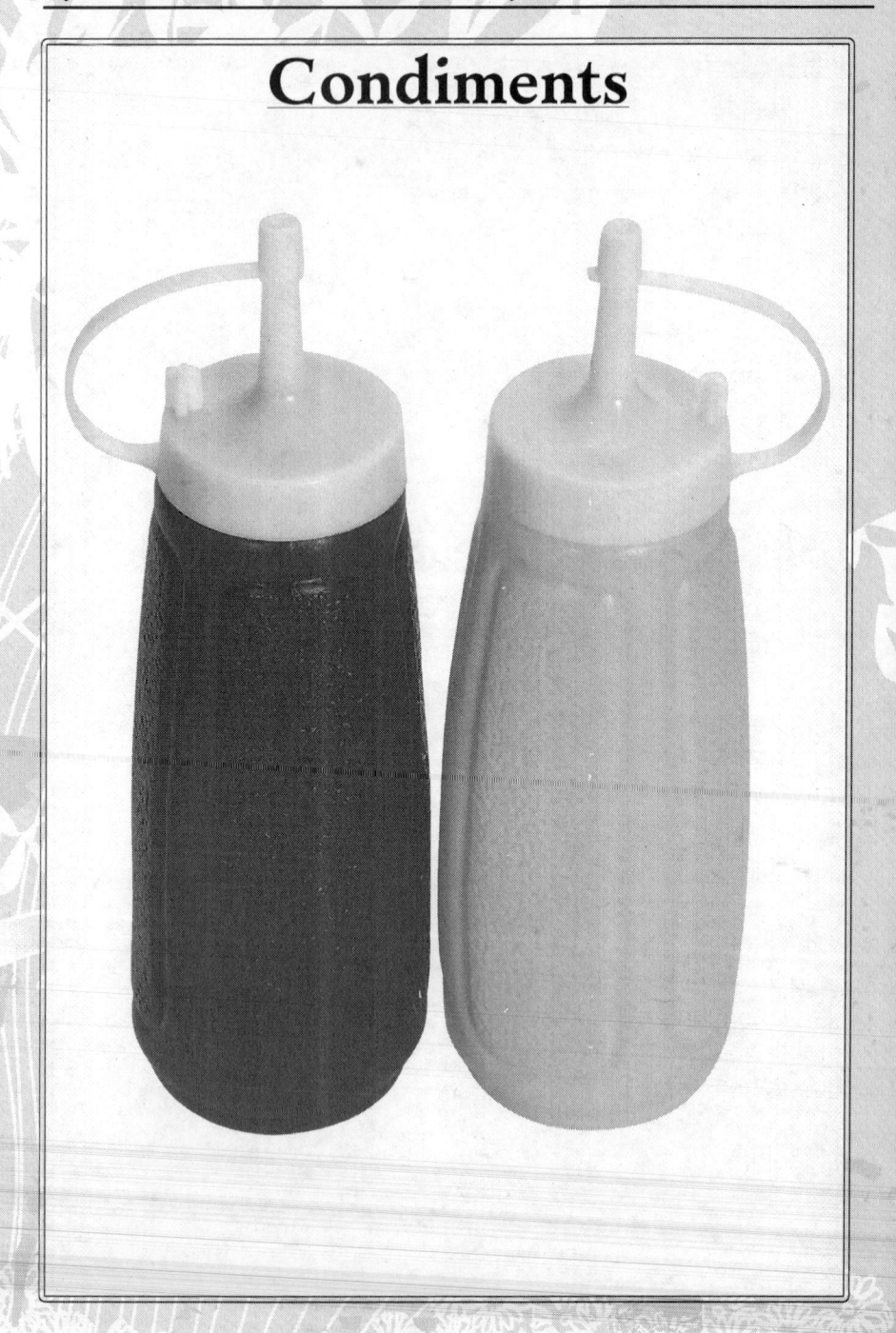

Condiments

Condiments

Baking Powder

Baking powder was perfected toward the end of the 19th Century, shortly after the invention of baking soda. A form of baking powder was used in the U.S. around 1790, and it had a bitter aftertaste. The first powder containing cream of tartar was developed around 1835. It was a mixture of sodium bicarbonate and residue of cream of tartar from the barrels in which the cream of tartar was made. This kind of baking powder was first sold commercially in 1850. At the end of the 19th century, the cream of tartar was replaced with the acid monocalcium phosphate, aluminum sulphate, and sodium sulphate. Fast acting begins bubbling immediately (pancakes). Slow acting bubbles during baking (cakes). Common brands are mixed. Avoid aluminum when possible (e.g., the Rumford Brand).

Energy: Warm
Taste: Salty
Post Digestion: Sweet
Indications: Appetite, saliva, sore throat gargle
Systems: No nutritional value

Dosha Affected:
Vata: Moderation
Pitta: Best (due to alkaline)
Kapha: Moderation
Mixes Well With: Grains

Bragg Liquid Aminos

This is a salt substitute made from soybeans. Bragg's formulated vegetable protein is made from certified non-GMO soybeans and purified water only. It contains no preservatives, no coloring agents, no alcohol, no gluten, no additives, and no chemicals. Bragg's is not fermented, and is very high in minerals.

Dosha Affected:

Good for all Doshas (Kaphas in moderation)

Breadcrumbs

6 pieces of 2- to 3-day-old bread (any kind)

¼ tablespoon Italian seasoning

In oven or toaster, toast bread crisply on both sides – do not burn. Cut bread in small pieces, put in blender on grind, and pulverize. Add seasoning. This can be made with any kind of bread, and the seasoning of your choice.

Chocolate

<u>Botanical Name:</u> *Theobroma cacoa*

Chocolate is an extraction of the bean of the cacao tree, a native of the tropical Americas. Cultivation of the cacao tree dates back some 3,000 years. The beans of this tree played a very important role in Mayan, Toltec, and Aztec cultures, where it was used as a food and for bartering (e.g., a slave could be bought for 100 cacao beans). When Cortez landed in Mexico, he was greeted with mountains of cacao instead of gold (which he was in search of), thus he began to take these beans to other parts of the tropics as a form of trade. Chocolate, by itself, is not sweet. It is a bitter substance that is high in minerals, particularly magnesium, when ingested in raw form. Sweet chocolate has much added sugar, palm oil, and milk products.

Energy: Warm

Taste: Bitter, Pungent

Post Digestion: Pungent

Indications: Calming nerves, sexual stimulation, depression, hypertension, muscle spasm

Systems: Nervous, Reproductive, Muscular

Dosha Affected:

Vata: Small amounts

Pitta: Avoid

Kapha: Small amounts (good without added sugar, milk or oil)

Mixes Well With: Fruits, sugars

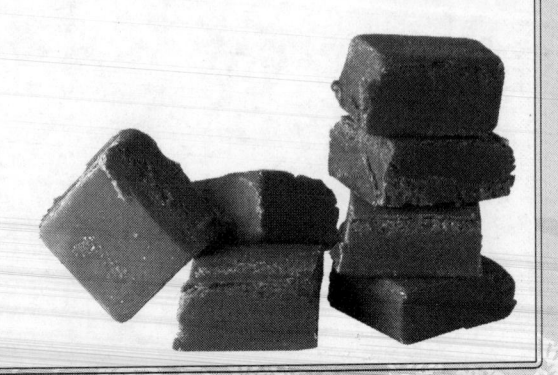

Chocolate Chip Cookies

- ¼ cup ghee
- ¼ cup almond butter
- ½ cup water
- 1 large egg, beaten (or egg substitute)
- 2 apples, grated
- 1 teaspoon vanilla
- ½ cup barley flour
- 1½ cups pastry flour
- ½ teaspoon baking powder
- ½ teaspoon baking soda
- 2 tablespoons sucanat or jaggary
- ¼ teaspoon salt
- ½ cup chocolate chips, unsweetened

Preheat oven to 350°. In a large bowl, mix ghee, almond butter, water, egg, grated apple, and vanilla. In separate bowl, mix flours, baking powder and soda, sucanat, salt, and chocolate chips. Fold dry mixture into wet mixture, stirring well. Drop by spoonfuls onto baking sheet. Bake for 20 minutes (or until brown).

Chocolate Banana Cream Topping

- 4 oz bitter chocolate
- 1 banana, large
- 2 tablespoons butter
- 1 teaspoon vanilla
- 2 tablespoons jaggary or raw sugar
- ½ teaspoon cardamom

In a double boiler, melt chocolate until smooth at low heat. Add other ingredients except the banana. Let cool down for 10 minutes. Mash banana and stir all ingredients together until creamy. Do not blend, it will become more liquid. Add topping to cakes, fruit salad, or yogurt. Use as a topping or fruit salad.

Guar Gum

<u>Botanical Name</u>: *Cyamopsis tetragonoloba*

This powder is made from the endosperm of the guar bean, a legume that grows mostly in India. It is high in fiber and sometimes used as a laxative, as well as a thickener for liquids.

Energy: Warming

Taste: Sweet

Post Digestion: Sweet

Indications: Weight loss, constipation, food thickener

Systems: All systems

Dosha Affected:

Vata: Moderation

Pitta and **Kapha**: Good

Mixes Well With: Fruits, vegetables

Kuzu / Kudzu

<u>Botanical Name: *Pueraria lobata*</u>

The kuzu or kudzu plant is native to Japan and China, and grows extensively (and invasively) in the southern U.S. Many parts of the plant are edible, but it is the starchy root that is ground into a powder and used as a thickening ingredient in Asian sauces, gravies, and stews. It is also known as "Japanese arrowroot," but is not related to the arrowroot plant (Maranta arundinacea). To keep the natural whiteness of this thickener, add cold water and sea salt for flavor, rather than tamari or soy sauce. Hot water and tamari will turn it brown. Stir quickly, adding cold water or broth to the kuzu powder to avoid lumps. Cooking time for gravy is 1 to 3 minutes.

Energy: Warm

Taste: Sweet

Post Digestion: Sweet

Indications: Intestinal problems, diarrhea, constipation.

Systems: Digestive

<u>**Dosha Affected:**</u>

Vata and **Pitta**: Good

Kapha: Avoid

Mixes Well With: Gravies, sauces, stews

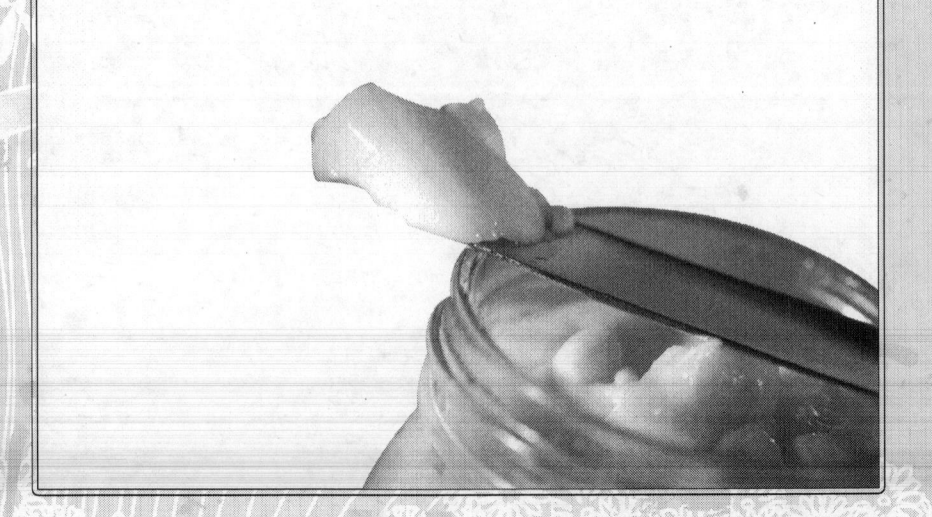

Mayonnaise

Mayonnaise is a combination of oils, vinegar, eggs, and sugar. The quality of this product depends upon the kind of oil used. It can also be made without eggs, and with lemon juice and honey instead of vinegar and sugar.

Energy: Warming
Taste: Sweet, Sour, Salty
Post Digestive: Sweet
Indications: Good for skin, hair and nails (due to the oil content), also weight gain
Systems: Skin, Skeletal

Dosha Affected:
Vata: Good
Pitta and **Kapha**: Moderation
Mixes Well With: Vegetables, starches

Eggless Mayonnaise

- 4 tablespoons sunflower oil
- 1 tablespoon arrowroot powder
- 2 tablespoons apple cider vinegar
- 2 tablespoons lemon juice
- ½ teaspoon honey
- ¼ cup water
- 1 teaspoon lecithin

Blend all ingredients together until smooth.

Miso

Miso is a product of the orient, a smooth, dark puree made from fermented soybeans, barley, or rice, and sea salts. It is an excellent addition to soups. Miso contains living enzymes, is highly nutritious, and loaded with minerals. In Japan, Miso is believed to be a gift from the gods.

Energy: Warming

Taste: Sour/Sweet

Post Digestive: Sweet

Indications: Aids digestion, blood and circulation, weight gain, promotes longevity, immune builder

Systems: Digestive, Epithelial (skin)

Dosha Affected:

Vata: Good

Pitta: Avoid or Reduce

Kapha: Small amounts (best as soup)

Mixes Well With: Vegetables, grains, legumes

Miso Nourishing Soup

- 2 cups water
- 1/3 cup grated ginger
- 1/2 bunch chives, chopped
- 4 sheets nori, cut in small pieces
- 2 tablespoons miso

Bring water to a boil; add ginger, chives, and nori. Remove from heat and add miso; mix in well, and serve.

Miso-Tahini Sauce

Makes 1 cup

- 1 tablespoon barley miso
- 2 tablespoons sesame tahini
- 2 tablespoons sesame oil
- 1 tablespoon unaboshi vinegar
- 1/4 cup water

Blend all ingredients until smooth.

Salt

Salt comes from mineral deposits from old sea beds and is then dried and commercially refined. Most commercial salt has been stripped of minerals, which are then sold to vitamin companies. They add dextrose to prevent the salt from absorbing water. Sea salt is best and is high in minerals from the sea. In excess, it causes nausea and increases the heat in food.

Energy: Warming

Taste: Salty

Post Digestive: Sweet

Indications: Increases appetite, aids saliva and gastric juices, draws moisture from the skin; in large amounts is emetic, helping to clear mucus from stomach, abdominal distension

Systems: Digestive, Epithelial (skin)

Dosha Affected:

Vata: Excellent

Pitta and **Kapha**: Avoid or reduce

Mixes Well With: Vegetables, (fruit for Vata), meats, grains

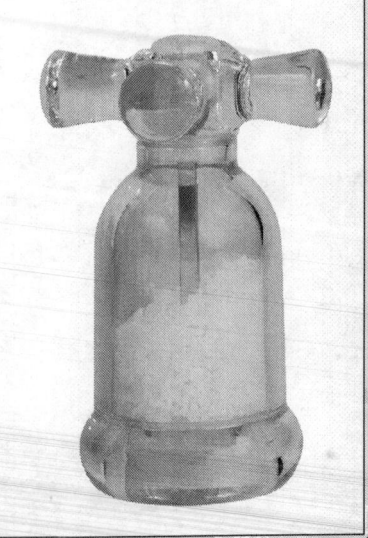

Soy Sauce

Soy sauce is made from fermented and aged soybeans. Most of the soy sauce that is available in America is processed with chemicals and artificially aged. Look for "naturally fermented" labels. The famous "Shoyu" is processed with chemicals and is not naturally fermented.

Energy: Warming
Taste: Salty, Sweet
Post Digestive: Sweet

Dosha Affected:
Vata: Good
Pitta: Moderation (in small amounts)
Kapha: Avoid or Reduce

Tamari

Tamari is a Japanese soy sauce that is naturally fermented from soybeans. It is a by-product of miso, the liquid that runs off miso as it matures.

Energy: Warming
Taste: Salty, Sweet
Post Digestive: Sweet

Dosha Affected:
Vata: Excellent
Pitta and **Kapha**: Avoid
Mixes Well With: Vegetables, proteins, grains

Umeboshi

This is the dried ume, a fruit similar to the apricot that grows in the cooler northern regions of Japan. The fruit is picked in early summer while it is still very acidic and cannot be ingested raw. It is then fermented with sea salt, enzymes, and bacteria for a period for 1 to 2 years, producing a strong medicinal product.

Energy: Warming
Taste: Salty, Pungent, Sweet
Post Digestion: Sour
Indications: Digestive aid for assimilation of meat and grains, immune builder
Systems: Digestive, Immune

Dosha Affected:
Vata: Good
Pitta and **Kapha**: Avoid or Reduce
Mixes Well With: Grains, meats

Vinegar

Vinegar is a fermented product made from grape, apple, or any other fruit that is fermented past the wine stage. Soaking herbs in vinegar extracts the alkaloids from the herb, making an herbal tincture. White vinegar has been bleached and refined; it is best to use apple cider or balsamic vinegar. The sourness is good to cut olive oil over salad or vegetables.

There are many kinds of vinegars: apple, rice, red wine, balsamic, umeboshi, Coconut, infused fig vinegar, and herbal vinegars

Energy: Warming

Taste: Sour

Post Digestive: Sour

Indications: Digestive aid, assists with production of hydrochloric acid, promotes menstruation

Systems: Digestive, Reproductive

Dosha Affected:

Vata: Good (unless yeast sensitive)

Pitta: Avoid (best used with lime or lemon)

Kapha: Moderation

Mixes Well With: Leafy green vegetables (best on salads or early in the morning to increase digestive enzymes)

Herbs & Spices

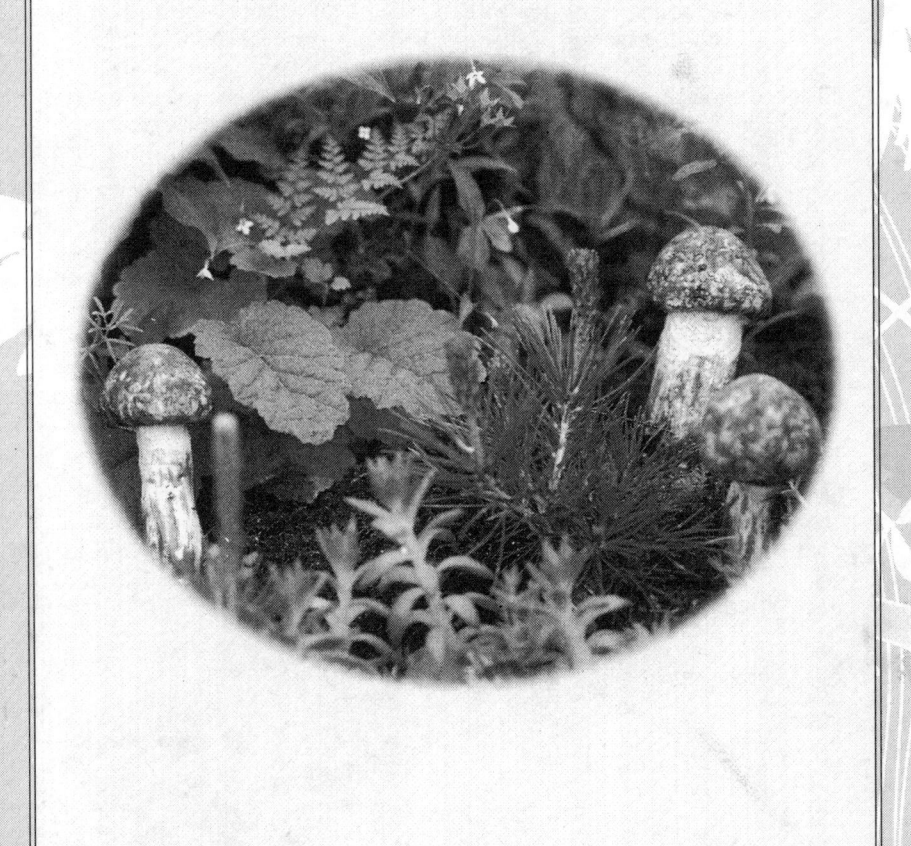

Herbs and Spices

General Considerations

Herbs and spices have been used since ancient times, not only for their flavoring, but also for the preservation of foods. Before refrigeration, spicing of meats and vegetables was an important form of preservation; salting, drying, and pickling were also used. Many spices can be consumed in fresh form in salads and cooked fresh in soups. They are found to be higher in food value than dried herbs. Due to the fact that the volatile contents of aromatic herbs are significantly destroyed in the grinding and drying process, it is best to purchase fresh herbs to obtain optimum value when available. Whole or flaked dried herbs will be superior to ground or powdered herbs. Some species carry strong pungent properties, and the energy properties last longer than other herbs.

Spices strengthen and regulate the appetite, improve digestion, prevent aging, and are an aid to the digestive tract assisting with assimilation of foods. They are useful in treating many diseases. Many pungent spices increase Pitta and so are particularly good for Kapha and Vata imbalance. Sweet, bitter, astringent, and/or cooling herbs are best for Pittas.

In treating imbalances (vikriti – disease), the use of spices (especially fresh) in foods can be an effective way to produce rapid change. Adding the "spice" into "life" often makes the patient come alive to the enjoyment of living. There is a form of Arabic medicine called Unani, where spices are the main medicine and it is a system also based on the tastes.

In Ayurveda, powdered spice mixtures are called churnas. They are traditionally prepared with mortar and pestle, then filtered through a linen cheesecloth. When cooking, pay attention to digestive herbs because they are the quickest way to get the digestive fire going and the most efficient way to increase health.

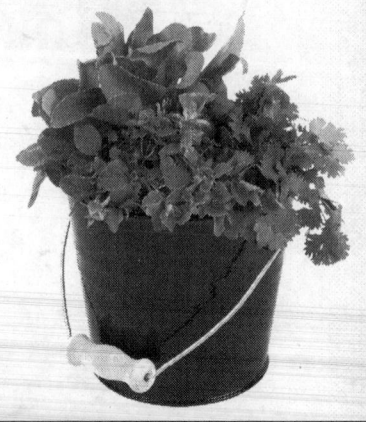

Ajwan (Ajwain)

Botanical Name: Trachyspermum copticum

Ajwan is sometimes called "wild celery seed." It is native to India, and was brought to Egypt and the Mediterranean in the 1500's. It has many medicinal uses in Ayurveda.

Energy: Warming

Taste: Pungent/Salty

Post Digestive: Pungent

Indications: Cold, bronchitis, digestive and arthritis, food poison, constipation, indigestion, uterine disorder, kidney and bladder problems

Systems: Digestive, Reproductive

Dosha Affected:

Vata: Good

Pitta: Avoid

Kapha: Moderation

Mixes Well With: Vegetables, soups, sauces, meats, beans, grains

Allspice

Botanical Name: Pimenta dioica

Allspice is native to India and Mexico. Today, some of the largest production comes from Jamaica, where it was introduced by the British. The Aztecs used the herb to flavor chocolate. The tree is a beautiful tropical evergreen with black or brown seeds.

Energy: Warming

Taste: Pungent

Post Digestive: Pungent

Indications: Lethargy, indigestion, flatulence, obesity

Systems: Digestive, Nervous

Dosha Affected:

Vata: Good

Pitta: Avoid

Kapha: Good

Mixes Well With: Vegetable dishes, fruits

Anise

<u>Botanical Name: *Pimpinella anisum*</u>

Anise is native to the western Mediterranean. This herb is mentioned in the Bible, and the Egyptians used it as an aphrodisiac. It was used for many digestive disorders in ancient times, and today it is frequently used in India. In the West, it is used to make the flavoring "licorice" (not related to the herb). When traveling on Indian Airlines, the flight attendant will always come before mealtime and offer you this delicious seed. When visiting an Indian restaurant, you will always see it mixed with candies and offered after the meal. The fresh plant may also be eaten as a vegetable. The dried herb is often confused with fennel. Anise is used frequently in Italian and Mexican cooking, as well as in many liqueurs, such as Anisette and Ouzo. Anise is a member of the parsley family.

Energy: Warming

Taste: Pungent, Sweet

Post Digestive: Pungent

Indications: Colds, dry cough, flatulence, digestive aid, halitosis, menstrual cramps

Systems: Digestive, Respiratory, Excretory

Dosha Affected:

Vata and **Kapha**: Good

Pitta: Moderation (small amounts)

Mixes Well With: All fruits, vegetables, starches, teas, drinks

Asafoetida (Hing)

Botanical Name: Ferula assafoetida

Asafoetida is a native of India; it did not extend to other parts of the world until the rebirth of Ayurveda. Some find the smell nauseating, vaguely reminiscent of garlic, very strong. It is great for preventing negative energies, and yet it has many medicinal properties to support the human body. It is one of the best antidotes for the gas produced when eating beans.

Energy: Hot

Taste: Pungent

Post Digestive: Pungent

Indications: Flatulence, stomach distension, fever, nervousness, fear, depression, headaches, PMS, angina, heartburn, joint disorders, rheumatism, parasites

Systems: All systems

Dosha Affected:

Vata: Excellent

Pitta: Avoid

Kapha: Excellent

Mixes Well With: Vegetables, legumes, meats

Basil

Botanical Name: Ocimum basilicum

Today the cultivated variety is different than the original variety in India, called "holy" or "Krishna" basil. Basil is cultivated today all over the world, especially in sub-tropic and tropical climates.

Energy: Warming

Taste: Pungent

Post Digestive: Pungent

Indications: Fevers, headaches, arthritic joints, sinuses, colds, lung cleanser

Systems: Immune, Muscular, Skeletal, Respiratory

Dosha Affected:

Vata: Good

Pitta: Small amounts

Kapha: Good

Mixes Well With: Vegetable dishes, salads, soups, grains, beans

Bay Leaf

Botanical Name: Laurus nobilis

Bay laurel is an herb native to ancient Greece and grown today on many of the Greek Islands. At one time, the Greeks burned an offering of this herb to Apollo, the God of Light. Bay leaves make great bug repellent and can be added to dried herbs and grains to preserve for long periods of time. They are an excellent addition when cooking beans, and can also assist with the elimination of phytates.

Energy: Warming

Taste: Pungent

Post Digestive: Pungent

Indications: Headaches, flatulence, dandruff, increases nail growth, congestion, cough, diarrhea

Systems: Circulatory, Respiratory, Excretory, Skeletal

Dosha Affected:

Vata & Kapha: Good

Pitta: Moderation (well cooked)

Mixes Well With: Legumes, soups, grains

Black Pepper

Botanical Name: Piper nigrum

Native to India, black pepper was brought to Europe by the Jesuits. At one time, it was used as a currency and for the payment of taxes during the time of the Roman Empire.

Energy: Heating

Taste: Pungent

Post Digestive: Pungent

Indications: Heart disease, flatulence, stomach problems, bowel disturbances, hiccups, weak memory, weight loss

Systems: Digestive

Dosha affected:

Vata: Moderation

Pitta: Good

Kapha: Good

Mixes Well With: Everything

Borage

Botanical Name: *Borago officinalis*

Borage is a beautiful plant with small blue and purple flowers that is worth growing just for the flower. They can be added to salads. A native of Europe, borage has many leaves and stems with alternate simple leaves. It grows well in almost any garden. In Europe, they produce a wonderful oil from the palms of this plant that is then used for skin care.

Energy: Cooling

Taste: Sweet

Post Digestive: Sweet

Indications: Eye infections, skin irritation and rejuvenation, gastric problems.

Systems: Ocular, Skin, Digestive

Dosha Affected:

Vata: Moderation

Pitta: Excellent

Kapha: Moderation

Mixes well with: All starches, vegetables and proteins.

Capers

Botanical Name: *Capparis Spinosa*

A native of the Mediterranean, this coppery bush is a prickly perennial plant. Capers are the flower buds of a creeper shrub. The plant was mentioned in the Old Testament. In modern times, capers are used as a spice in condiments. In this country, capers are rarely used. Traditionally, they are used in Mediterranean foods.

Taste: Pungent, Sweet

Post digestive: Sweet

Indications: Digestive aid, good skincare

Systems: Digestive, Excretory; helps with breakdown of starches, constipation, infections, and food flowing.

Dosha Affected:

Vata: Good

Pitta: Moderation

Kapha: Moderation

Mixes Well With: Grain starches, vegetables

Rice with Capers

Serves 2

- ½ onion, well chopped
- 1 tablespoons ghee
- 1 cup grated carrots
- 2 cups cooked rice
- 1 cup capers

Sauté onions in ghee until caramelized. Add carrots, rice, and capers; stir until heated.

Caraway Seeds

Botanical Name: Carum carvi

Caraway is native to Egypt and the Middle East, and is now cultivated all over the world. This plant is mostly cultivated because of its seeds, even though the stems and leaves can also be used. Roots are wholesome and edible raw or cooked. It will do well in almost any garden. Caraway seeds are used to add flavor to bread, especially rye. They aid in digestion of starches. The oil is used for parasites.

Energy: Warming
Taste: Sweet, Pungent
Post Digestive: Pungent
Indications: Gas, colic, nervous condition, parasites
Systems: Nervous, Digestive

Dosha Affected:
Vata: Moderation
Pitta: Avoid
Kapha: Good
Mixes Well With: Starches, vegetables, breads, soups

Cardamom

Botanical Name: Elettaria cardamomum

Cardamom is a native of India and was introduced to Europe by Alexander the Great. Many Europeans believe that it is a native of Northern Europe as it is used extensively in their pastries and desserts. Today, cardamom is cultivated in Sri Lanka, Madagascar, and Guatemala. The essential oil is used as a flavoring and in perfumes. In Ayurveda, this herb is considered Sattvic. Cardamom is an antidote to caffeine; add 2 drops of essential oil to a cup of brewed coffee, or 1 teaspoon of ground cardamom when brewing your own.

Energy: Heating, Moisturizing
Taste: Pungent, Sweet
Post Digestive: Pungent
Indications: Circulation disorders, menopause, heart disorders, indigestion, fevers, flatulence, ulcer, cough, mucus expeller, weak eyesight
Systems: All systems

Dosha Affected:
Vata: Good
Pitta: Moderation
Kapha: Excellent
Mixes Well With: Vegetables, starches, cookies, coffee, cakes

Cayenne

<u>Botanical Name: *Capsicum annuum*</u>

Cayennes are hot red chili peppers. They were used by the Aztecs for purification and cleansing. The name came from Greek, meaning "bite." Christopher Columbus introduced to Europe these hot peppers that were much hotter than people were used to. There are many varieties today, all belonging to the same family. Cayenne is available as fresh peppers, as dried flakes, or ground into powder.

Energy: Heating
Taste: Pungent
Post Digestive: Pungent
Indications: Infection, flues, colds, constipation, weight reduction
Systems: Digestive, Respiratory

<u>**Dosha affected:**</u>
Vata: Moderate
Pitta: Avoid
Kapha: Good
Mixes Well With: All foods

Pico de Gallo

- 6 tomatoes, well chopped
- 3 green peppers, chopped
- 1 tablespoon olive oil
- 2 small cayenne peppers, chopped
- ½ cup cilantro, chopped
- salt to taste

Mix all ingredients in a bowl. Serve with chips, guacamole, tacos, or over grains.

Hot Mile Sauce

Makes about 2 cups

- 1 ½ cup onion, chopped
- 3 large tomatoes, chopped
- 3 tablespoons cayenne pepper, chopped
- 1 cup raisins
- 1 cup almonds, finely ground
- ½ cup cashews, finely ground
- 1 banana, ripe, mashed
- 2 garlic cloves, well chopped
- 3 tablespoons olive oil
- 2 oz chocolate, unsweetened
- ¼ teaspoon clove powder
- ½ cup sesame powder
- ½ teaspoon cumin powder
- ½ teaspoon coriander powder
- ½ teaspoon cinnamon powder
- 3 tablespoons water

Soak the raisins in water. In a skillet, saute garlic, cayenne, and onions. Then add tomatoes. Reduce mixture to low heat and melt in chocolate. Stir. Add nuts and seeds.

Blend soaked raisins and all the water. Add blended raisins & spices. Mash the banana. Whisk everything together with a whisk until smooth. For a smoother consistency, can be put in a blender.

Cilantro / Coriander

<u>Botanical Name</u>: *Coriandrum sativum*

The seed of this wonderful herb is called coriander and is a delightful aromatic from Asia and Central America. Today, cilantro is gaining great recognition in the West because of the high nutritional value in the green leaves and the seeds. It is also very high in phytoestrogen components. Cilantro is the antidote to hot, spicy foods. The Germans have also used it as a bug repellent.

Energy: Cooling, Moisturizing

Taste: Bitter, Pungent, Sweet

Post Digestive: Pungent

Indications: Indigestion, liver disorders, piles, emaciation, intestinal parasites, dysentery, fever, cold, kidney disorders

Systems: Digestive, Urinary, Endocrine, Urinary, Excretory

<u>**Dosha Affected:**</u>

Vata: Neutral

Pitta: Good

Kapha: Excellent

Mixes Well With: Starches, vegetables, proteins, juices, soups

Cilantro Mint Chutney

- 2 cups cilantro, leaves and tender stems, loosely packed
- 1 cup mint leaves, loosely packed
- 1 cup chopped onion
- ½ teaspoon minced garlic
- ½ teaspoon minced ginger
- ½ teaspoon cumin, ground
- 1 teaspoon minced green chili (serrano, Thai, or jalapeño)
- 1 teaspoon jaggary
- ½ teaspoon salt
- 2 tablespoons fresh lemon juice
- 3 tablespoons plain low-fat yogurt

In food processor or blender, combine all ingredients and process to a smooth puree, adding more or less yogurt as needed to obtain creamy (not watery) consistency.

Cilantro Quesadillas

Serves 4

- 2 cups cilantro, well chopped
- 2 cups mashed potatoes
- 1 cup salsa
- 2 tablespoons ghee
- ½ pound of Mexican cheese of your choice, grated
- 8 tortillas

Mix cilantro with mashed potatoes. Add half of the ghee. Mix well. Baste each tortilla, on both sides, with ghee. Fill the center of the tortilla with potato-cilantro mix. Add one teaspoon of salsa and 1 teaspoon cheese. Fold tortilla in half. Place in skillet. Add remaining ghee and press them with a spatula until crispy on each side. Continue until they are all done. Serve with salad or Spanish rice.

Cinnamon

Botanical Name: Cinnamomum species

Cinnamon is a very old and ancient herb, actually the dry bark of the cinnamon tree. It dates as far back as 2,800 B.C., and is one of the spices mentioned in the Bible. There are over 100 different varieties cultivated today in Asia, India, and South and Central America. A close relative of true cinnamon is Cassia (Cinnamomum aromaticum); it is cheaper and has a less delicate flavor than true cinnamon.

Energy: Warming / Neutral (depending on the spices, with Cassia being hotter)

Taste: Pungent, Sweet, Astringent

Post Digestive: Sweet

Indications: Digestive stimulant, flatulence, diarrhea, circulatory disorders, menopause, sinus congestion, bronchitis, sexual stimulant, impotency

Systems: All systems

Dosha Affected:
Vata: Excellent
Pitta: Good
Kapha: Excellent
Mixes Well With: All foods

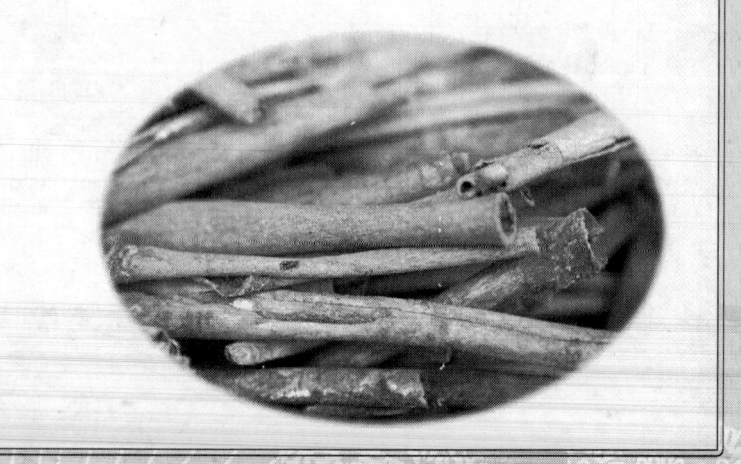

Cloves

Botanical Name: Eugenia aromatica

Cloves are native to the Maluku (Spice) Islands, and were introduced throughout the world by Jesuit Priests. They have been used for over 2,000 years in the East, and were introduced to Europe in the fourth century. The tree can grow as high as 50 feet. The cloves are the dried flower buds of the tree. Excellent in Chai.

Energy: Heat

Taste: Pungent

Post Digestive: Pungent

Indications: Vomiting, nausea, chronic colds, toothache, flu, blood sugar regulator, infections

Systems: Digestive, Skeletal, Immune

Dosha Affected:

Vata: Moderation

Pitta: Avoid

Kapha: Excellent

Mixes Well With: Starches, fruits

Dill

Botanical Name: Anethum graveolens

Dill is an annual herb, native to Asia and Europe. It is related to the carrot family. Both the fresh dill and dried dill weed are used as herbs in cooking, and the dried seeds are used as spices.

Energy: Cooling (the seed is Warming)

Taste: Pungent, Bitter

Post Digestive: Pungent

Indications: Good for lactation, flatulence, digestive aid, gastric pain, flatulence, eye sight, muscular problems, arthritis, bone break, pain relief

Systems: Digestive, Muscular, Excretory, Reproductive

Dosha Affected:

Vata: Moderation

Pitta: Good

Kapha: Excellent

Mixes Well With: Vegetables, proteins, starches, soups, breads

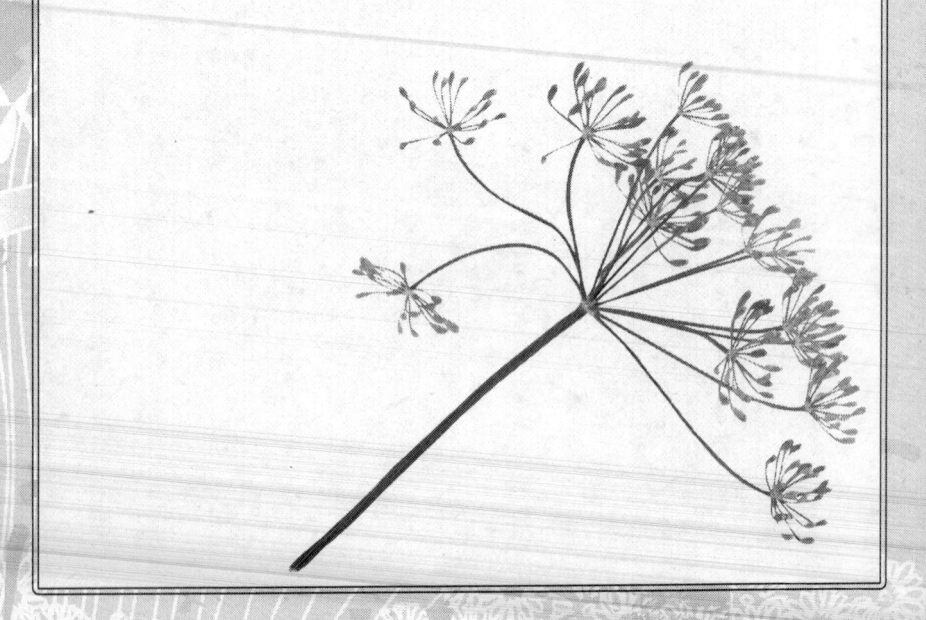

Dill Almond Dressing

- 2 tablespoons olive oil
- 1 bunch dill, chopped
- 1 cup almonds (raw, soaked overnight)
- 2 tablespoons Bragg's

Place all ingredients in blender, and mix until smooth. Serve with your choice of salad or vegetables.

Dill Millet

Serves 2

- ½ cup dill, well chopped
- 1 cup millet
- 2 cups water
- ½ tablespoon ghee or olive oil
- Bragg's or salt to taste

Use 1 cup millet to 2 cups water. Bring water to boil, add millet, and cook for 20 minutes. When cooked, add dill, and onions. Cover. Lower flame and simmer for 15 minutes. Add Bragg's or salt.

Fennel

Botanical Name: Foeniculum vulgare

Fennel is a perennial European herb mostly cultivated because of its seeds and oil. The plant requires plenty of sunshine, but it's easy to grow (as most herbs are). It grows wild, as all over the South. In many parts of Europe, it is used as a vegetable and, today, is available in many of our Western markets. Its origin is from the Mediterranean. Greeks and Romans used this plant for many festivities and after dinner as a digestive aid. In Europe, it is cooked like asparagus. When fasting, it is an excellent addition for flavoring and food value. The stalk can grow as big as 6 feet high.

Energy: Cool

Taste: Sweet

Post Digestive: Sweet

Indications: Gastric pains, flatulence, eyesight, muscular problems, arthritis, bone break

Systems: Nervous, Digestive, Muscular, Endocrine

Dosha Affected:

Vata: Good (best cooked or added to foods)

Pitta: Good

Kapha: Good

Mixes well with: Proteins, all vegetables

Group Veggie Combo

1 tablespoon ghee
4 green onions, chopped
⅓ cup grated ginger
¼ cup grated turmeric (fresh)
1 bunch kale, chopped
1 bulb fennel, chopped
¼ cup fresh cilantro, chopped
½ head of red cabbage, chopped
¼ cup fresh basil, chopped
¼ cup unsweetened vanilla almond milk

In large wok or skillet, melt ghee. Sauté green onion, ginger, and fresh turmeric for 1 to 2 minutes. Add kale, fennel, cilantro, cabbage, and basil, and continue cooking for 10 minutes. Add almond milk and sauté for 2 more minutes. Serve with Green Tara Dressing (see page 384).

Fennel Soup

Serves 2

1 cup coconut, fresh, soft meat
 OR 1 cup coconut milk
1 tomato, chopped
½ onion, chopped
¼ cup cilantro, well chopped
¼ cup mint, well chopped
1 cup water
¼ cup olive oil
2 tablespoons coconut amino acids

Blend all ingredients until smooth, except the mint & cilantro. Sprinkle mint & cilantro on top when serving.

Fenugreek

Botanical Name: Trigonella foenum-graecum

Fenugreek is a native of India and Southern Europe, and is now becoming quite popular in health food markets (the seeds are sold for sprouting). It is also a major ingredient in curries. Egyptians consumed this food as a vegetable. The food industry uses it in artificial preparation of maple syrup. This is a wonderful spice and is in many varieties of curry. It can also be sprouted and Added to salad or stir fry.

Energy: Warm

Taste: Bitter, Pungent

Post Digestive: Pungent

Indications: Loss of appetite, bowel disorders, parasites, fever, swelling, eye inflammation, joint pain, diabetes, longevity, allergies, increases milk flow

Systems: Excretory, Digestive, Muscular, Skeletal

Dosha Affected:

Vata: Good

Pitta: Moderation (small amounts; best sprouted)

Kapha: Excellent

Mixes Well With: All vegetables, starches and proteins

Ginger

<u>Botanical Name: Zingiber officinale</u>

Ginger is native to India and South Asia, where it has been used for over 2,000 years. It was introduced to Europe in the thirteenth century. Today, ginger is cultivated in Indonesia, South America, Hawaii, Mexico, and South America. For cooking, the ginger root is used extensively in the orient, Caribbean, and South America. In Ayurveda, this herb is considered to be Sattvic.

Energy: Warm

Taste: Pungent, Sweet

Post Digestive: Sweet

Indications: Flatulence, headaches, loss of appetite, digestive aid, earache, chronic bowels, abdominal distension, excess mucus, sore throat, cough

Systems: All systems

Dosha Affected:

Vata: Good

Pitta: Small amounts (best fresh, mixed in foods)

Kapha: Excellent

Mixes Well With: All foods

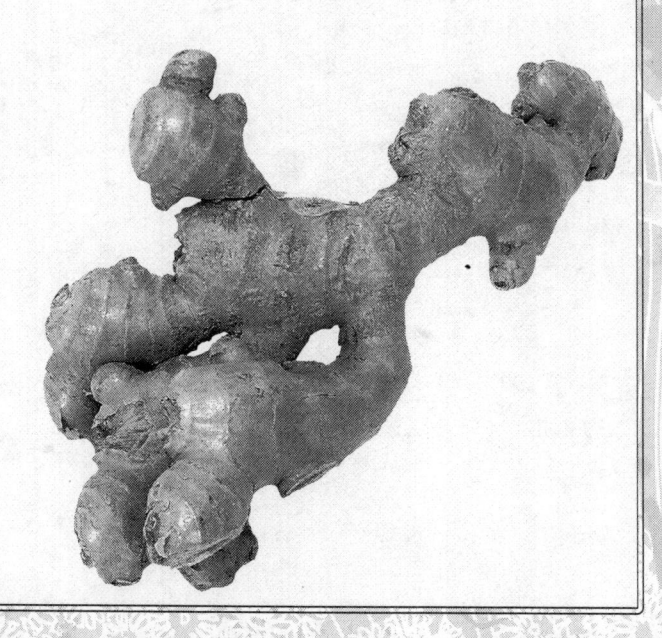

Ayurvedic Curative Cuisine for Everyone

Ginger Rice Balls

- 2 cups green onions, well chopped
- ½ cup ginger, chopped
- ¼ cup ghee
- 3 cups cooked rice
- 1½ cups rice flour or rice breadcrumbs
- 2 eggs (or 1 tablespoon lecithin)
- 2 cups cilantro, well chopped
- 1 tablespoon coriander
- 1 tablespoon agave syrup

Sauté onions and ginger in ghee. Put rice in a large bowl, and add onion mixture. Add flour, eggs (or lecithin), cilantro, and coriander. Form into 1½-inch balls and place on baking sheet. Bake at 350° for 10 minutes.

Ginger Mint Chutney

Makes 1 cup

- 1 cup ginger, fresh, well chopped
- 2 tablespoons lemon juice
- 2 teaspoons turmeric powder
- 1 tablespoon fennel
- 1 cup mint, well chopped
- ¼ cup cilantro, well chopped
- 1 teaspoon cumin
- 2 tablespoons jaggary
- 2 tablespoons ghee
- ¼ cup water
- ¼ teaspoon salt

In a skillet, add ghee and saute ginger at low heat until soft. Add spices, lemon juice, water, mint, salt, and cilantro. Mix well. Add jaggary and mix again. Cover. Cook for 10 minutes until it is like jam.

Raw Tip: This recipe can be done raw in the blender.

Horseradish

Botanical Name: Armoracia rusticana

Horseradish is a member of the mustard family. The root of this plant is long and similar to the parsnip; it has a sharp, peppery taste, and is used mainly as a condiment. The plant was cultivated in Greece and Egypt and traded all over Europe, Scandinavia, and Russia. In Egypt, at one time, it was treasured as much as gold. Arriving in the United States with the colonists, it was used medicinally to kill parasites in fish and beef. In Scandanavian countries it is used as a condiment or relish. The Japanese variety always accompanies pan fish. Horseradish is very high in vitamin C. Very high in minerals, particularly calcium and potassium. The root, by itself, has very little aroma. When the cell wall is cut, grated, or chopped, the cell wall enzymes break down releasing the chemical constituent called sinigrin (glucosinate). This causes a strong mucousal irritant, especially to the eyes and sinuses. As soon as the horseradish is cut, it needs to IMMEDIATELY be added to, or stored in, vinegar. Horseradish is a kidney stimulant, thyroid stimulant and is highly antibiotic.

Energy: Warming

Taste: Pungent

Post Digestive: Pungent

Indications: Aggressive emotions, chronic fevers, heartburn, fever, skin eruptions, blood purifier, immune builder, poor protein digestion

Systems: Circulatory, Endocrine, Digestive

Dosha Affected:

Vata: Avoid

Pitta: Moderation

Kapha: Excellent

Mixes Well With: Proteins and vegetables

Horseradish Sauce

- 2 tablespoons sesame oil
- 1 tablespoon soy sauce
- 1 tablespoon red wine vinegar
- 2 tablespoons parsley, chopped
- 1 medium horseradish root, peeled and grated

Put all ingredients in blender and IMMEDIATELY blend until smooth. Serve on fish, roast beef, or meats.

Horseradish Vegan Mayonnaise

- 3 tablespoons vegan mayonnaise (See page 345 to make your own)
- 1 tablespoon balsamic vinegar
- ¼ cup cashews, chopped
- 1/3 cup dill, well chopped
- ¼ cup water
- ½ tablespoon tamari or Bragg' Amino Acids
- ½ teaspoon jaggary or raw sugar
- ½ teaspoon mustard oil
- 1 horseradish, medium size, fresh, well chopped

Place all ingredients in blender and blend until smooth.

Juniper Berries

Botanical Name: Juniperus communis

This evergreen is a native of North America and Asia, and the fruit (berry) is a grayish, greenish, deep purple color. Juniper berries are excellent as a food flavoring, and the seeds are used in sauerkraut, soups, and sauces. To add great flavor to steamed vegetables, the berries can be added to the water.

Add ½ cup berries to 2 cups of water for steaming veggies.

Energy: Warming

Taste: Pungent, Bitter, Sweet

Post Digestive: Pungent

Indications: Lumbago, edema, joint problems, diabetes, immune builder, bladder infections, menstrual disorders, swollen glands, infection

Systems: Urinary, Muscular, Reproductive, Endocrine, Lymphatic

Dosha Affected:

Vata: Small amounts in food

Pitta: Moderation

Kapha: Excellent

Mixes Well With: Vegetables, starches, pickles

Sauerkraut

- ½ cup juniper berries
- 1 large onion, well chopped
- 1 large cabbage, grated
- 2 carrots, grated
- 4 tablespoons apple cider vinegar
- 2 ounces hiziki, crushed
- 1 tablespoon salt
- 2 tablespoons lemon juice

Put all ingredients in a ceramic crock. Cover, and let sauerkraut ferment for a few days. Drain the liquids off, and transfer sauerkraut to container. Refrigerate.

Serve with proteins.

Infused Juniper Berry Vinegar

Makes 16 ounces

- ½ cup Juniper Berries, dry
- 16 ounces rice vinegar or apple cider vinegar
- ¼ cup coriander seeds

Add juniper berries and coriander to vinegar bottle. Shake. Let sit for 2 weeks.

Serve on salad or vegetables.

Leeks

Botanical Name: Allium ampeloprasum

There is much confusion as to the origin of the leek plant; some say from Northern Europe, others speak of it as a native of Egypt. Belonging to the onion family, this delicate and tender plant produces stems up to 2 inches in diameter when mature, and grows to 12 inches in height. Leeks are similar to scallions, not as strong as onions or garlic. Leeks are great in soups and salads.

Energy: Warming

Taste: Pungent, Sweet

Post Digestive: Sweet

Indications: Flues, colds, ear aches, fluid reduction, parasites, joint problems

Systems: Respiratory, Urinary, Skeletal

Dosha Affected:

Vata: Moderation (well cooked)

Pitta: Moderation (only when sweet)

Kapha: Good

Mixes Well With: Vegetables, starches, proteins

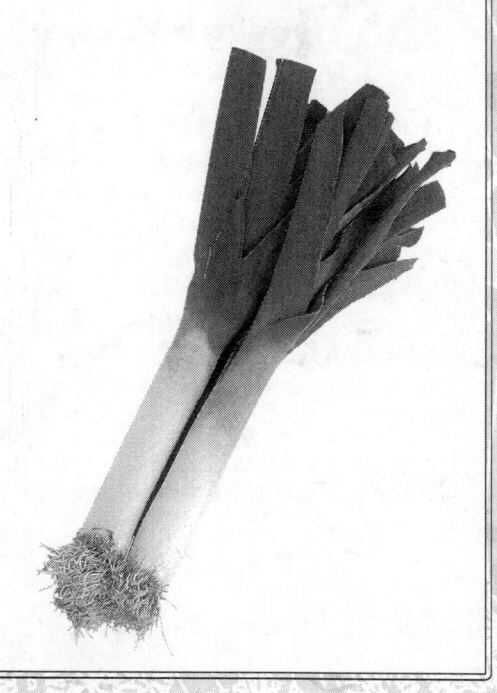

Potato Leek Soup

Serves 6

- 6 potatoes, cut into cubes
- 8 cups water
- 1 medium onion, well chopped
- 2 large leek, thinly sliced
- 1 tomato, chopped
- ½ cup dill weed
- 2 tablespoons Bragg's

Boil the cubed potatoes in water, and let them cool. In a skillet, sauté onions, leek, tomatoes and half of the dill. Add Bragg's, and blend all the ingredients together in blender until smooth. Garnish with other half of dill.

Serve with salad and crackers.

Baked Leeks With Broccoli & Cauliflower

- 1 cauliflower, medium
- 1 cup broccoli
- 2 leeks, large, sliced into rings
- ¼ cup pecans
- 1 tablespoon ghee
- ¼ teaspoon rosemary, well chopped

Cut all flowerettes into small sections. Cut stalks of broccoli and cauliflower into rings and set aside. Lightly steam cauliflower and broccoli for about 15 minutes – do not overcook – they should remain firm and slightly raw. In a skillet, caramelize the leeks.

Preheat oven. In a baking pan put the rest of the ghee, pecans, broccoli & cauliflower rings, rosemary, and remaining leeks. Bake at 300 for 10-15 minutes.

Lemongrass

Botanical Name: Cymbopogon citratus

Lemongrass is native to Malaysia, and a member of the grass family. Today, it is highly cultivated in Africa, although it grows well in any sub-tropical or tropical climate. This plant multiplies quickly, like a weed. Lemongrass is used in Thai food, and small slices can be added to soups and sauces. It is highly nutritious and filled with beta-carotene, making for a great food flavoring. This is traditionally used in Thai recipes, particularly in soups. When cooking with lemongrass, use the fresh grass and remove before serving. In Israel today, it is used in teas and soups as a cancer preventative.

Energy: Cooling

Taste: Pungent, Bitter

Post Digestive: Pungent

Indications: Muscle pain, infections, night blindness, bladder and kidney infections, lymphatic congestion, edema, varicose veins, digestive aid

Systems: Urinary, Circulatory, Muscular, Immune

Dosha Affected:

Vata: Avoid (or use tiny amounts)

Pitta: Good

Kapha: Excellent

Mixes Well With: Soups, sauces, teas

Lemongrass Coconut Soup

½ cup chives, chopped

2 tablespoons grated ginger

2 tablespoons ghee

½ cup carrots, sliced

8 sprigs of lemongrass

4 key lime leaves

6 cups water

1 cup baby corn

1 teaspoon coriander

1 cup coconut milk

salt to taste

Sauté chives and ginger in ghee. Add carrots, lemongrass, key lime leaves and water; bring to a boil. Lower heat and add baby corn, coriander, salt, and coconut milk. Let steep for 10 minutes, then remove lemongrass.

Making Coconut Milk - Split a fresh coconut and take out coconut meat. This is called a fresh, Thai, or green coconut.

Place in blender with 1 cup water. Blend until smooth.

When using the brown coconut, break into half, ply the white hard meat from the brown shell with a knife, cut the white flesh into small pieces, add 2 cups water and blend.

Marjoram

<u>Botanical Name: *Origanum majorana*</u>

This small aromatic shrub grows 2 ft. high. Marjoram is a native of North Africa, and today is cultivated in the Mediterranean and all sub-tropical climates. Marjoram has a relaxing effect for Vata and Kapha. Good in soups, rice, quinoa, and potatoes. Can be useful with weight loss, and the breakdown of carbohydrates.

Energy: Warm
Taste: Pungent
Post Digestive: Pungent
Indications: Cough, anti aphrodisiac
Systems: Digestive

<u>**Dosha Affected:**</u>
Vata: Good
Pitta: Moderation
Kapha: Good
Mixes Well With: starches, proteins, vegetables

Marjoram Dressing

- 2 tablespoons marjoram
- 2 tablespoons olive oil
- ¼ cup lemon juice
- 1 teaspoon agave syrup
- 1 tablespoon Bragg's

Mix all ingredients in blender until smooth. Serve with salad.

Marjoram Cheese Dip

- ¼ cup cream cheese
- ½ cup water
- 1 tablespoon marjoram
- ½ teaspoon Bragg's or Tamari

Place all ingredients in food processor or blender until smooth.

Marjoram Rice or Quinoa

Serves 2

- 1 cup grain - rice or quinoa
- 2 cups water
- 1 tablespoon marjoram

Cover and let steep for 20 minutes. Serve.

Marjoram can be useful for weight loss and the breakdown of carbohydrates.

Mint

Botanical Name: Mentha (various species)

Mint plants are some of the most widely used plants in the herbal kingdom, with over 500 varieties throughout the world. This herb is mentioned in the Bible, and is native to the Mediterranean and North America. Today, it is used extensively in flavoring and for medicinal purposes. Mint grows well indoors, as well as in outdoor gardens where it requires shade with plenty of water. The most common varieties are spearmint, peppermint, wild mint, and horsemint. Great in sauces, potatoes, and fruit salads.

Energy: Cooling

Taste: Pungent

Post Digestive: Pungent

Indications: Cold, fever, stomach disorders, sore throat, earaches, asthma, hiccoughs.

Systems: Digestive, Immune, Respiratory, Nervous

Dosha Affected:

Vata: Reduce

Pitta and **Kapha**: Excellent

Mixes Well With: Curries, sauces, jellies, salads, drinks

Green Tara Mint Dressing

¼ cup fresh mint

½ cup fresh stevia (or 1 teaspoon agave)

½ cup fresh cucumber (peeled, seeded, and chopped)

2 tablespoons peanut oil

juice of one medium lime

Blend all ingredients together in a blender until smooth. Serve with vegetables.

Mint Sauce

Makes 1 ½ cups

1 cup mint, chopped

¼ cup tamarind pulp

¼ cup coconut milk

1 tablespoons sunflower oil

Add ingredients together in blender and blend until smooth.

Mint-Raspberry Lemonade

Makes 35 ounces - Serves 4

1/8 cup lemon juice, fresh

4 cups water

½ cup raspberries

1 tablespoon jaggary

2 tablespoons of maple syrup

In blender, add the lemon juice, berries, mind and 1 cup of water. Blend. Strain the mixture. Place back in blender, add remaining water, jaggary, and maple syrup. Blend until well mixed.

Mustard Seeds

<u>Botanical Name</u>: *Sinapis alba (white mustard) Brassica nigra (black mustard)*

Mustard is native to the Mediterranean, with the black mustard seeds being natives of India. Throughout the world, there are over forty species today.

Energy: Heating

Taste: Pungent

Post Digestive: Pungent

Indications: Back problems, massage oil, stimulating digestive aid

Systems: Muscular, Digestive

Dosha Affected:

Vata: Moderation

Pitta: Avoid

Kapha: Moderation

Mixes Well With: Vegetables, proteins, and starches

Nettles

<u>Botanical Name</u>: *Urtica dioica*

Nettles are herbaceous plants originating in Eurasia and growing wild in Northern Europe and the U.S. This plant is covered with stinging hairs, and can be found in temperate climates, growing along roadsides or along the waterfront. Despite its reputation for bad stinging and itching, it is an incredible plant with a peppery flavor. The dark green, oval leaf (like spinach) is delicious when cooked or used in soups. There are a few varieties like Great Nettle and Stinging Nettle, which can grow as high as 5 feet. Dog Nettle is also called Burning Nettle. One must wear gloves when harvesting all of these varieties. After nettles are dried or cooked, the stinging sensation is lost.

Energy: Warm

Taste: Bitter

Post Digestive: Pungent

Indications: Highly nutritious, kidney tonic, menopause liver tonic, aids lactation, rheumatism, infection and dandruff, anemia, very high in calcium disorders

Systems: Urinary, Circulation, Skeletal, Endocrine

Dosha Affected:

Vata: Avoid

Pitta: Good

Kapha: Excellent

Mixes Well With: Starches, dairy beverages

Ayurvedic Curative Cuisine for Everyone

Nettle Soup

½ cup onions, chopped

2 tablespoons ghee

3 cups nettles, chopped

6 cups water

1 bunch cilantro, chopped

1 cup cream or thick nut milk

Bragg's or salt

Sauté onions in ghee; add nettles and water, and bring to a boil. Lower heat; add cilantro, mint, cream or milk, and Bragg's to taste.

Nettles & Potatoes

Serves 2

2 cups potatoes, cubed

2 cups nettles, dried

¼ cup parsley, chopped

2 tablespoons ghee

2 teaspoons black or green mustard seeds

¼ cup water

Salt to taste or aminos

In a skillet, roast mustard seeds until aromatic. Add ghee & mix. Then add potatoes, nettles, and remaining ingredients. Add salt to taste or Braggs. Serve.

Nutmeg

Botanical Name: Myristica fragrans

Nutmeg is native to the Maluku (Spice) Islands. Since the thirteenth century, it has been traded in Europe, where it became well known and was added to cakes and pastries. The tree grows wild today in tropical climates. In large amounts, it can cause dulling of the mind.

Energy: Heating

Taste: Pungent

Post Digestive: Pungent

Indications: Impotence, headaches, cough, chest pain, influenza, TRP, bowel disturbances, bloating, pneumonia, vomiting, parasites

Systems: Nervous, Excretory, Digestive

Dosha Affected:

Vata and **Kapha**: Good

Pitta: Avoid

Mixes Well With: Starches, fruits

Nutmeg-Almond Drink

Serves 1

- 1 cup almond milk – or milk of your choice
- 1 teaspoon jaggary or raw sugar
- 1 tablespoon slippery elm
- ½ teaspoon nutmeg

Bring milk to rolling boil. Add slippery elm, stir well, steep for 15 minutes. Strain slippery elm from milk. Add nutmeg and jaggary or raw sugar.

Ayurvedic Curative Cuisine for Everyone

Onions

<u>Botanical Name: Allium cepa</u>

Onions are one of the oldest vegetables known to man, as references in Sanskrit and Hebrew literature indicate. The onion is a hardy, biennial herb usually grown for its firm, ripe, white bulbs and its stem, which is eaten as a relish or in salads. Numerous varieties exist, with the Yellow Globe, Ebenezer, and White Pearl being favorites. Onions grown in warm climates have a milder flavor than those grown in cold climates. The strong odor and flavor is due to the presence of a pungent mustard oil. Close allies to onions are chives, garlic, leek, shallots, scallions, and the Welsh onion. Research has documented that an abundant use of onions has a tendency to reduce the number of red cells and lower hemoglobin.

Energy: Heating

Taste: Pungent, Sweet

Post Digestive: Sweet

Indications: Sweating, stimulant, sexual debility

Systems: Urinary, Reproductive

Dosha Affected:

Vata: Good

Pitta: Avoid

Kapha: Good

Mixes Well With: Vegetables, starches, proteins

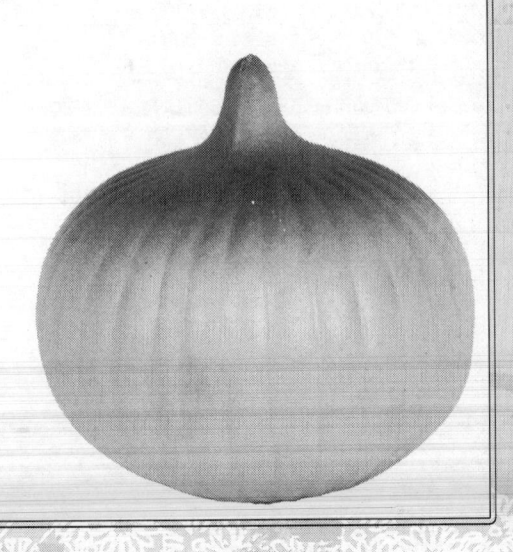

Parsley

<u>Botanical Name: *Petroselinum crispum*</u>

Parsley is a native of Southern Europe and ancient Greece, where it was offered to the Gods in ceremonies. The Greeks believed that when they ate this food, joy and fertility would come to them. It was also served at funerals and feasts. Many varieties are available in the market today, with the most common ones being Curly and Italian. Parsley is easy to grow in gardens and does very well indoors during the winter. Unfortunately, parsley is commonly used in restaurants as a decoration on the plates, and most people do not eat it. An herb so rich in minerals definitely needs to be acknowledged and used. It is an antidote to garlic and a breath freshener. Parsley is very rich in minerals, chlorophyll, and vitamin A. add as a garnish to grains after cooking. A small amount can be helpful for adrenal and thyroid glands.

Energy: Warming

Taste: Pungent, Bitter

Post Digestive: Pungent

Indications: Kidney stones, immune builder, scoliosis, edema, breath cleanser, swollen glands

Systems: Urinary, Endocrine, Muscular

Dosha Affected:

Vata and **Pitta**: Moderation

Kapha: Good

Mixes Well With: Vegetables, proteins, starches

Parsley Tomato Dressing

- ¼ cup parsley, chopped
- 2 teaspoons mustard seeds
- 2 tablespoons olive oil
- 2 tomatoes, sliced
- ½ cut water
- ¼ cup balsamic vinegar
- 1 teaspoon coriander
- ½ cup water

Mix all ingredients in blender until smooth. Serve with salad or steamed vegetables.

Infused Parsley Oil or Vinegar

- 1 quart olive oil
- ½ bunch parsley, chopped medium
- ½ bunch green onions, chopped

Add cut greens and onions to olive oil. Infuse for 3-5 days, shaking daily. Ready to use.

Poppy Seeds

Botanical Name: Papaver somniferum

The Chinese were some of the first people to use poppy seeds, as early as the second century. The Egyptians used them in food flavoring and other preparations. There are many varieties of poppy seed, and one must never use seeds bought from a flower shop.

Energy: Warm

Taste: Pungent/Astringent

Post Digestive: Pungent

Indications: Muscle pain, poor assimilation, cramps, diarrhea, digestion of starches

Systems: Digestive, Excretory

Dosha Affected:

Vata: Good

Pitta: Avoid

Kapha: Good

Mixes Well With: Starches, fruits

Rosemary

Botanical Name: Rosmarinus officinalis

Rosemary is a perennial herb native to the Mediterranean region, and called "Dew of the Sea." The Romans used the garlands to improve their memory, and the herb was used in many festivities and weddings to bring good fortune and fertility. In Europe, this herb is used medicinally far more than any other herb.

Energy: Heating, Drying

Taste: Pungent, Bitter

Post Digestive: Pungent

Indications: Headaches, mental clarity, blood cleanser, flu, cold, asthma, gallstones, liver disorders, joint pain, hair loss, dandruff, dispels phlegm

Systems: All systems

Dosha Affected:

Vata: Small amounts in soup or sauces

Pitta: Moderation

Kapha: Excellent

Mixes Well With: Vegetables, proteins, starches

Rosemary Potatoes

- 3 tablespoons olive oil
- ½ cup fresh rosemary
- 2 teaspoon Bragg's or salt
- 6 medium-size potatoes, cut in half

To make marinade, mix olive oil, rosemary, and salt in blender. Marinate potatoes in this mixture, or baste the potatoes as they bake. Bake at 300° for 35 minutes.

Rosemary Tomato Sauce

Makes 8 ounces

- ¼ cup rosemary, chopped
- 1 cup tomatoes, fresh, chopped
- 1 tablespoon olive oil
- 1/3 cup of lemon juice, fresh
- ½ teaspoon raw honey or sweetener of choice
- ¼ cup water

Place all ingredients in blender until smooth. Use in various recipes.

Saffron

Botanical Name: Crocus sativus

Saffron is one of the most valuable and exquisite spices available in the world. It is the most ancient of all spices of the East, and was introduced to the Egyptians and Romans in 1,500 B.C. The Moors introduced it to Spain in the eighth century, and saffron became known throughout Europe by the twelfth century. Today, it can be found primarily in Spanish and Indian markets, and it is often substituted with turmeric. It is also frequently used as a coloring agent on fine silks. Saffron is one of the most harmonious (Sattvic) of all spices. Used in rice, sauces, and desserts.

Energy: Neutral

Taste: Pungent, Bitter, Sweet

Post Digestive: Sweet

Indications: Nervousness, mental confusion, anemia, chronic back pain, rheumatism, depression, hysteria, meditation, enlarged liver, asthma

Systems: All systems

Dosha Affected:
All doshas good (very Sattvic)

Mixes Well With: Vegetables, starches, grains, dairy

Saffron Yogurt Sauce

- 1 cup plain yogurt
- ½ teaspoon saffron threads
- ⅓ cup sesame oil
- 1 tablespoon lemon juice
- 1 teaspoon agave syrup

Mix all ingredients in blender until smooth. Serve over fruits or salads.

Saffron Drink

- 1 cup milk or nut milk
- 5 threads of saffron
- 1 teaspoon jaggary or maple syrup

Warm milk. Add the saffron. Steep for 15 minutes. Remove Saffron threads. Drink.

Savory

Botanical Name: Satureja hortensis, Satureja montana

Savory is an herb native to the Mediterranean region and used by the Romans to flavor vinegars, as well as being used an aphrodisiac. It was introduced to the new world in colonial times, and is now cultivated primarily in Europe. Today, it is highly used for canned foods, especially sauces and pickles.

Energy: Heating

Taste: Pungent, Bitter

Post Digestive: Pungent

Indications: Hearing loss, abdominal, distension, flatulence, weight loss

Systems: Excretory, Nervous, Digestive

Dosha Affected:

Vata: Good

Pitta: Avoid

Kapha: Good

Mixes Well With: Vegetables, starches, proteins

Tarragon

Botanical Name: Artemisia dracunculus

Tarragon is an herb native to Asia and Northern Europe. It was used in ancient times as a blood cleanser as well as a food preservative. Today, it grows wild and can be used fresh or dried.

Energy: Heating

Taste: Bitter, Pungent

Post Digestive: Pungent

Indications: Digestive aid, parasite, menstrual irregularity, builds female organs, poor circulation, rheumatism

Systems: Reproduction

Dosha Affected:

Vata: Good

Pitta: Moderation (avoid in excess)

Kapha: Good

Mixes Well With: Vegetables, protein, starches

Tarragon Sauce

- ¼ cup fresh tarragon, chopped
- 2 tablespoons yellow mustard
- 1 tablespoon mayonnaise
- ½ tablespoon sunflower oil
- 1 tablespoon lemon juice
- salt to taste

In blender, blend all ingredients together until smooth. Serve on halibut or any other fish.

Savory Sauce

- ½ cup savory
- 1 cup pine nuts
- 1 tablespoon almond oil or vegetable oil of choice
- ½ tablespoon apple cider vinegar
- ½ teaspoon jaggary, honey or maple syrup
- ½ cup water

In blender, place all ingredients together. Blend until smooth. Great with vegetables.

Thyme or Oregano

<u>Botanical Name:</u> *Thymus (various species)*

Thyme is a perennial herb native to the Mediterranean; it grows 4 to 12 inches high. It was used by the Egyptians for embalming and for the preservation of meats. It was also frequently used medicinally in the southern Mediterranean region. Thyme is used in many canned foods, and grows well in home gardens. Many varieties exist of this plant – about 350 different species. Highly antiseptic and anti-bacterial. Useful for fungal infections.

Energy: Heating

Taste: Pungent

Post Digestive: Pungent

Indications: Brackets, flu, whopping cough, cellulite, rheumatism, halitosis, indigestion, flatulence, menstrual cramps, fungus, wounds

Systems: Digestive

<u>Dosha Affected:</u>

Vata: Good

Pitta: Avoid

Kapha: Moderation

Mixes Well With: Vegetables, proteins, starches

Thyme Sauce

- ½ cup green onions, chopped
- 1 tablespoon ghee
- 2 tablespoons thyme
- 2 tomatoes, well chopped
- 1 tablespoon salsa
- 1 cup grated zucchini
- Bragg's to taste

Sauté onions in ghee. Add remaining ingredients, cover pan, and cook for 5 minutes. Serve on vegetables or meat.

Baked Thyme Rice

Serves 4

- ½ cup fresh thyme or 1 tablespoon dry thyme
- 1 tablespoon ghee
- 2 eggs – or 4 tablespoons egg replacer
- 3 tablespoons water
- 2 carrots, chopped in squares
- ½ cup string beans
- 2 cup tofu in cubes
- 1 onion, small
- ½ cup mozzarella cheese, grated
- 1 cup basmati rice, cooked
- 2 cups water
- Salt to taste or Bragg's

Cut carrots, onions, string beans and steam. Remove from heat. Oil baking pan with ghee. Add remaining ingredients and mix well. Place rice and all ingredients in baking pan. Cook for 15 minutes. Then sprinkle with cheese and bake another 5 minutes. Serve with salad.

Turmeric

Botanical Name: Curcuma Longa

A perennial plant native to Indonesia and Malaysia and related to ginger, turmeric was brought to India by early traders. Today, much research has been done with this plant. It is said to relieve cancer and AIDS patients from pain. It also assists in building a healthy immune system whereby the body can start healing itself. In certain seasons, fresh turmeric root (a rhizome) may be bought in supermarkets or in Asian Markets. Probably one of the most common ingredients in Indian and Ayurvedic cooking. A common ingredient in most Indian curries. Can be grated in salad or added to chutneys, vegetable dishes, and rice. Regarded as one of the primary herbs of Ayurveda. In today's market, fresh turmeric is available.

Energy: Warm

Taste: Pungent, Bitter

Post Digestive: Pungent

Indications: Immune builder, reduces tumors or aid to cancer, infections, lymphatic congestion, blood clots, inflamed breasts. Liver cleanser helping with fat metabolism, liver cleanser helping with fat metabolism, Alzheimer's, inflammation

Systems: Immune, Digestive, Nervous

Dosha Affected:

Vata: Good

Pitta: Neutral

Kapha: Good

Mixes well with: Vegetables, all starches

Turmeric Sauce

- 2 tablespoons fresh turmeric (or 1 tablespoon dried)
- 2 tablespoons grated ginger
- 1 sprig fresh mint (or 1 tablespoon dried)
- 1 cup fresh cilantro, chopped
- 2 tablespoons olive oil
- 4 stevia leaves (or drops)
- 1 tablespoon Vata churna or mild curry powder
- lecithin granules (optional)

Blend all ingredients in blender until smooth. This can be used on a daily basis if desired – as a sauce for meats, steamed vegetables, etc.

Yellow Rice & Turmeric

- 3 cups basmati rice, cooked
- 6 cups water
- 1 tablespoon turmeric, fresh, chopped
- 1 tablespoon paprika
- ¼ cup green onions, sliced
- 1 carrot, sliced
- ¼ cup capers
- ½ cup green beans, chopped
- ½ cup cilantro, chopped
- ¼ cup olive oil

Cook rice with water and turmeric. Cook for 15 minutes. Add carrots & green beans. Cover. Lower flame. Simmer. When cooked, add cilantro, olive oil, and capers. Mix well. The rice will be yellow due to the turmeric.

Nuts & Seeds

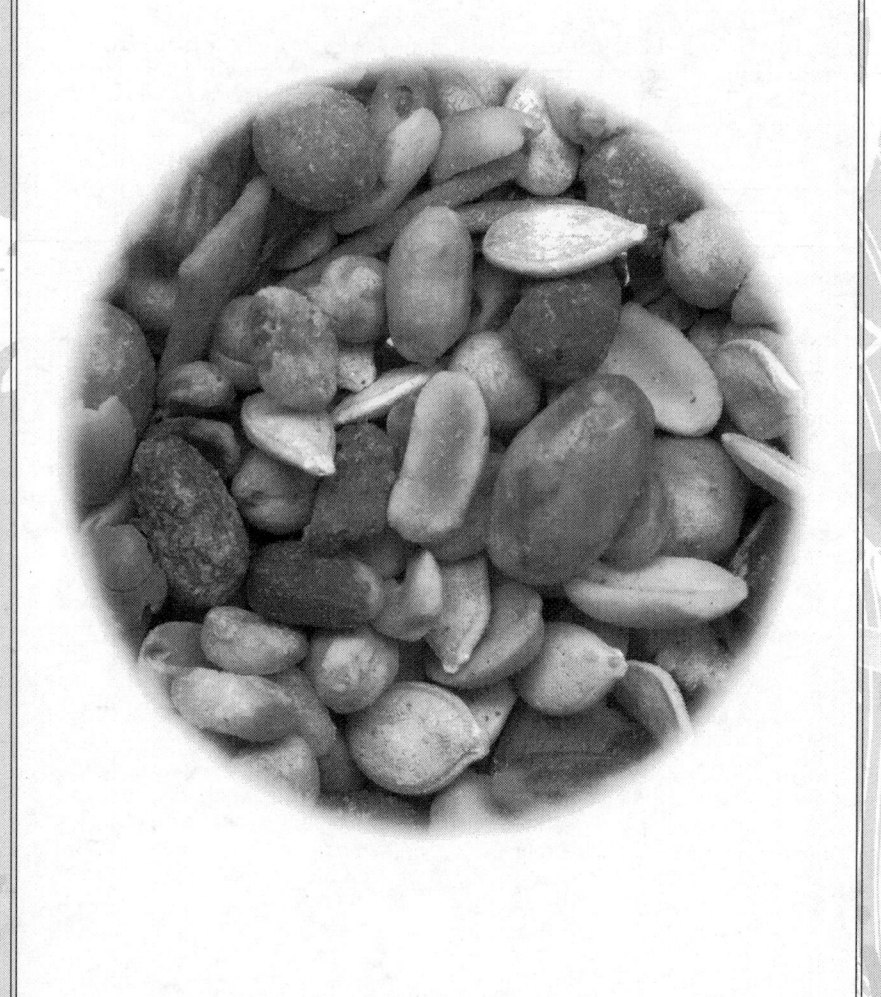

Nuts and Seeds

General Considerations

According to paleontologists, man was a nut eater. Then, as he wandered away from the fruitarian habits to which he was instinctively and physiologically adapted, nuts were discarded and neglected. At the present time, nuts and seeds are given the role of a confection rather than that of the very good staple article of the diet they rightfully deserve.

Normally, nuts have a hard outer shell enclosing a kernel (the nut). The market is flooded with halved, broken, and sliced nuts which more easily turn rancid due to being exposed to oxygen. Therefore, when storing whole nuts, pick out the ones with broken shells and store them in vacuum-sealed glass jars to prevent rancidity.

In nutritive value, nuts are superior to any foodstuffs per pound that we know. According to scientific investigation, the proteins in nuts are superior to those of animal origin.

Nuts are sweet, high in fat and calories. An average nut contains between 3 to 10 grams of protein, 17 to 37 grams of fat, and 8 to 16 grams of carbohydrates. Nuts and seeds, being of plant origin, contain no cholesterol, and are good sources of manganese, potassium, copper, pantothenic acid, iron, and riboflavin.

For vegetarians, nuts are probably the best source of protein and fat available. Normally, they help increase fat, marrow, and nerve tissue. They increase ojas (the essence of immunity) and are excellent for memory and creativity. Nuts are tonic, nutritive, strengthening, and rejuvenative.

Thorough mastication of nuts cannot be underrated. Being a dense, concentrated, and highly nutritious food, it is important that every particle be thoroughly crushed and emulsified before it is swallowed. Even small particles pass through the alimentary canal undigested because of the inability of the digestive fluids to penetrate hard substances. Mastication is a function half forgotten. Insufficient chewing is one of the many causes of indigestion and other digestive disorders. Chewed well and in good combination, nuts should be a prominent part of the daily diet, not as an appetizer. To assist the process of digestion, nuts are best soaked from 5 to 8 hours or overnight, which expands and softens their density and increases the food value.

Nuts can also be made into yogurt or cheese. First soak 1 cup of wheat berries (or barley or rye) in 2 cups of water overnight. Then pour off the water and place the berries in a warm area or thermos for 8 hours (or overnight). This produces a culture called "rejuvelac." For yogurt: grind nuts, add rejuvelac, and allow to culture for 12 hours; then strain off berries. For making cheese: soak this mixture for approximately 24 hours, then strain in cheesecloth or a colander. This firmer substance is called nut cheese.

For those unable to thoroughly chew, nut butter made from fresh raw nuts can be a wonderful dietary supplement. Refrain from nut butters made from roasted, salted nuts, because they are made indigestible by the processing. In reference to feeding nuts to children, finely ground and emulsified nuts have proven to be the very best substitutes for milk when the mother's milk fails and the child is sensitive to cow's milk. Nut milks are excellent with fresh or dry spices added; nut milks may be added to teas, like cream or milk. (See below for recipe to make nut or seed milks.)

The best time to eat nuts and seeds is in the winter, because their energy is warming and moisturizing. They go well with spices such as cardamom, nutmeg, and ginger. They are best to be combined with green leafy vegetables, but they also combine well with acid fruits. It is best not to combine with starches or sugars as the sugar can cause putrification in the warm stomach.

In Ayurveda, nuts are used to strengthen the weak and are added to other natural preparations and formulas for health enhancement.

Dr. J. H. Kellogg has this to say of the superiority of nuts over flesh foods:

   1. Nuts are free from waste products, uric acid, urea, and other tissue wastes which abound in meats.

   2. Nuts are aseptic, free from putrefactive bacteria, and do not readily undergo decay either in the body or outside of it. Meats as found in markets, on the other hand, are practically always in an advanced stage of putrefaction. Ordinary fresh, dried, or salted meats contain from three million to ten times that number of bacteria per ounce, and such meats as hamburger steak often contain more than a billion putrefactive organisms to the ounce. Nuts are clean and sterile.

   3. Nuts are free from trichinae, tapeworm, and other parasites, as well as other infections due to specific organisms. Nuts are in good health when gathered and usually remain so until eaten.

Seeds are generally easier to digest than nuts and are lighter in oil content. What is the difference between Nuts and Seeds? From the Whole Foods Market website: "Botanically speaking, a nut is a dry fruit with a seed that is encased in a hard, woody shell. While all nuts are seeds (the fruit is the seed – think pecans), not all seeds are nuts (the seed can be separated from the fruit and is not one in the same – think pumpkin seeds). Most people think of nuts in culinary terms – a very loose and unrestrictive category that includes any oily kernel that grows inside a shell and is used for food. So, botanically speaking, all nuts are seeds but only those seeds that are produced by plants in the order Fagales are true nuts. Edible true nuts include: walnuts, butternuts, hickory nuts, pecans, chestnuts, hazelnuts and filberts. What about the rest of what we commonly call nuts? While these are seeds, they are not true nuts in the botanical sense because they are not produced by plants within the order Fagales. Culinary nuts include: almonds, pistachios, Brazil nuts, cashews, peanuts, pine nuts and macadamia nuts. Peanuts are not nuts at all, nor do they grow on trees. They are legumes whose curious growth on low vines forces the shell into the ground. Finally, we have a small group of seeds – pumpkin seeds, sesame seeds, sunflower seeds – that are not considered nuts, even in the culinary sense, but are eaten like nuts and used in recipes like nuts."

Nut or Seed "Milk"

1 cup nuts or seeds

6 cups water (divided)

cinnamon, cardamom, nutmeg, or turmeric (great for joints)

1 teaspoon vanilla

agave, honey, maple, or sucanat to taste

1 teaspoon lecithin (optional – to emulsify)

Soak nuts or seeds overnight in 3 cups of water; drain the next day. Put nuts or seed in blender with 3 cups of fresh water, and blend well. Strain through fine mesh strainer or folded piece of cheese cloth (about 9 inches); squeeze well, discard pulp. Put liquid back into blender, add spice, vanilla, sweetener of choice, and lecithin.

To make nut "cream," cut down on the amount of water.

Drink as a milk substitute:

- Sesame Milk
- Sunflower Milk
- Almond Milk
- Coconut Milk
- Hazelnut Milk
- Cashew Milk

Almonds

Botanical Name: Prunus dulcis

The almond tree is native to Africa and Asia. The Old Testament mentions the almond tree seventy-five times. In ancient times, almonds were an important product of commerce and carried from Syria and Israel to Egypt. The Greeks were the first to cultivate this tree, which grows 20 to 30 feet. The almond tree is related to the peach tree, and very sensitive to cold, preferring temperate climates like that of the Mediterranean. It has a beautiful pink and white flower, and an oval fruit with a fibrous green covering which breaks open when mature, leaving a hard beige-brown covering. It is usually opened by machines, exposing the seed. Today, almonds are grown in California, South America, and Australia. The increased production and improved methods of cultivation now make it possible for western society to find this food in the marketplace year-round.

Caution: As of September 2007, "raw" organic almonds purchased in stores are not really raw. All almonds commercially grown in the U.S. (for purchase in North America) are now required by law to be "pasteurized," either by steaming or by fumigation with propylene oxide (a chemical recognized as a probable carcinogen by the EPA, and banned from use on foods in Canada, Mexico, and the European Union). The only way you can be sure that steam rather than the chemical was used, is by buying organic almonds. And these almonds may still be labeled as "raw," but because of the high heat they were treated with, are no longer raw. Conventional almonds have been fumigated and/or steam-treated.

Energy: Warming

Taste: Bitter, Sweet

Post Digestive: Sweet

Indications: Dry cough, increases marrow and semen, strengthens kidneys, reproductive organs

Systems: Circulatory, Reproductive, Respiratory, Endocrine, Nervous

Dosha Affected:

Vata: Excellent

Pitta: Avoid or reduce

Kapha: Moderation

Mixes Well With: Ginger, cinnamon, greens and non-starchy vegetables

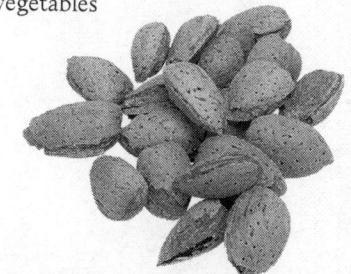

Almond Nut Milk

Makes about 1 quart

- 1 cup raw almonds
- 3 cups water
- 1 teaspoon vanilla
- 1 teaspoon lecithin
- agave syrup (or other sweetener)

Soak almonds over night; drain the next day. Put almonds in blender, and add 3 cups of fresh spring water. Blend until smooth. Pour the almond mixture into a nylon or cheesecloth bag; squeeze liquid out, being careful not to let pulp through. Discard pulp. Pour liquid back into the blender, add vanilla, lecithin, and sweetener to taste. Blend and enjoy.

Variation: use with other nuts or seeds, such as cashews or sesame seeds.

Almond Croquettes

- 1½ cup almonds, well ground
- ½ cup quick oats
- ½ onion, well chopped
- 1 tablespoon ghee or olive oil
- ¼ cup water
- 1 tablespoon nutritional yeast (Kapha only)
- 1 tablespoon lecithin
- 1 teaspoon sage
- 1 teaspoon rosemary

Combine and knead all ingredients, then form into burger-size patties. Sauté in ghee, or bake at 275° for 20 minutes.

Cashews

Botanical Name: Anacardium occidentale

The cashew tree is a native of the Amazon regions, and in the same family as mango, pistachio, and poison ivy. It grows in tropical climates, with the major producers being Brazil, India, and Nigeria. The fleshy fruit, called a cashew "apple" or "pear," is bright orange-red in color, and the nut (actually a seed) grows suspended below the fruit. In Brazil, the fruit is used in beverages and wines. The skin of the fruit can cause blisters and skin rashes. Cashews were once thought to be toxic. Today many people eat "raw" cashews with no problem at all, because they are not really raw. In order to shell them and remove the toxic liquid contained within the shell, they are steamed and/or boiled. Cashew butter is a great source of protein and can be used as a substitute for peanut butter. Used with crackers, vegetables, bread, and salad dressings.

Energy: Warming

Taste: Sweet

Post Digestive: Sweet

Indications: Lung disorders, chronic skin diseases, anemia, impotency

Systems: Reproductive, Circulatory, Respiratory

Dosha Affected:

Vata: Good

Pitta: Moderation (watch for allergies)

Kapha: Avoid

Mixes Well With: Green vegetables, non-starchy vegetables

Cashew Salad Dressing

- 2 tablespoons olive oil
- 1 cup raw cashew pieces
- 1 cup chopped basil
- ¼ bunch cilantro, chopped
- 2 tablespoons lemon juice
- 1 teaspoon coriander
- ½ teaspoon maple syrup
- ½ cup water

Place all ingredients in blender, and mix until smooth. Serve with your choice of salad or vegetables.

Cashew Cream

- 1 cup raw cashews
- ½ cup sunflower oil
- ½ cup almond milk
- 1 teaspoon vanilla
- 2 teaspoons agave syrup or jaggary

Blend cashews in blender on "chop" (low speed). Slowly add sunflower oil, turning speed to "whip" (high speed). Blend until creamy, slowly adding almond milk, vanilla, and sweetener of your choice. Use as a topping on fruit, cookies, or pie.

Cashew Nut Loaf

- 1 bunch green onions, chopped
- 1 clove garlic, finely chopped (Kapha only)
- 2 tablespoons olive oil
- 1 tablespoon ginger, grated
- 3 medium tomatoes, chopped
- 2 cups raw cashews, ground
- 1½ cups freshly made breadcrumbs
- 1 egg, beaten (or egg substitute)
- 1 tablespoon Italian seasoning
- 1 teaspoon black pepper
- 1 teaspoon salt

Sauté onions and garlic in olive oil until translucent. Add ginger and tomatoes. Cook until tomatoes are soft and mushy. Transfer to a mixing bowl; add cashews, breadcrumbs, egg, and seasonings. Mix well. Press into a greased loaf pan, making sure to eliminate any air bubbles. Bake in a pre-heated moderate oven (275°) for 30 to 45 minutes. Use tin foil on top until the last stage of cooking, then remove to brown top of loaf.

Coconut

Botanical Name: Cocos nucifera

The coconut palm is a native of all tropical lands. There is argument as to its origins, whether it was in India, South America, or the Pacific Islands. Today the palm is cultivated and grown wild, producing a smaller coconut which, when ripened, is used for the production of coconut oils and butters. Coconut margarine is a substitute for dairy butter in older countries. Almost all parts of the coconut palm tree are useful; its leaves are used to make ropes, baskets, brushes, carpets, and fabric. The liquid inside the immature coconut is called "coconut water;" it is highly alkaline, sweet, refreshing, and high in minerals. The soft meat – called coconut pudding or coconut jelly – is also nutritious. As the coconut matures, the water is gradually absorbed into the edible meat, which becomes firmer and drier. "Coconut milk" is made by mixing shredded or grated coconut meat with water or milk, and then straining out the pulp.

Energy: Cooling

Taste: Sweet

Post Digestive: Sweet

Indications: Fevers, lung disorders, skin problems, suntanning, infectious diseases

Systems: Respiratory, Circulatory, Urinary Tract (liquid)

Dosha Affected:

Vata: Excellent

Pitta: Good (because of cooling properties)

Kapha: Avoid

Mixes Well With: Green vegetables, non-starchy vegetables

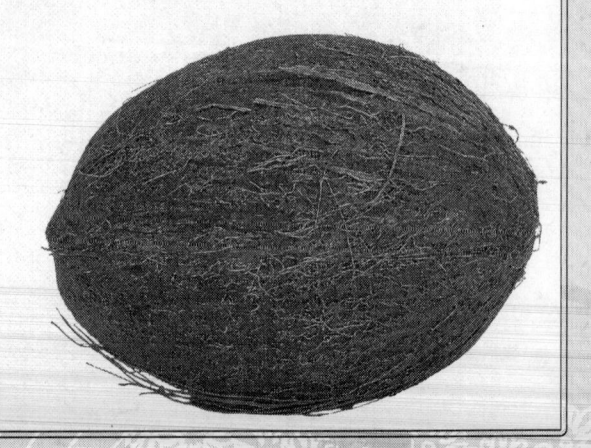

Coconut Custard

Serves 4

- 2 cups coconut milk
- 2 teaspoons cinnamon
- 1/8 cup jaggary or maple syrup
- 4 tablespoons arrowroot or cornstarch

Put coconut milk in a saucepan with cinnamon and jaggary or maple syrup; bring to a boil, stirring quickly and consistently. Lower heat and add arrowroot, stirring quickly until custard thickens. Let cool and refrigerate. Sprinkle top with cardamom.

Note: When using jaggary, it must be grated because it comes in a large cube.

Coquito

Makes about 1½ gallons

- ½ cup raisins
- 2 cups water
- 6 cans (13.5 oz) coconut milk, unsweetened
- 4 egg yolks, well beaten
- 3 teaspoons nutmeg
- 2 teaspoons cinnamon
- 1 teaspoon vanilla
- agave syrup or honey

Soak raisins in 2 cups of water overnight; do not drain. Pour coconut milk into a large bowl, and mix in egg yolks. Add raisins and water they soaked in; then add nutmeg, cinnamon, vanilla, and desired sweetener to taste. Blend in small batches in blender, then refrigerate.

Optional: add rum

Hazelnuts and Filberts

Botanical Name: Corylus (various species)

Hazelnuts and filberts, close cousins, are native to North America, Asia, and Europe. There are approximately 100 different varieties. This nut is even mentioned in the ancient manuscripts of China. The nuts are round or oblong, growing in pairs, and are covered with a foliage membrane.

Energy: Warming
Taste: Sweet, Slightly Bitter
Post Digestive: Sweet
Indications: Alzheimer's, headaches, senility, to gain weight
Systems: Circulatory, Endocrine

Dosha Affected:
Vata: Good
Pitta: Avoid
Kapha: Moderation
Mixes Well With: Green vegetables, non-starchy vegetables

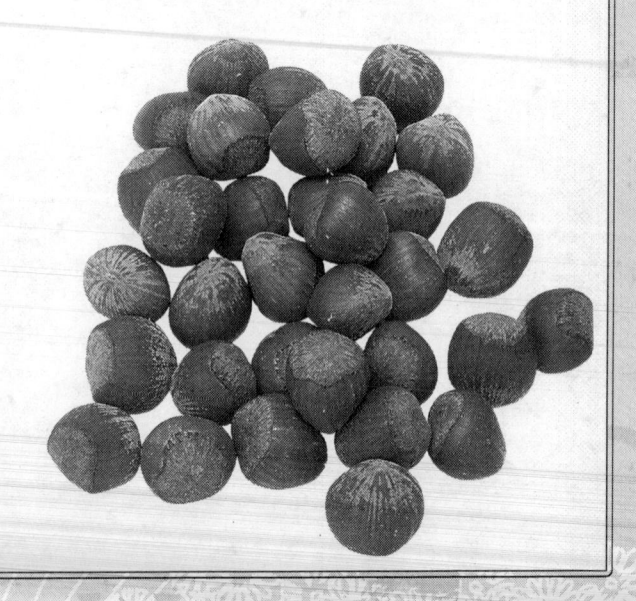

Hazelnut Dressing

- 1 tomato, chopped
- ½ cup hazelnuts
- juice of 1 lemon
- ¼ cup water
- 2 tablespoons sunflower oil
- 2 tablespoons parsley, chopped
- Bragg's to taste

Put all the ingredients in blender; blend until smooth. Serve with your choice of salad or vegetables.

Hazelnut Stuffing with Cranberries

Serves 4

- 1 cup hazelnuts, crushed
- ½ cup cranberries, chopped
- 2 cups bread crutons
- 2 eggs, well beaten – or egg substitute
- ½ cup almond milk
- ½ cup celery, chopped
- ½ onion, chopped
- ½ cup cilantro, chopped
- 1 tablespoon Italian seasoning
- 2 teaspoons sage

In a bowl, mix all ingredients together. Oil baking pan. Preheat oven to 325. Bake for 40 minutes at 325.

This is a good recipe for turkey stuffing.

Pecans

<u>Botanical Name: *Carya illinoensis*</u>

Pecans, a species of hickory tree, are native to south-central North America. The Spaniards brought the pecan into Europe, Asia, and Africa during the 16th century. Pecans were not commercially grown in the U.S. until the late 1800's; now, we produce 80–95% of the world's pecans. Nutritionally, pecans are a good source of protein and unsaturated fats. The antioxidants and plant sterols found in pecans reduce high cholesterol by reducing the "bad" LDL cholesterol levels. Pecans make a nice addition to salads, smoothies, or steamed vegetables.

Energy: Warming

Taste: Sweet

Post Digestive: Sweet

Indications: Nerve disorders, muscular debility, to gain weight

Systems: Nervous, Muscular, Endocrine

Dosha Affected:

Vata: Excellent

Pitta: Moderation

Kapha: Avoid

Mixes Well With: Green vegetables, non-starchy vegetables

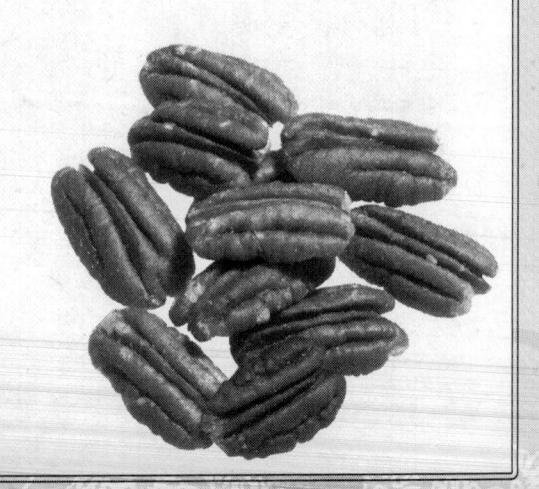

Pecan Salad Dressing

- 1 cup sunflower oil
- 1 cup pecans
- 2 tablespoons coriander, ground
- 1/3 cup balsamic vinegar (Pitta – omit)
- 2 lemons, freshly juiced (Pitta – use limes)
- 1/2 bunch basil or cilantro
- 1/4 teaspoon honey
- 3/4 cup water
- Bragg's to taste

Place all ingredients in blender, mix until smooth. Serve with your choice of salad or vegetables.

Pecan Balls

Serves 4

- 2 cups pecans, ground
- 3 tablespoons sunflower oil
- 1/4 cup carrots, grated
- 1 tablespoon nutritional yeast
- 1 cup green onions, chopped
- 1 cup cilantro, well chopped
- 1 cup dry coconut
- 2 teaspoons Vata, Pitta, or Kapha churna
- Salt to taste

Mix all ingredients together, except coconut. Mix well. Roll into balls. Roll each one of them into coconut. Serve with salad.

Pine Nuts

Botanical Name: Pinus (various species)

Also known as pignolias or pinōns, pine nuts are the seeds of various pine trees. These pines are native to southern Europe and found today in the U.S., Siberia, Australia, and Mexico. The bible mentions the pine nut and its attributes. This nut is quite expensive as hand harvesting is required, and because it takes 25 years for the tree to bear fruit and 50 more years before they can be harvested for commercial sales. Pine nuts are covered with a hard shell, elongated, creamy in color, with an average length of one-half inch. They are considered sattvic in nature and are highly nutritious.

Energy: Warming

Taste: Sweet

Post Digestive: Sweet

Indications: Anemia, female tonic, convalescence, lung tonic

Systems: Respiratory, Circulatory, Reproductive

Dosha Affected:

Vata: Excellent

Pitta and **Kapha**: Moderation

Mixes Well With: Green vegetables, non-starchy vegetables

Pine Nut Eggplant Bites

Serves 6

2 eggplants

1 cup olive oil

½ cup balsamic vinegar

1 teaspoon agave syrup

1 tablespoon Bragg's

½ cup basil, finely chopped

1 cup pine nuts, ground

½ cup pecans, ground

½ cup parsley, finely chopped

½ bunch basil, finely chopped

1 tablespoon Italian seasoning

Cut eggplants lengthwise into very thin slices, and place in a flat baking dish. Marinate overnight in a mixture of oil, vinegar, agave, and Bragg's. The next day, bake at 250° for 30 minutes. (This step is optional for those who want a raw dish.) Put ground nuts, parsley, basil, and Italian seasoning into a bowl. Remove eggplant slices from marinade, and place on a paper towel to absorb extra moisture. Pour the marinade into the nut mixture, and stir well. Put a tablespoonful of this filling on each eggplant slice, and roll up like a jellyroll. Serve with salad.

Pumpkin Seed

<u>Botanical Name: *Cucurbita (various species)*</u>

There are as many varieties of seeds as there are varieties of squash. The seeds of gourds are all highly nutritious and are best roasted, but may also be eaten raw. Pumpkin seeds, sometimes referred to as pepitas, are anti-parasitical, and especially good for expelling worms. They have also been shown to be supportive of prostate health. They can be eaten raw or lightly toasted as a snack. Pumpkin seeds can be grounded and added to salads. They are very high in zinc. They make an excellent butter.

Energy: Warming

Taste: Sweet, Astringent

Post Digestive: Sweet

Indications: Blood tonic, edema, excess sweating, inflammations, worms, excess Kapha, prostate cancer

Systems: Excretory, Digestive, Urinary, reproductive

<u>Dosha Affected:</u>

Vata: Moderation (due to its lightness)

Pitta and **Kapha**: Good

Mixes Well With: Green vegetables, non-starchy vegetables

Pumpkin Seed Squares

- 1 cup raisins
- 1 cup dried figs
- 3 cups water
- 2 cups pumpkin seeds
- 1 cup apple juice
- 1 teaspoon jaggary or sucanat
- 1 teaspoon agave syrup
- 1 teaspoon salt
- 2 teaspoons cinnamon
- 1 teaspoon nutmeg
- ¼ cup shredded coconut

Soak raisins and figs in water overnight. Grind pumpkin seeds into a powder in a food processor, and pour into bowl. Mix raisins, figs, water, and apple juice in blender (into a paste), then add to ground seeds. Add sweeteners, salt, and spices. Oil a square pan, spread out the pumpkin mixture, and sprinkle coconut on top. Place in the refrigerator for 20 minutes. Cut into squares before serving.

Pumpkin Seed Salad Dressing

- 1 cup pumpkin seeds (raw)
- 2 tablespoons olive oil
- ½ cup water
- 1 clove garlic (for Kapha)
- ½ tablespoon fresh ginger, chopped
- 1 tablespoon coriander
- ¼ cup cilantro
- ¼ cup lemon juice
- ¼ teaspoon raw honey
- 1 tablespoon Bragg's

Place all ingredients in blender, mix until smooth. Serve with your choice of salad or vegetables.

Sesame Seeds

<u>Botanical Name:</u> *Sesamum indicum*

Sesame is a tropical herb native to Asia, Africa, Palestine, and Syria. Sesame was introduced to America by the African slaves. Today, it is primarily cultivated in India, China, and Mexico. It grows as a thick bushy plant averaging two feet in height, with pink flowers from which the pods develop. When mature, the pods burst open. ("Open sesame," the famous phrase from the Arabian Nights, reflects this distinguishing feature of the sesame seedpod.) The seeds can be white, yellow, reddish, cream, or black in color. Sesame seeds are one of the oldest foods known to man, and a staple for many ancient people. The seeds are a commonly used food in Ayurvedic medicine; they are one of the first condiments and the first plant used as an edible oil. Ground sesame seeds make a butter called tahini in the Middle East. Sesame seeds are one of the highest sources of calcium available; one teaspoon of sesame seeds equals more calcium than a glass of milk. Sesame is known for its rejuvenative properties.

Energy: Warming

Taste: Sweet

Post Digestive: Sweet

Indications: Dry skin, digestion, liver/gall bladder disorders, nutritive (high in vitamin E), tonifies blood, constipation, bone disorders (high in calcium), anorexia, hemorrhoids

Systems: Good for all tissues and systems

Dosha Affected:

Vata: Excellent

Pitta: Avoid

Kapha: Avoid

Mixes Well With: Green vegetables, non-starchy vegetables, legumes

Sesame Dressing

- 1 cup sesame seeds (soaked overnight)
- 2 tablespoons sesame oil
- ¼ sweet onion, chopped
- ½ tablespoon fresh ginger, chopped
- 2 tomatoes, chopped
- 2 tablespoons coriander, ground
- ¼ cup balsamic vinegar
- ½ teaspoon sucanat or jaggary
- ½ cup water

Place all ingredients in blender, mix until smooth. Serve with your choice of salad or vegetables.

Joy Balls

- 1 cup raw almonds
- ½ cup sesame seeds
- 1 cup raw cashews or sunflower seeds
- 1 cup sesame seeds
- 1 cup shredded coconut, (divided) unsweetened
- ½ cup carob powder
- ½ cup honey

Grind nuts and seeds to a powder. Place in a bowl, and add all remaining ingredients – except for ½ cup coconut (to be set aside). Mix well. Form into 1-inch balls (or use a small ice cream scoop). Roll each ball in the coconut. They should look like snowballs.

Sunflower Seeds

Botanical Name: Helianthus annuus

Sunflowers are an annual plant native to the Americas, and believed to be one of the first cultivated crops in the U. S. Sunflowers were brought to Europe in the 15th century by the Spaniards. Ancient people cultivated the plant for over 5,000 years because of its nutritional properties. This plant is of great importance because of the oil that is produced in Argentina, France, China, and the U.S. Sunflower seeds are high in vitamin E, vitamin B-1, and many minerals. They may be purchased in the shell or shelled, and eaten roasted, raw, or sprouted. Since raw sunflower seeds have a high fat content and are prone to rancidity, it is best to store them in an airtight container in the refrigerator or freezer. To sprout sunflower seeds for use as salad greens, use raw seeds still in the shell.

Energy: Cooling

Taste: Sweet, Bitter

Post Digestive: Sweet

Indications: Nail growth, strengthens bones, diabetes, fevers, infectious diseases, lymphoedema, boils and carbuncles, inflammations

Systems: All systems

Dosha Affected:

Good for all doshas, especially Pittas

Mixes Well With: Green vegetables, non-starchy vegetables

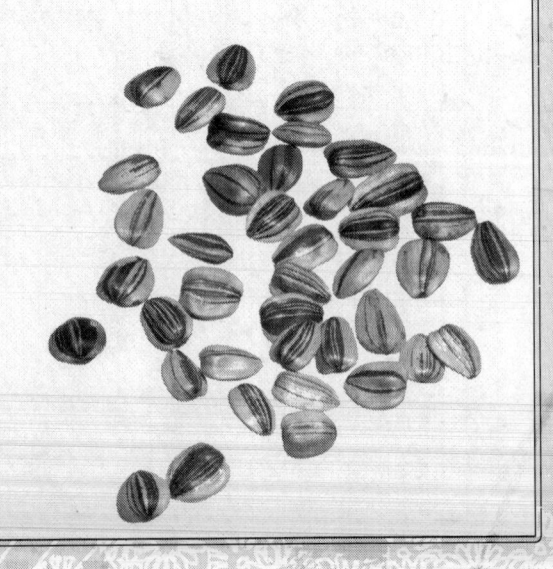

Sunflower Seed Dressing

- 1 cup raw sunflower seeds (soaked overnight)
- ½ cup cilantro
- ½ cup sunflower oil
- ¼ cup lime juice
- 1 teaspoon coriander, ground
- 1 teaspoon fennel, ground
- ½ cup water

Place all ingredients in blender, and mix until smooth. Serve with your choice of salad or vegetables.

Roasted Nuts & Seeds

Makes 1 pound

- 1 cup ginger, fresh, well chopped
- 2 cups sunflower seeds -OR other nuts or seeds
- 1 tablespoon Bragg's aminos or salt

Spread all seeds and ginger into a large baking pan. Sprinkle with Bragg's amino liquid – or salt to taste. Mix well.

Bake at 350 for 20-30 minutes. Every so often, stir seeds around in pan.

Walnuts

Botanical Name: *Juglans regia, Juglans nigra*

Walnut trees are native to Northern India and were introduced in Europe by the Romans in the 4th century to the Americas by the 17th century. Today, many varieties of walnuts are cultivated around the world: the most common edible species are English or Persian walnuts (J. regia) and black walnuts (J. nigra). Butternut (J. cinerea) is an edible type of walnut as well. In California, there are trees that are over 150 years of age, and some have lived for as long as 300 to 400 years. The hulls of the nuts are used as an anti-parasitical, and the leaves are good for skin sores. The walnut is regarded as a sacred tree.

Energy: Warming

Taste: Sweet

Post Digestive: Sweet

Indications: Sexual stimulant, constipation, nerve disorders, infertility, parasites, leukorrhea, open sores, diabetes, vision

Systems: Excretory, Reproductive, Nervous, Circulatory

Dosha Affected:

Vata: Excellent

Pitta and **Kapha**: Avoid

Mixes Well With: Green vegetables, non-starchy vegetables

Walnut Loaf

Serves 4

2 cups ground walnuts

½ cup grated zucchini

1 cup green onions, chopped

1 cup parsley, finely chopped

1 tablespoon Italian seasoning

1 tablespoon fennel

1 teaspoon sage

2 tablespoons sesame tahini

2 tablespoons walnut oil

½ cup tomato sauce

1 tablespoon Bragg's

Put walnuts in a large bowl, and mix in zucchini, green onions, parsley, and seasonings. Add tahini, oil, and tomato sauce, mixing well. Add Bragg's as you begin to mold mixture into a loaf. Refrigerate loaf to firm it up. Serve with salad or steamed vegetables.

Ayurvedic Curative Cuisine for Everyone

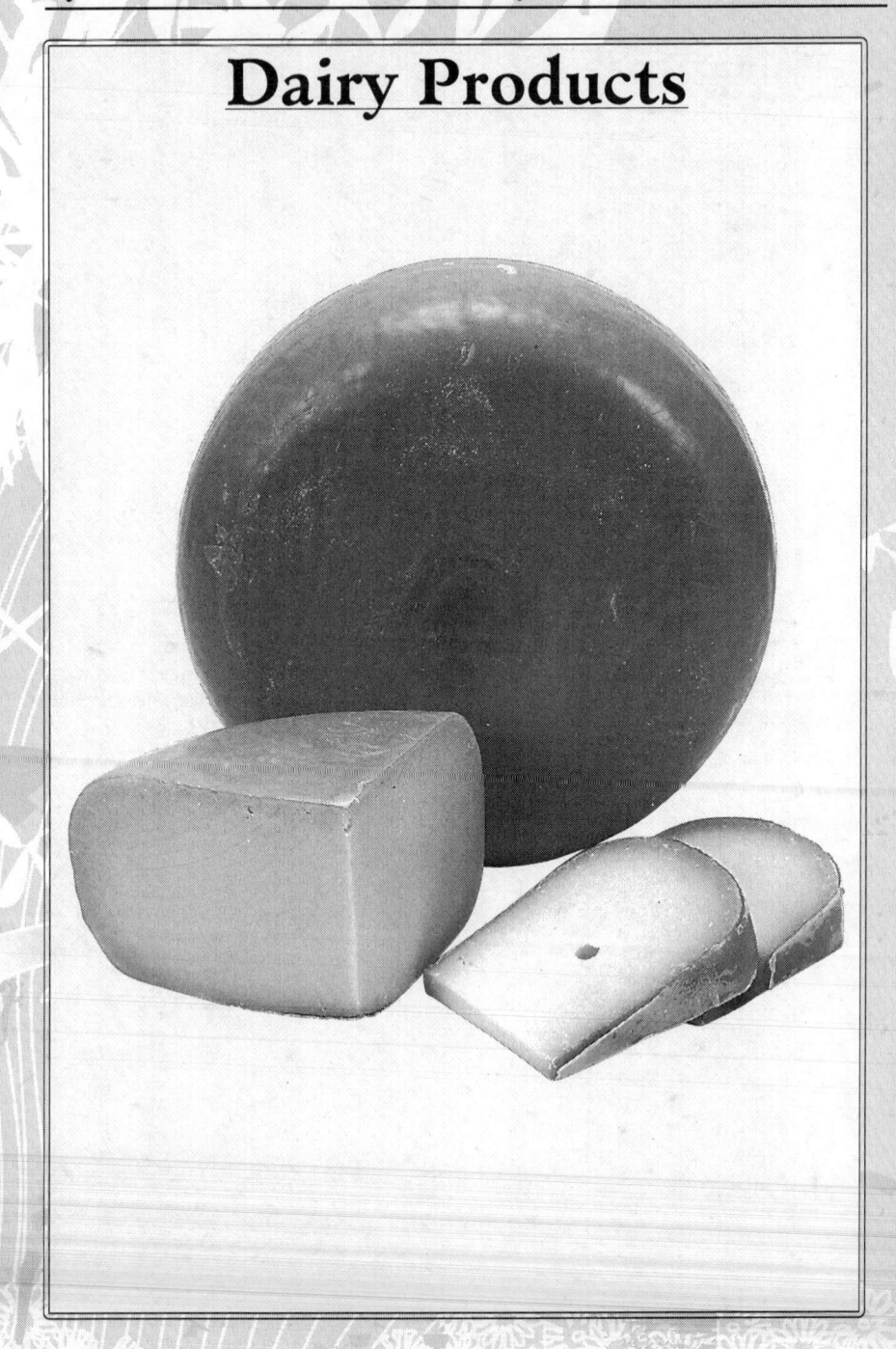

Dairy Products

Dairy Products

General Considerations

In Ayurveda, the use of dairy is considered Sattvic. In India, the quality of milk is good, because cows are considered sacred and loved. The milk is purchased fresh, then brought to a boil and served immediately or used to make yogurt.

In the west, the quality of milk is very poor due to the conditions under which cattle are raised. They live in crowded conditions, are fed grains and hormones to increase production, and often need antibiotics to stay disease. These drugs show up in the milk and, therefore, affect us. Cow's milk is the most common variety of milk in this country, but in many other countries, milk is obtained from buffalo, sheep, and goats.

The ability to digest lactose (the sugar found in milk) after early childhood, is a genetic adaptation among milk-consuming populations. Asians, Africans, and African-Americans generally have some difficulty digesting lactose as well as do people from the Middle East and Northern Africa. Lactose intolerance is caused by a deficiency in lactase, a digestive enzyme that transforms lactose into a glucose which can be absorbed through the intestines. Within two hours of consuming milk, those with a lactose intolerance experience symptoms of bloatedness, abdominal pain, diarrhea, flatulence, nausea, and sinus problems.

The above symptoms are rarely associated with the consumption of yogurt or aged cheeses, because the lactose in yogurt is decomposed or hydrolyzed and there is little or no lactose in cheese. Cottage cheese, cream cheese and cheese spreads, however, do contain a certain amount of lactose and may provoke some symptoms.

It appears that whole milk is harder to digest than skim milk. Most lactose intolerant adults can digest milk from which 50% of the lactose has been removed, and it is possible to buy dairy products that contain only 10% of the lactose normally found in milk.

All dairy is made from milk; therefore, most of the quality of our dairy consumption is loaded with pesticides and hormones fed to the cows. The excessive use of hormone treatment stimulates growth, resulting in products getting to the market faster.

Most dairy is best ingested while warm or at room temperature. When buying dairy products, make sure they're from animals that eat organic feed and are free of antibiotics and hormones.

Types of Milk

Pasteurized: This process was named for its inventor, the famous French chemist and microbiologist, Louis Pasteur. Milk is heated to a temperature below the boiling point, then rapidly chilled, thereby destroying most of the pathogenic bacteria and extending the shelf life. This process also destroys some of the nutritional value and produces a milk which causes more mucous in the body.

Ultra-pasteurized: This process uses even higher temperatures to pasteurize the milk, in order to extend the shelf life. Boxed milk (and even some organic milk) is ultra-pasteurized, and has a shelf life of 6 to 9 months. While this process makes milk available to people who do not have access to fresh milk, it is not advisable for daily consumption.

Homogenized: This means that the fat content has been whipped into tiny particles which remain suspended in the liquid. The cream remains in the milk in tiny globules instead of rising to the top. Some researchers think that homogenization makes the fat harder to digest and may cause arteriosclerosis and hormone imbalance.

Raw: This is untreated milk. It is illegal to sell raw milk in many of the United States, Canada, and numerous European countries, because it is regarded as a health risk. Raw milk can easily become contaminated and drinking it can cause illnesses such as tuberculosis and salmonella (food poisoning). In areas where it is legal, it is usually found in health food stores. Healthy animals generally produce healthy milk. Sanitary dairy conditions and handling prevent contamination.

Whole: This milk contains 3.25% to 3.7% fat, and may be homogenized or not. Whole milk is fortified with vitamin D (by law).

Lowfat or Partially Skimmed Milk: This milk contains 1% to 2% fat and tastes slightly less rich than whole milk. It has comparable nutritional value as whole milk but contains less fat and calories. Extra vitamins A and D are added to lowfat milk.

Nonfat or Skim Milk: This milk contains no more than 0.3% fat. Vitamins A and D are added to compensate for lost nutrients when the fat is removed.

Buttermilk: Nonfat or low fat milk with added bacteria that provide a tangy-sour flavor. It is slightly thicker than whole milk.

Acidophilus Milk: This is whole, lowfat, or nonfat milk containing lactobacillus acidophilus – bacteria that benefit the digestive system.

All Milk

Energy: Cooling

Taste: Sweet

Post Digestive: Sweet

Indications: Rejuvenative, builds bones, builds muscle, dry cough, fever, thirst, immune builder, laxative, dizziness, weak mind, tuberculosis, anemia, fatigue, tiredness, hemorrhoids, urinary tract, infections

Systems: All systems

Dosha Affected:

Good for all doshas (small amounts for Kapha)

Mixes Well With: Milk should be taken alone; sometimes with spices

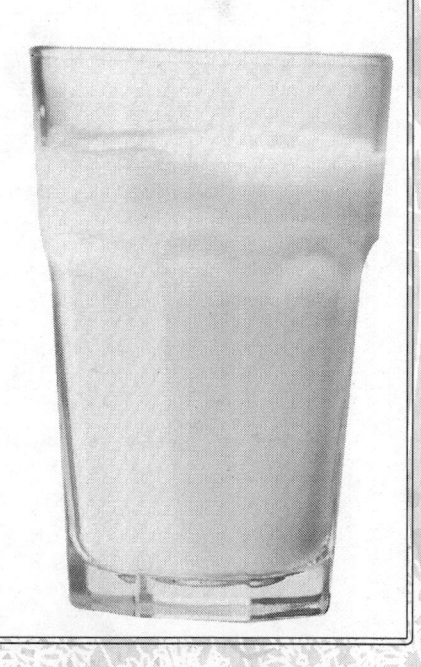

Ayurvedic Curative Cuisine for Everyone

Paneer
(Recipe provided by the Chopra Center for Wellbeing)

yields about 2 cups

Prep Time: 20 minutes to make cheese; 2 hours to compress; 20 minutes to fry

- 2 quarts whole milk
- ¼ cup lemon juice
- olive oil for sautéing

Heat milk in large, deep pot over medium-high heat. As soon as it reaches a full boil and foams up, remove from heat and stir in lemon juice. Milk will split into curds and whey. Pour contents of pot into cheesecloth or dishtowel placed inside a colander. When cool enough to handle, gently twist cloth to squeeze out most of the liquid. Scrape milk solids together into ball. Keeping it wrapped in cloth, flatten ball into ½-inch disc and set on a cookie sheet. Place heavy pan partially filled with water (2 to 3 pounds) on top of disc. Let stand for 2 hours at room temperature until cheese becomes a flat slab. In a wok or deep saucepan, heat oil to 350°. While oil heats, unwrap slab and cut into roughly ½-inch square cubes. Sauté the cheese cubes, half at a time in oil, until light golden. Remove with a slotted spoon to paper towels to drain any excess oil.

Longevity Shake

Serves 2

- 2 cups milk of your choice – or fruit or Vegetable juice
- 1 teaspoon ashwagandha
- ½ tablespoon spirulina
- ½ tablespoon bhrami
- ¼ teaspoon cinnamon
- ¼ thumb size, fresh ginger, chopped
- ¼ teaspoon cardamom

Place all ingredients in blender until smooth. Drink.

Butter

This is produced by churning cream and is a smooth, fatty substance. Churning causes the fat in the cream to separate from the liquid (known as buttermilk). Before it can be churned, the cream has to be separated from the milk, because the fat is the only part of the milk that can be made into butter. Butter is usually made from cow's milk but can be made from the milk of other mammals. It takes about 10 quarts of milk to make 1 pound of butter. The word "butter" also refers to creamy, fatty substances derived from a variety of sources with the names of these butters specifying the source, such as peanut butter, almond butter, cocoa butter, etc. In ancient times, butter was used in religious ceremonies and as a medication – such as applying a plaster to an infection or burned skin. The ancient Romans and Greeks rarely cooked with butter; however, they did use it medicinally. Today, North African and Arab cooks rely on a type of clarified butter (called smen or smeun), which fares much better than regular butter in hot climates. When purchasing, be aware that artificial coloring and salt are added to some brands of butter.

Energy: Sweet

Taste: Cold

Post Digestive: Sweet

Indications: Burns, nourishes all tissues, extreme Vata, weight loss

Systems: All systems are nourished

Dosha Affected:

Vata and **Pitta**: Good

Kapha: Avoid

Mixes Well With: Grains, vegetables

Buttermilk

This milk is a whitish, slightly sour-tasting liquid which separates from cream during the production of butter. Somewhat creamy, buttermilk separates into two layers when left undisturbed. The relatively light top layer is comprised of lactoserum, and the bottom layer consists of fine lumps of coagulated casein. The buttermilk sold today is not a by-product of the traditional butter-making process but, instead, is made by adding a bacterial culture to skim, or partially skim, milk. In chemistry, it is the closest type of cow's milk to human milk.

Energy: Warm

Taste: Sour, Astringent

Post Digestive: Sour

Indications: Digestive aid, and same indications as for milk

Systems: All systems

Dosha Affected:

Vata: Good

Pitta: Avoid

Kapha: Moderation

Mixes Well With: Eat alone

Buttermilk Salad Dressing

- 1 cup buttermilk
- 2 teaspoons fennel, ground
- 2 tablespoons olive oil
- 1 teaspoon mustard seed
- 1/8 cup lemon juice
- 1 teaspoon ginger, grated
- 1 teaspoon agave syrup

Place all ingredients in blender, mix until smooth. Serve with your choice of salad or vegetables.

Buttermilk Pancakes

- 1 ½ cups buttermilk
- 1 cup barley flour
- 1 cup pastry flour
- 2 eggs – OR ½ cup of egg substitute
- 2 tablespoons maple syrup
- 2 tablespoons ghee
- 2 teaspoons vanilla
- 1 teaspoon salt

In a large bowl, beat eggs with 1 tablespoon ghee. Add remaining ingredients and beat until batter is smooth. Using a skillet or griddle on medium heat, add 1 tablespoon ghee. Pour a small amount of batter to make each pancake. When pancake begins to bubble, turn to the other side. Continue with remaining batter.

Cheese

Cheese is known to be mucous-forming in the body, more so than any other dairy product, and tends to clog the channels, especially if not digested well. Raw cheeses may be better for you.

Energy: Warming
Taste: Sweet
Post Digestive: Sweet
Indications: Same as milk
Systems: Same as milk

Dosha Affected:
Vata: Good
Pitta and **Kapha**: Avoid
Mixes Well With: Salads

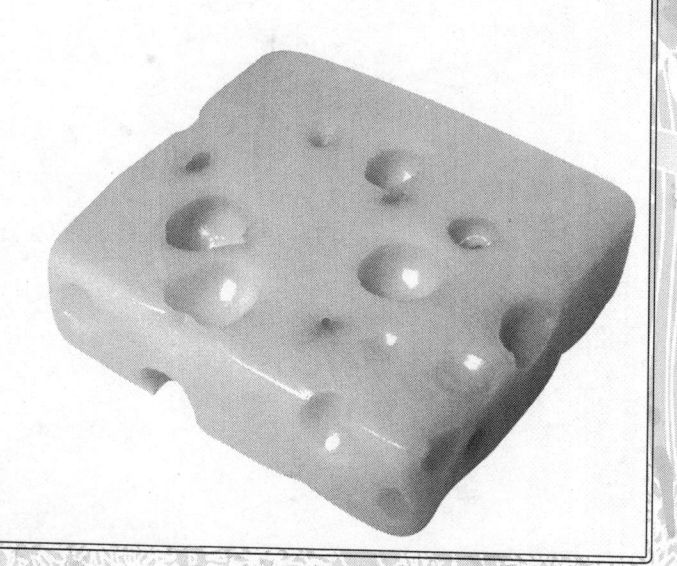

Cheese Blintzes

- 1 cup ricotta cheese
- ½ cup chives, well chopped
- 1 teaspoon coriander, ground
- 1 cup pastry flour
- ¼ teaspoon baking powder (aluminum-free)
- 2 eggs, well beaten
- 2 teaspoon agave syrup
- 3 cups water
- 2 tablespoons ghee

Mix chives and coriander into the ricotta cheese; set aside. In another bowl, mix flour and baking powder together; add eggs and agave, then water, and mix until smooth. Heat ghee in a skillet. Scooping batter with a ladle, make very thin pancakes. Stuff each pancake with a spoonful of cheese mixture, roll up, and add your favorite sauce.

Spinach-Mozzarella Sauce

- 2 cups steamed spinach
- 2 tablespoons olive oil
- ¼ lb. mozzarella cheese
- ½ onion, chopped
- 1 tablespoon curry powder
- ½ tablespoon cumin
- 1 tablespoon Bragg's

Place all ingredients in blender, mix until smooth. Serve on vegetables, proteins, grains.

Cottage Cheese

This is a fresh cheese with very low heat applied to it. Cottage cheese is milder and is easier to digest than other cheeses, because it is not fermented; it also has a shorter life span.

Energy: Cooling

Taste: Sweet

Post Digestive: Sweet

Indications: Rejuvenative, strong bones, dry cough, fever, thirst, immune builder, laxative, dizziness, weak mind, tuberculosis, anemia, fatigue, tiredness, hemorrhoids, urinary tract infections

Systems: All systems

Dosha Affected:
Good for all doshas

Mixes Well With: Fruit, salads

Cottage Cheese Supreme

Serves 2

- 8 ounces cottage cheese
- ¼ cup pineapple chunks
- 1-2 tangerines, peeled and sectioned
- 1 cup sunflower seeds, ground
- ¼ cup fresh mint, chopped
- ¼ cup cilantro, chopped

Place cottage cheese in bowl. Add pineapple chunks and tangerine sections; then add sunflower seeds, mint, and cilantro. Mix all ingredients and serve.

Cream

Cream is very much like milk, only heavier and richer with a higher fat content.

Energy: Cooling
Taste: Sweet
Post Digestive: Sweet
Indications: Rejuvenative, strong bones, dry cough, fever, thirst, immune builder, laxative, dizziness, weak mind, tuberculosis, anemia, fatigue, tiredness, hemorrhoids, urinary tract infections
Systems: All systems

Dosha Affected:
Good for all doshas
Mixes Well With: Should be taken alone

Cream Cheese

Cream cheese has similar properties to milk, yet is harder to digest.

Energy: Cooling
Taste: Sweet
Post Digestive: Sweet
Indications: Rejuvenative, builds bones, builds muscle, dry cough, fever, thirst, immune builder, laxative, dizziness, weak mind, tuberculosis, anemia, fatigue, hemorrhoids, urinary tract infections
Systems:
Vata: Moderation
Pitta: Good
Kapha: Avoid

Dosha Affected:
Good for all doshas (in small amounts for Kapha)
Mixes Well With: Green leafy vegetables; avoid using in rich foods.

Cream Cheese Celery

- ¼ lb. cream cheese
- ½ cup chives, finely cut
- ½ cup cilantro, chopped
- 2 tablespoons mild salsa
- 6 stalks celery, cut in 6-inch pieces

Mash cream cheese in a bowl, then add chives, cilantro, and salsa. Spread mixture in celery sticks.

Curried Cream Cheese & Herbs

Makes 10 ounces

- 1 (8 oz.) cream cheese
- 1/3 cup heavy cream
- 1 tablespoon mild curry – or Vata, Pitta, or Kapha churna
- 2 teaspoons coriander
- ¼ cup basil, fresh, well chopped
- 1/3 cup water

Place all ingredients in blender. Blend on low, then liquefy. Serve over vegetables or as a spread on crackers or bread.

Eggs

Eggs are high in protein and cholesterol but contain lecithin, which allows for the metabolism of the cholesterol. They are treated as a high protein. Modern industrial farm production often uses feeds with pesticides, antibiotics, and occasional hormone additives. The chickens are caged and de-beaked, and their eggs concentrate the chemicals that they are fed. Natural eggs from free-range chickens that are fed organic grain and greens would be the ideal. For karmic considerations, unfertilized eggs don't mean taking a life; however, some experts feel the fertilized eggs contain more life force and nutrients. Tough call! Eggs are less Tamasic than meat.

Energy: Warming

Taste: Sweet

Post Digestive: Sweet

Indications: Infertility, convalescence, weight loss

Systems: Reproductive, Immune, Muscular, Skeleton

Dosha Affected:

Vata: Excellent

Pitta: Moderation (egg white is best)

Kapha: Moderation

Mixes Well With: Vegetables, starches, proteins

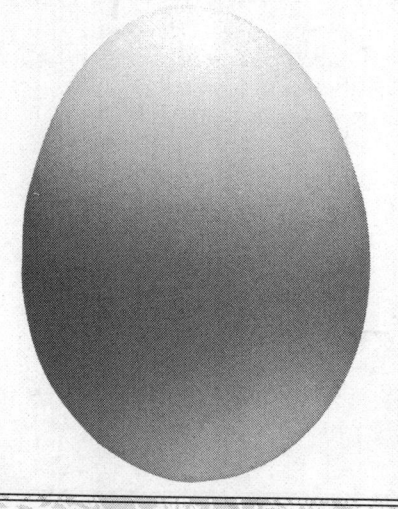

Eggs of the Sea

- 3 cups water
- 1 tablespoon vinegar
- 4 eggs
- 1 teaspoon ghee
- 1 sheet nori,
  cut into small pieces and softened with several teaspoons of hot water

In a saucepan, bring water and vinegar to a boil. Crack open eggs, and slowly drop into water to poach. Remove from water, place on plate, place ghee and nori on top, and serve. Season to taste.

Vanilla Flan

Makes 8

- 4 egg yolks, well beaten
- 2 ½ cups arrowroot or cornstarch
- 2 cups raw sugar
- 1 teaspoon agave or maple syrup
- 1 teaspoon vanilla
- 3 cups half-and-half, organic
- 2 cups water

Mix together egg yolks, sugar, milk, and vanilla. Whip in the arrowroot. Using custard cups, place some agave (or maple syrup) in bottom of each cup. Pour mixture onto the agave. Place the custard cups in a large baking dish holding 2 cups water on bottom. Bake at 400 for 35-45 minutes.

Ghee

Ghee is butter that has been clarified and purified. There are many ways to make ghee; we suggest one way below. Ghee does not need refrigeration. In cooking, ghee does not burn like butter or other oils. For some people, the taste may take getting used to, and for others it is immediately enjoyed. The aroma and flavor is exquisite. It is used in Ayurveda as a remover of toxins. Ghee is highly nutritious and is used in India as a vehicle for many herbal medications. Very Sattvic in nature, ghee is one of the best foods for human consumption.

Energy: Cooling

Taste: Sweet

Post Digestive: Sweet

Indications: Dryness in the body, makes skin glow, bone tonic, muscular pain in joints, mental disorder, tonic to the liver/spleen/kidney, clear vision

Systems: All systems

Dosha Affected:
Good for all doshas

Mixes Well With: Vegetables, starches

Home Preparation of Ghee

Ghee is easy to make and rather than buying expensive prepared products, it's always more empowering to make your own ghee. In the West, convenience is everything. But ancient wisdom says the more involvement you have in your own healing or food preparation, the more beneficial that healing or that food will be for you. So the ghee you make yourself will have your personal energetics added to it, and will be much more helpful and healing to you than the ghee you buy. It is best to make ghee with unsalted butter, although the salt will, to a large extent be removed, if you do not have unsalted butter available. Into a large pot or skillet, slowly melt one pound of unsalted butter. Bring it to a light boil and a white foamy material will rise to the surface, which you can scoop off with a spoon or ladle and set to the side. Continue for about fifteen minutes until the liquid becomes clear. The foam can be discarded and, after it is a little cooler, the golden liquid in the pan can be strained through a cheesecloth into a jar. As it cools, it will become more firm. The milk solids in the bottom of the pan should be discarded.

Goat's Milk (and Cheese)

Goat's milk is whiter than cow's milk, has a stronger taste, and contains slightly less cholesterol. It has been consumed by humans since prehistoric times. Unlike cow's milk, it does not have to be homogenized because its fat globules, which are very small in diameter, tend to remain suspended in the milk. Goat's milk is easier to digest because it contains more short-chain fatty acids than cow's milk. This milk is rich in potassium, calcium, phosphorous, vitamin A, magnesium, niacin, pantothenic acid, thiamin, zinc, vitamin B-12, vitamin B-6, and copper, and is a good source of riboflavin. It is more similar to human milk than cow's milk, and often tolerated better by babies or those allergic to cow's milk.

Energy: Warm

Taste: Sweet

Post Digestive: Sweet

Indications: Same as milk

Systems: All systems

Dosha Affected:

Vata: Good

Pitta: Avoid

Kapha: Moderation

Mixes Well With: Best to use by itself

Goat Cheese Quesadilla

1 tablespoon ghee
8 tortillas
1 lb. firm goat cheese, grated
½ cup black olives, finely chopped
1 avocado, thinly sliced
¼ cup salsa
1 cup cilantro, well chopped

In a skillet, melt small amount of ghee and warm tortillas one at time. Sprinkle cheese and olives on each tortilla, fold in half, press with a spatula, and flip over to warm other side. Keep finished quesadillas warm while making the others. Top with avocado, salsa, and cilantro.

Goat Cheese & Spinach

Serves 10

2 teaspoons cumin seeds
1 tablespoon ghee
1 tablespoon fresh ginger, finely chopped
1 large or 2 medium onions, chopped
1½ teaspoons red chili powder
½ teaspoon turmeric
2 tablespoons coriander
1½ teaspoons salt
1 package fresh spinach
750 grams goat cheese, cut into cubes (about 3 cups)
1 teaspoon garam masala
butter

Roast cumin seeds for 5 minutes in skillet; add ghee. Add ginger and onions, and sauté until brown. Add chili powder, turmeric, coriander, and salt, and continue sautéing. Add spinach and cook until it wilts. If necessary, add ½-1 cup water if sauce is too thick. Pour it on goat cheese cubes and serve garam masala and butter on top for garnish. Serve with rice or chapattis.

Ice Cream

Ice cream should be used in moderation as a treat, not as a food. It clogs all tissues, thereby weakening the digestion, spleen, and pancreas. It is also Ama-producing. Large consumption may cause diabetes. It is best to use tasty substitute products such as Rice Dream, soybean ice cream, etc. The best time to eat ice cream is during the summer months. As a substitute, frozen fruit can be mashed, blended, or run through a juicer to make fruit sorbet.

Energy: Cold

Taste: Sweet

Post Digestive: Sweet

Indications: No recommended usage for any condition.

Systems: Can be harmful

Dosha Affected:

Not recommended for any (too cold for Vata; too rich for Kapha and Pitta)

Mixes Well With: Nothing

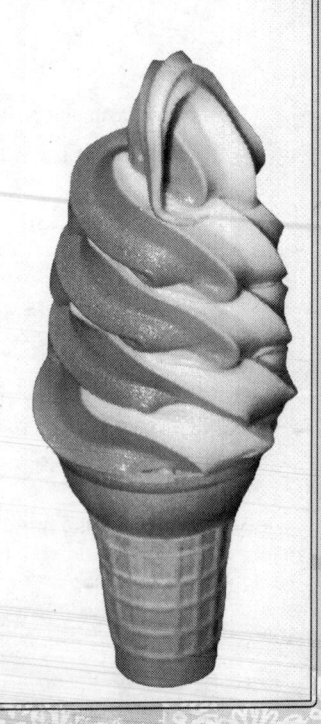

Ice Cream with Cinnamon

- 6 cups cream
- 2 tablespoons agave
- 1½ teaspoons cinnamon

Mix all ingredients together in blender, put in ice cube tray and freeze. After the cubes are frozen, blend again. For best results, use a Green Machine, Vitamix, or Champion. (If using a regular blender, use on lowest speed.)

Serve over fruit as a dessert.

Kefir

Kefir is made from a different bacteria than that of yogurt (which is primarily lactobacillus bulgaricus), and is more liquid than yogurt.

Energy: Warming

Taste: Sour

Post Digestive: Sour

Indications: Improves digestion and absorption, improves appetite, helps to gain weight

Systems: Digestive

Dosha Affected:

Vata: Good

Pitta and **Kapha**: Avoid

Mixes Well With: Sour fruits

Sour Cream

Sour cream, or soured cream, is an acidic tasting cream. The sour cream sold today is pasteurized cream that has been soured with a bacterial culture. "Cultured" and "acidified" sour cream are slightly different. "Cultured" sour cream is homogenized pasteurized cream that is soured with Streptococcus lactic at 71° F until the level of acidity reaches at least 0.5%. "Acidified" sour cream is pasteurized cream that has been soured with bacteria that produce lactic acid. The cream is left to ferment for 12 to 14 hours, much like yogurt. It is sometimes stabilized with additives (gelatin, sodium, carrageen) and may contain milk solids or whey, buttermilk, and salt. It is thick, uniform, and smooth.

Energy: Warm

Taste: Sweet, Sour

Post Digestive: Sour

Indications: Vata conditions

Systems: All systems

Dosha Affected:

Vata: Good

Pitta and **Kapha**: Avoid or reduce

Mixes Well With: Spices, salads

Sour Cream Dressing

- ⅓ cup sour cream
- 2 tablespoons olive oil
- 1 cup chives, chopped
- ¼ cup lime juice
- 1 teaspoon agave syrup

In blender, mix all ingredients together until smooth. Serve on salads, vegetables, or crackers.

Sour Cream Pineapple Dressing

Makes about 6 oz dressing

- 4 oz sour cream
- 1 cup pineapple, fresh
- 2 tablespoons almond oil
- 1 teaspoon honey
- 1 tablespoon orange juice
- ½ cup cilantro, fresh, chopped

Serve with fruit salads

Ayurvedic Curative Cuisine for Everyone

Yogurt

Yogurt is thought to have originated in Bulgaria, where people eat yogurt on a regular basis and where an unusually high number of people live to be 100 years of age. Yogurt is a fermented dairy product obtained by adding lactic bacteria to milk. The words yogurt, yoghurt, yoghourt are derived from the Turkish word yoghurmak, meaning, "to thicken". The two lactic bacteria used to make yogurt are Streptococcus thermophilus and Lactobacillus bulgaricus; ideally used in equal amounts. Yogurt is a traditional food in the Balkans, Greece, Turkey, Mongolia, India, the Middle East, and certain parts of Asia. During the 1970-1980 decade, yogurt finally began to gain acceptance in the United States and has increased dramatically in recent years. However, Europeans still consume 3 to 5 times as much yogurt as North Americans. Yogurt is thought to be cold and mucus-forming. Ayurveda reduces this by making a drink called Lassi (lah'see) by blending equal parts of yogurt and water with fruit and spices. Vatas get heating fruits and spices (like mango and ginger); Pittas get cooling additives like mint and strawberry; and Kaphas get to lick the blender. The best time to eat yogurt is during Pitta time, which is late morning to early afternoon.

Energy: Warming

Taste: Sweet, Sour

Post Digestive: Sweet

Indications: Fevers, stomach disorders, flatulence, anemia, dizziness, fatigue, hemorrhoids, kidney and bladder disorders, edema, weak mind, tuberculosis, leprosy

Systems: Urinary, Circulation, Immune, Digestive

Dosha Affected:

Vata: Good

Pitta and **Kapha**: Avoid or reduce

Mixes Well With: Spices, salads

Homemade Yogurt

Items Needed

3 tablespoons organic yogurt

1 quart raw milk

4 quart pot

2 or 3 quart pot

Put the small pot inside the larger pot. Put boiling Water in large pot until it reaches halfway up the smaller pot. Place milk in small pot. Add yogurt and stir with wooden spoon. Put both pots in over, cover, and cook at 150-185 for 8 hours. For a thicker consistency, add a tablespoon of powdered milk. Cool. Refrigerate.

Note: Be sure that the plain yogurt has an expiration date at least 10 days ahead.

Fruit Lassi

Serves 1

½ cup plain yogurt

¾ cup water

1 teaspoon coriander, ground

3 cardamom seeds

¼ cup fresh fruit (mango)

1 tablespoon rosewater

Blend yogurt and water; add rest of ingredients and blend again. Drink at room temperature.

Ayurvedic Curative Cuisine for Everyone

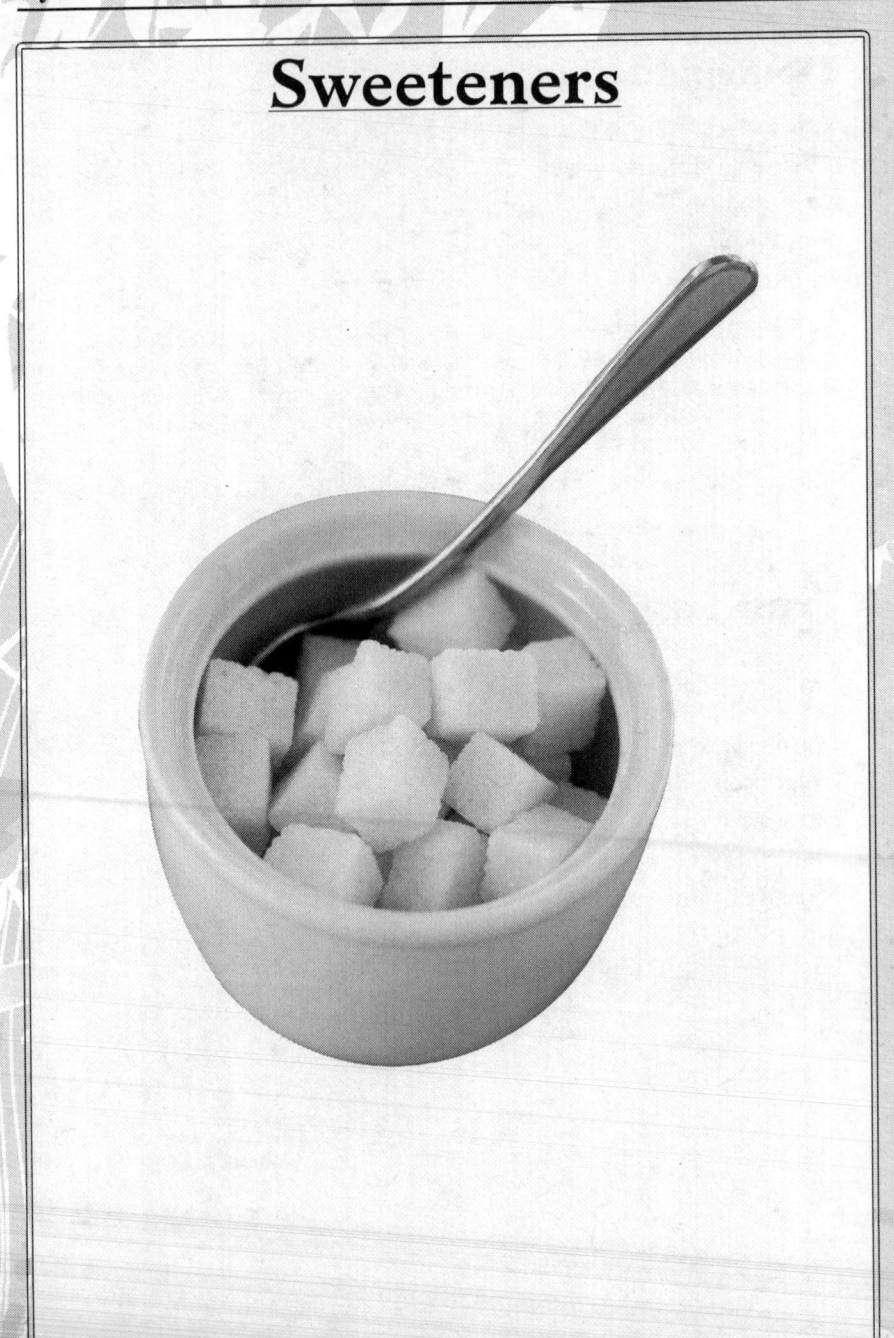

Sweeteners

Sweeteners

For proper tissue development, the body requires a certain amount of sweeteners in the diet because "sweet" is the body's basic taste. Refined sugars are ama producing, particularly white sugar, because the nutrients of the sugar cane have been removed in processing. Refined sugars create many health disorders within the body and are the main cause of allergies which weaken the immune system. Including a small amount of sweets into the diet is fine, however, too much sweets will derange the doshas. Sweet spices can satisfy the desire for sweet tastes, i.e., cinnamon, cardamom, ginger, fennel, and mint. Sweets, in general, are tonic for the body, working as a laxative and as a preservative and can be used with herbal tonics and jellies. Sweets combine well with milk, fruits, and nuts. They are very good for rejuvenation and debility. The right kind of sweets produce kapha and this can be helpful for children and for an emaciated condition. Natural raw sugars are beneficial for relieving bleeding diseases, burning, vomiting, fainting, and thirst. Sweets can be consumed when there is a healthy digestive system and no obstruction of the tissue. Most sugars are hard to combine and they should never be combined with salty taste. Sugars are best used with nourishing drinks, ghee, and spices such as nutmeg, cinnamon, cardamom and ginger.

Bitter taste is an antidote to sweet cravings, i.e., green leafy vegetables, spirulina, blue green algae, and bitter herbs such as gentian, barberry, turmeric, neem, and kutki (bitters).

These bitter herbs do not readily combine well – it is better to take in capsule form. Ayurvedic medicine has an herb called jymena sylvestrie, known as gurmar or shardunika. When having extreme desire for sweets, you can use this herb on the tip of the tongue to stop the craving of sweets. This herb is also very good for diabetes.

Agave Nectar

This sugar is made from the same sweet cactus nectar that tequila is made from. It is a naturally extracted sugar from the pineapple shaped core of the blue agave with a 90% fruit sugar content and only 10% glucose. Agave absorbs into the tissues and blood slowly creating no harmful side effects and maintains balanced sugar levels with no highs and lows. When your body doesn't make enough insulin (diabetes), eating white sugar increases the sugar in your blood to unhealthy levels. Agave does not do that when consumed in very small amounts.

In today's market there is much research stating that the process of making agave is the same as corn syrup and may affect the body in the same way. However, some companies process this sweetener in a way that does not affect glucose levels. Listen to your body. Some of my clients who have diabetes use agave with no problem. I personally have no problem with it, however, I cannot use corn syrup because it changes my blood sugar. Some people have no reaction to agave. For diabetics, use with caution.

Best used in cereals, fruits, teas, decoctions, and all baked goods.

This sweetener has recently been introduced to the US market.

There is a lot of propaganda about agave today. Some of the most recent research shows that agave is heavily adulterated. Others say that it is heavily processed and is almost as bad as corn syrup. Yet, I find that many diabetic people with blood sugar problems use it with no ill effect. I am very sensitive to sugar and I do very well with it. Use with care and monitor your condition to see what effect it has on you.

Energetics: sweet, cold

Action: astringent, demulcent

Indications: cold, flu, cough, weight loss

Dosha Affected:

Dosha: Good for all doshas (Kapha in moderations)

Contraindications: None

Brown Sugar

Brown sugar, in most cases, is simply white sugar with a small amount of molasses added. This should be used in small quantities, if necessary. Many people think that brown sugar is more nutritious, however, its nutritive value is no better than that of white sugar. The amount of molasses in brown sugar is so low it doesn't contribute enough of any vitamin or mineral to count on a food label.

Energetics: this is white sugar with molasses added.

Action: astringent, demulcent

Indications: not recommended

Dosha Affected:
Good for Vata avoid for Pitta and Kapha

Sugar Cane

Sugar cane produces a balanced source of energy. Sugar cane juice is one of the highest sources of vitamins and minerals. The juice is good for quenching thirst. In Thai and Chinese neighborhoods of New York or other large cities (Caribbean Islands, Puerto Rico), sugar cane can often be bought fresh. In the Indian markets its called jaggary, in the mexican market it is called pilonllo. This product is pretty pure. In excess it can cause ama toxicity. When you purchase this product be sure it is organic.

Energetics: sweet/cold/sweet

Action: astringent, demulcent

Indications: builds body tissue, increases Kapha, increases urine output, Aphrodisiac, strengthens urinary tract, jaundice, anemia, constipation, strengthens heart muscles, sexual stimulant

Dosha Affected:

Vata: good

Pitta: reduce

Kapha: Avoid

Corn Syrup

Avoid. Toxic. Probably one of the most refined and processed sugars on the market.

Make sure you read labels it is one of the most used sugars on the market.

Fruit Sugar

Today there is a great demand for fruit sugar. It is definitely better than white sugar but due to the bleaching process it looses most of its mineral content (like white sugar) and can derange all doshas when taken in excess, particularly digestion. Fruit juices derange sugar metabolism, weaken digestion, and promotes excessive ama.

Two of the more beneficial fruit sugars are grapes and dates. It is important to know the source of the fruit sugar that you purchase because many of the fruit sugars sold in America have been made from fruit that has been sprayed in 'third world' countries with the American banned pesticides.

Use only when organic.

Vata- good

Pitta-good

Kapha - avoid

Honey

This is one of the best sweeteners to use. Purchase and use in raw form only; it should never be bought pasteurized nor cooked in foods – this creates ama.

Honey provides energy and is versatile in its qualities. It enhances the value of foods -particularly when consumed with milk. Useful for treating sore throats, improves digestion, asthma, hemorrhoids, tuberculosis, blood disorders, urinary tract, nausea, vomiting, hiccups, and constipation. It is very good for skin care. There are many contradictions about honey and babies, however, Ayurveda says that honey should not be given to babies until the age of one, Aged honey should be not be given to babies till the age of three. Honey aggravates Vayu. Becomes toxic when cooked. Becomes toxic for Pitta diseases when used in hot climate. Do not use with HOT foods. Use warm raw honey. It is best to eat honey in its raw form.

Energetics: sweet/hot/sweet

Action: tonic, rejuvenative, expectorant, nutritive, emollient, demulcent

External: astringent, antibiotic, demulcent.

Indications: relieves Kapha, poison, hiccup, diabetes (in small doses), heals the eyes, heals skin conditions, diarrhea, cough, wounds, difficult breathing, cleans wounds, sores, decoction enemas, burns, and can be used in weight reduction

Dosha Affected:

Vata: Moderation

Pitta: Avoid

Kapha: Good

Contraindications: medicinal properties destroyed by heat, can create subtle toxins so do not cook or bake with honey; aggravates Pitta. It is subtly toxic and produces ama when taken with equal amounts of ghee (better to make the portions 1:2 or 2:1). Feeds fevers, tumors, and infections.

Jaggery
(Guda)

This is an Indian raw, natural sugar which contains vitamins and minerals and is consumed with meals. Also known by the name of pinlon cillo. Sucinate cane sugar is similar, but cooler for Pitta. Older, washed jaggery increases Kapha only slightly and helps with the elimination of urine and feces.

In this form of sugar, all vitamins and minerals are kept intact. It is only available for purchase in Spanish and Indian stores.

At health food stores we can purchase something similar – Sucanat – which is Similiar to jaggary. It is best to buy it in whole form and grated it yourself. This sweetener is similar to molasses and is very high in B vitamins. Commonly used in Indian cooking. Best to use grated or chopped. It can be boiled down into a syrup to add to desserts.

Energetics: sweet/hot/sweet

Action: tonic, stimulant

Indications: anemia, debility, rejuvenation, urine disorders or irregularity, heart, nervous system disorders

Dosha Affected:

Vata: good

Pitta: moderation

Kapha: very small amounts

Contraindications: excess Kapha, diabetes, Lactose

Lactose

Lactose sugar comes from milk and is a derivative of whole milk. It is used in many prepared and processed foods. When using bitter herbs, lactose can be mixed with them.

Energetics: milk sugar

Action: tonic empowers herbs, headache, chest pain, lung disorders, vomiting, illnesses

Dosha Affected:

Vata: good

Pitta: good

Kapha: neutral

Contraindications: Do Not Overuse

Maltose/Malt Syrup

Maltose is made from grains (barley, rice or a combination of the two grains) and is good for gaining weight. It is also good for children, long term illnesses, and a good source of energy.

Energetics: sweet/cold/sweet

Action: analgesic, tonic, demulcent Indications: stomach, lungs, chronic colds, intestinal spasms, abdominal spasms, colic, convalescence, cough

Dosha Affected:

Vata: good

Pitta: good

Kapha: moderation only

Contraindications: Do not use if diabetic – or with a candida condition.

Maple Sugar

Maple sugar should not be confused with any commercial maple syrup (which is artificially made). Pure maple sugar is expensive. It is naturally harvested from maple trees and is probably one of the best and most nutritious sugars available. [Do] not use when there is fever, cough, burning, infections, poor circulation or candida high Pitta disorders.

Energetics: sweet/cold/sweet

Action: nutritive, demulcent, one of the best natural sweeteners.

Dosha Affected:
Vata: moderation
Pitta: good
Kapha: moderation

Molasses

Molasses is made during the first stage of sugar refining. The result is a dark, thick, nutritious product which is high in B vitamins and minerals, particularly iron. It is good for all gynecological disorders.

Energetics: sweet/hot/sweet

Action: tonic, nutritive, iron

Indications: pregnancy, postpartum, builds blood, debility, muscles, heart, blood, circulation, anemia

Dosha Affected:
Vata: good
Pitta: good
Kapha: in excess avoid
Contraindications: Do not use on high Pitta during fever or inflammation.

Rock Candy

(Mishri)

Better than molasses. Used in spiritual ceremonies and eaten as spiritual food (prasad). It is not readily available in the U.S. Used in India for celebrations, puja offerings, religious rituals, and taken as Prasad in small amounts. This product use with can be found in Indian grocery stores.

Energetics: provides energy. It is made from sugar.

Action: demulcent

External: astringent, antibiotic, demulcent.

Indications: emaciation, reducing vayu, burning in chest, cough, aphrodisiac, relieves Pitta when taken with ginger in water

Dosha Affected:
Vata: good
Pitta: moderation
Kapha: avoid

Contraindications: do not use with swelling, edema, or candida

Stevia

This is a sweet plant native of South America and cultivated in Japan. It is an herb in the chrysanthemum family, extremely sweet tasting but with no calories, and rich in minerals. Documented research indicates that stevia produces a healing effect within the pancreas. When used as a white powder, it has a bitter after taste. In plant form it has no after taste. Can be brewed in tea and cooked in fresh form.

Energetics: astringent, bitter, sweet

Action: balances pancreatic functions Indications: diabetes, low blood sugar

Dosha Affected:
VPK-

Contraindications: None known

White Sugar

Tamasic. Toxic. Refining removes the nutritional value (vitamins & minerals) as well as the life force and leaves only a sterile product that produces incomplete metabolism when consumed. This sugar creates ama in the body.

White sugar is not recommended because it has no nutritive value. Within the body, sugar leaches minerals from the tissue, thereby, increasing the need for a greater vitamin and mineral intake in order to remain healthy. Degenerative conditions may result from prolonged sugar consumption, such as calcium depletion of bones and teeth, enlarged liver, compromised brain and memory capacity, overabundance of white blood cells, and a compromised immune system.

Best to avoid. White sugar is the main cause of diabetes throughout the world. It's overconsumption leads to many health problems. Many people wake up with edema after eating white sugar. This form is hard to digest and has laxative properties.

Energetics: sweet/cold/sweet

External: astringent, antibiotic, demulcent.

Indications: AVOID

Dosha Affected:
All doshas should avoid.

Action: None

Contraindications: Do not use with serious illnesses, cancer, immune disorders, or candida

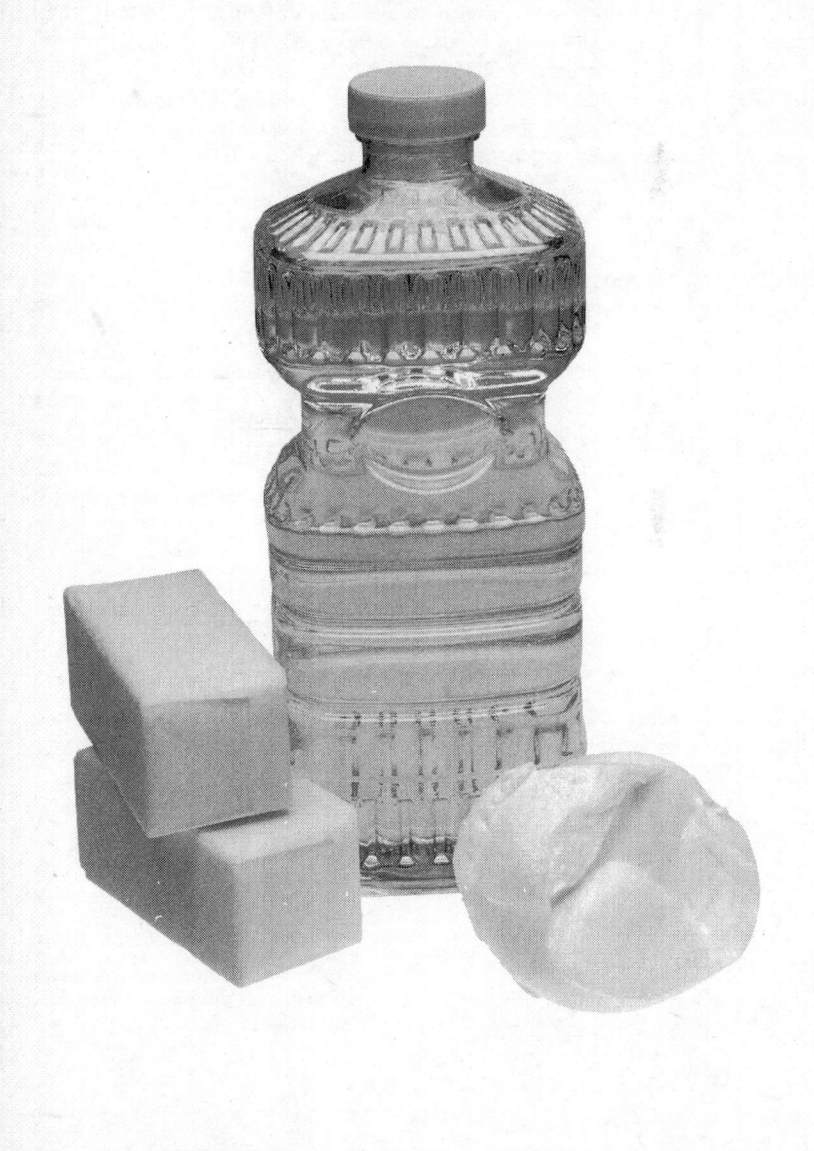

Oils

All vegetables oils are best used heat.

Always use cold pressed oil because it is best to maintain healthy joints.

Oils

Oils are excellent for healthy skin, hair and organs. They have multiple uses and can be added to cooking, salad dressings, soups, dips, massage oils, face creams, and salves. When used to extract herbs (medicated oils), they strengthen the cell walls, support the capillaries and add mobility to the joints. Oils can be used for frying or sautéing; one tablespoon is sufficient for cooking noodles, grains, and sautéing vegetables. Vegetable oils are not high in cholesterol, are easy to digest, easier to assimilate than animal fats, and are high in vitamins E and A which are essential for a healthy body. Many oils are high in essential fatty acids which are important in hormone balance.

All oils are produced from seeds, beans, and nuts. There are many varieties and grades of oils; keep away from refined oils because they may have been pressed or extracted with solvents. In this type of processing, all nutrients are lost. Always use cold pressed, unrefined oils. Keep stored in cool, dark places (refrigeration is best) in order to preserve freshness.

For more information on oils, consult the book, "Ayurveda and Aromatherapy," by Doctors Bryan and Light Miller.

In general, oils slow down digestion, requiring up to six hours to process (with large amounts). Oils are best with all vegetables, in sauces, or dressings. They are OK with bread, starches, or proteins. Generally, avoid combining oils with fruits.

Avocado Oil

This oil is pressed from Kapha: Moderation the seed of the avocado fruit and is very high Mixes Well With: in vitamin E. It is an Vegetables excellent oil for the face and body.

Energy: Warming

Taste: Sweet

Post Digestive: Sweet

Systems: All systems

Indications: Weak liver, dry skin, lack of vitamin E, weak tissues

Dosha Affected:

Vata: Good

Pitta: Moderation (avoid excess)

Action: None

External: astringent, antibiotic, demulcent.

Canola Oil

Canola oil is produced more today than at any other time in history it is one of the most available oils. Be careful when purchasing this oil as it is one which is often pressed with the use of solvents. Low in saturated fats and a member of the mustard family. This oil is a hybrid-GMO (genetically modified organisms) developed by the Canadian government and have never been tested for human consumption. It is derived from rape seed oil, which is known to produce hair and feather loss in animals. The FDA approved the sell of this product after receiving one million dollars from the Canadian government to avoid testing.

Energy: Warming

Taste: Sweet

Post Digestive: Sweet

Systems: Epithelial, Muscular, Endocrine

External: astringent, antibiotic, demulcent.

Dosha Affected:

Vata: Avoid

Pitta and **Kapha**: Good

Action: None

Mixes Well With: Vegetables

Indications: Dry skin, high cholesterol, obesity

Castor Oil

Castor oil packs were originally recommended by Edgar Cayce and their use has been well documented. Primarily used medicinally for constipation, both externally and internally. The taste of this product is pungent it is not normal to use for food preparation. In ayurveda it is use for purging with purganive herbs.

Energy: Warming

Taste: Bitter, Sweet

Post Digestive: Pungent

Systems: Epithelial, Muscular, Nervous

Dosha Affected:

Vata and **Pitta**: Moderation (use in compress)

Kapha: good

Indications: Purgative, constipation, muscle spasms, epilepsy, pain, tumors, swelling, sores, stimulates lymph movement

Corn Oil

The oil has a buttery flavor and is smooth. The dark oil is from the kernel and the lighter colored oil is from the germ. Not generally well thought of. It is not a great oil for human consumption because it is heated and heavily processed. Today it is generally a GMO (genetically modified organism) product. However, a good quality oil can provide benefits.

Energy: Warming

Taste: Sweet

Post Digestive: Sweet

Systems: Urinary, Epithelial

Indications: Good for kidneys, urinary tract infections, skin moisturizer, lowers high cholesterol

Dosha Affected:

Vata: Avoid

Pitta: Moderation

Kapha: good

Mixes Well With: Vegetables

Coconut Oil

It is commonly believed that coconut oil has an aroma, but true coconut oil does not. Many cultures use this oil in cooking and they have no problem with cholesterol. This is one of the oils which needs to be heated above room temperature because it is solidified. High in saturated fats. Best to use externally. Some of the latest research shows that cold pressed coconut oil can help improve many illnesses particularly auto immune.

Energy: Cooling

Taste: Sweet

Post Digestive: Sweet

Systems: Epithelial

Dosha Affected:

Vata and Pitta: Good

Kapha: Moderation

Indications: Suntan lotion (reflects radiation), dry skin, skin infections, liver disorders and hair growth.

Flaxseed Oil

Also known as Linseed Oil and is high in essential fatty acids. Most often taken as a supplement. It is too expensive, and nutrients are wasted in cooking.

Energy: Warming

Taste: Sweet, Pungent

Post Digestive: Pungent

Indications: Excellent detoxifier, expectorant for lungs, stops coughing, lubricating laxative, loosens congestion, excellent for internal use, cancer prevention, immune stimulation

Dosha Affected:

Vata and Pitta: Good

Kapha: Moderation

Mixes Well With: Cottage cheese, green juices

Systems: All systems

Lard

This is the fat of animal products and is one of the most difficult for humans to digest. It is extremely heavy producing toxicity in the body, increasing cholesterol, and promoting obesity. Used extensively in Chinese, Korean, and Mexican food. Avoid the use of this product entirely.

Energy: Warming

Taste: Sweet

Post Digestive: Sweet

Indications: Not recommended

Margarine

The development of margarine came about in 1869 as the result of a contest initiated by Napoleon III to find an alternative to butter, which was quite rare and expensive during the 19th Century. The winning product had to be capable of being stored without going rancid, so was initially made from refined tallow. At the beginning of the 20th Century, science discovered a process that prevented vegetable fat from oxidizing too quickly, called hydrogenation (solidifying liquid fats); hence, margarine was born.

Hydrogenated vegetable oil is difficult for the body to process, as it is different from all other fats consumed. Therefore, it is suspected of leaving deposits of fats congested in the arteries and interfering with hormone balance.

Hydrogenation is combining hydrogen atoms with fatty acid molecules, which has a solidifying effect on oil. This process raises the melting ability, prevents spoiling, and can improve the consistency of food when added. Overall, this process of hydrogenation destroys the many valuable components of vegetable oils and is not recommended as part of an Ayurvedic diet. It was once touted as safer than butter; however, the American Medical Society changed its mind several years ago. Butter is better.

Energy: Warm

Taste: Sour

Post Digestive: Sweet

Indications: Depending on what oil is used - generally hard to digest. Externally, skin and hair care.

Dosha Affected:

Vata: Avoid

Pitta: Avoid

Kapha: Avoid

Mixes Well With: Grains

Mustard Oil

Mustard oil is most Vegetables commonly used in Eastern and Oriental cooking. Effective massage oil for Kaphas.

Energy: Warming

Taste: Pungent

Post Digestive: Pungent

Indications: Breaks down congestive tissue, good compress, abdominal pain

Systems: Respiratory, muscular

Dosha Affected:

Vata and **Kapha**: Good

Pitta: Moderation (in small amounts)

Mixes Well With: Vegetables

Olive Oil

This oil is polyunsaturated which makes it heavier than other oils and has a longer shelf life. Requires no heating above room temperature. The highest quality is from the first pressing called "extra virgin," and all olive oil on the market is cold pressed. This oil is great for cooking.

Energy: Slightly cooling

Taste: Sweet

Post Digestive: Sweet

Indications: Softening gallstones, decongests bile, antiseptic, rheumatic joints, infections, liver disorders, good for healthy hair and skin

Systems: Immune, Epithelial, Skeletal, Muscular

Dosha Affected:

Vata and **Pitta:** Good

Kapha: Avoid (in excess)

Mixes Well With: Vegetables

Peanut Oil

Another oil recommended by Edgar Cayce because of its curative properties, (especially externally). It has an aroma that is difficult to cover up in a massage blend. When using this product make sure it is cold pressed.

Energy: Warming

Taste: Sweet

Post Digestive: Sweet

Indications: Constipation, joint pain, urinary tract

Systems: Urinary, Epithelia, Muscular, Skeletal

Dosha Affected:

Vata: Good

Pitta and **Kapha:** Moderation (use small amounts)

Mixes Well With: Vegetables

Safflower Oil

This is a relative of sunflowers and is a mid-range quality oil.

Energy: Warming

Taste: Sweet, Pungent

Post Digestive: Pungent

Indications: Detoxifier, promotes circulation, heart disorders, blood, laxative, promotes menstruation

Systems: Circulatory, Reproductive, Excretory

Dosha Affected:

Vata and **Kapha:** Good

Pitta: Avoid

Mixes Well With: Vegetables

Sesame Oil

The most commonly used in Ayurvedic medicine because of its nutritional value due to the high vitamin and mineral content. Has many healing properties with many natural preservatives which delay rancidity. There are two kinds of sesame oil: dark oil, in which the seeds have been roasted, with a nutty flavor and a smoky aroma; and a light oil, which is produced from raw, white sesame seeds, and has a milder flavor. This is a good oil for nourishing and protecting the skin from the sun because it blocks 45% of the suns UV rays.

Energy: Warming

Taste: Sweet

Post Digestive: Sweet

Indications: Strengthens all tissues, helps anxiety, muscle spasms, dry skin, muscle tension

Systems: All systems

Dosha Affected:

Vata: Good

Pitta and **Kapha:** In very small amounts

Mixes Well With: Vegetables

Soy

One of the most commonly used in Oriental cooking. Contains vitamins A and E, and preserves a healthy glow of the skin. Considered a low grade oil. When purchased make sure it is cold pressed and not GMO (genetically modified organism.)

Energy: Cooling

Taste: Sweet, Astringent

Post Digestive: Sweet

Indications: Kidney disorders, inflammations, ulcers, colitis, diarrhea

Systems: Urinary, Digestive, Excretory

Dosha Affected:

Vata: Good

Pitta and **Kapha:** Excellent

Mixes Well With: Vegetables

Sunflower Oil

Made from pressing sunflower seeds. Considered a higher grade oil.

Energy: Cooling

Taste: Sweet, Astringent

Post Digestive: Sweet

Indications: Skin rashes, diabetes, infections, diarrhea

Systems: Epithelial, Endocrine, Excretory

Dosha Affected:

Vata: Avoid

Pitta: Excellent

Kapha: Moderation (in small amounts)

Mixes Well With: Vegetables

Immune System

Currently, there is a health care crisis within this country, even though millions of dollars are spent for medical care. There are many dis-eases today; such as aids, cancer, chronic fatigue syndrome, ect. which impact the immune system, leading to poor quality of life. Because of the complexity and expense of the medical system, many people are turning to alternative therapies.

In order for us to maintain a healthy immune system we most be aware of foods that enhance and boost our immune system. A strong immune system is like the guardian angel of the body, it keeps a person healthy and resilience to many diseases. Through the use of foods that are rich in vitamin C and anti oxidants we can create a healthy immunity. The system relies on good nutrition to keep the cells and organs in a state of balance. As we learn about foods, this knowledge and application, everyone can keep their immune system in optimal health. Ayurveda recommends and teaches that variety in ones diet, a life style, herbal therapy, yoga and meditation, is a way of maintaining a healthy body and avoiding allergies.

Here is list of some other best immune boosters:

Amalaki, avocado, apples, blueberries, apricots, apricot seeds, beets, cabbage, cauliflower, broccoli, grapefruit, shitake mushrooms, sweet potatoes, wheat grass, celery, parsley, dang shen, ashwaganda, grape seeds, hazel nuts, walnuts, snow peas, evening prim rose, cherries, raspberries, melons, passion fruit, guava, papaya, pineapple, arugula, sea weeds, mustard seeds, peppers, ginger, black cumin, rosemary, sage, chamomile, peppermint, duck, soy beans, oats, sesame seeds, avocado oil, flax seed oil, savoy cabbage, acai berry, goji berries, tumeric, pipli, echinacea, cardimon, osha, nettles, artichokes, astralaguas,

Super Foods for Shakes:

Zrii (a liquid nutritional product), Barley Greens, Super Greens, Chatavari Powder, Chyavan Prash, Chlorella

Immune Broth for Pitta and Kapha

Makes large pot of soup

- 1 onion, chopped
- 4 cloves garlic, chopped (Kapha only)
- 1 cup carrots, sliced
- 1 cup cabbage, sliced
- 1 cup broccoli, cut in pieces
- ½ cup shitaki mushrooms (optional)
- 3-inch piece wakame or kombu, cut in small pieces
- 4 pieces astralagus
- 4 roots dang shen
- 2 roots ashwagandha (pieces)
- 6 roots shatavari
- ½-inch piece ginger, well chopped (Kapha only)
- ½ bulb fennel
- 2 tablespoons cumin seeds
- ½ teaspoon ajwan seeds
- 1 tablespoon coriander
- 8 cups water
- ½ bunch cilantro, chopped
- ½ bunch parsley, chopped

In a large pot, add all ingredients to water except cilantro and parsley; bring to a boil, then turn heat to low and simmer for 1 hour. Add herbs (cilantro, spinach, parsley) to soup pot just before serving. Remove astralagus and dang shen roots – do not eat. Place ingredients in blender and blend until smooth.

Immune Broth for Vata

Serves 10
Makes large pot of soup

1 onion, chopped

2 cloves garlic, chopped

1 cup carrots, sliced

1 cup sweet potatoes, cut up

1 cup broccoli, cut in pieces

3-inch piece wakame or kombu

4 pieces astralagus

4 dang shen roots

4-6 roots ashwagandha (pieces)

6 roots shatavari

½-inch piece ginger, well chopped

2 tablespoons cumin seeds

2 teaspoons ajwan seeds

10 cups water

1 cup cilantro

2 cups spinach

½ cup of parsley

In a large pot, add all ingredients to water except cilantro, spinach, and parsley; bring to a boil, then turn heat to low and simmer for 1 hour. Add herbs (cilantro, spinach, parsley) to soup pot just before serving. Remove astralagus and dang shen roots – do not eat. Place ingredients in blender and blend until smooth.

Green Immune Soup

Serves 8-10

- 10-15 cups water
- ½ head broccoli, cut up
- ½ head cauliflower, cut up
- 5 stalks celery, chopped
- ½ celery root (celeriac), chopped
- ½ cup green onions (green tops only), chopped
- 6 large leaves and stems of curly kale, chopped
- 1 cup cilantro, chopped
- 2 sheets kombu, cut in small pieces
- ½ bulb fennel, chopped (do not use the stalks, only the bulb portion)
- 1 thumb-size turmeric rhizome, chopped
- 1 thumb-size piece ginger root, chopped
- 6 pieces astralagus dried root
- 8 medium size (about 3") sulfur-free ashwagandha root
- 4-inch piece burdock, chopped
- 1 tablespoon ajwan seeds
- 1 tablespoon cumin seeds
- 2 tablespoons coriander
- 2 tablespoons ghee
- 1 tablespoon miso, add at end just before serving so as not to destroy enzymes by cooking
- Add Bragg's to taste

Cook hardy vegetables and herb roots first. Bring to boil and immediately turn down to simmer. Add lighter vegetables and seaweed. Sauté spices in ghee briefly, then add to pot.

Resource List

CHINESE HERBS
May Way Corporation 800-2-mayway Astragalus Dan Shen

AYURVEDIC HERBS & SUPPLEMENTS
Banyan Trading Co. 800-953-6424 P.O. Box 13002 Albuquerque, NM 87192 Email: www.banyanbotanicals.com Toll free: 800-953-6474 spices. vegetabe oils organic whole sale and retail
Bazaar of India 800-261-7662 Ashwagandha -Whole Shatavari - Whole Good selection of Ayurvedic herbs and spices

SPICES - CUT & SIFTED
St. John's Herb Garden, Inc. 301-262-5302 7711 Hillmeade Rd (FAX) 301-262-2489 Bowie, MD 20720 Email: vallentyne@aol.com

FRONTIER HERBS
PO box 299 Norway.IA52318 www.frontiercoop.com

StarWest Botanicals
11253 Trade Center Dr Rancho Cordova, CA 95742 800-800-4372 or 916-853-9354 www.starwest-botanicals.com herbs & herb supplies

ESSENTIAL LIVING FOODS, INC
12304 Santa Monica Blvd., #218 Los Angeles, CA 90025 310-571-3272 www.essentiallivigfoods.com raw cacao, coconut oil, lycii berries, and the very best superfoods ever.

AYURVEDIC-HEALERS.COM
Bodytype herbal blends for Immune soup. Special blends for Vata, Pitta and Kapha. Essential oils. Books. Pancha Karma. Kaya Kalpa. Guru Kula. Spa Treatments. Ayurvedic Correspondence Course. Contact Blaire at 941-894-8678 or 941-400-9758 or AyurvedicHealers.Blaire@gmail.com Contact Light Miller at 941-806-7760 or Earthess@aol.com www.AyurvedicHealers.com

Food Resources

USE EWG'S SHOPPER'S GUIDE TO REDUCE YOUR PESTICIDE EXPOSURES

http://www.foodnews.org/

CENTER FOR FOOD SAFETY

Works to protect the environment and human health.

Non-GMO Product Chart

http://truefoodnow.org/

TIPS ON STORING FRUITS & VEGETABLES

http://www.ecologycenter.org/factsheets/veggie-storage.pdf

AN AMAZING 11-YEAR OLD TEACHING IMPORTANCE OF ORGANIC FOOD

http://www.youtube.com/watch?v=F7Id9caYw-Y

Ayurvedic Curative Cuisine for Everyone

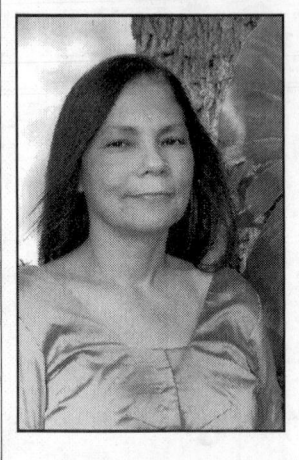

Z. Light Miller - Light (Jyoti) Miller travels throughout the world teaching Ayurveda, Aromatherapy, Herbology, Goddess, Tantra, Pancha Karma Trainings, Kaya Kalpa Trainings, as well as other specialized seminars. Light's Eastern heritage gives her a strong Ayurvedic background which connects her to the roots of Indian philosophy and healing. She has been teaching Ayurveda for 22 years and her mission has been to create a greater global awareness of the science of Ayurveda and to spread this knowledge throughout the world.

Light is one of only a few practitioners in the world who practices Kaya Kalpa and was the first woman trained in this ancient art. She offers Pancha Karma rejuvenation programs as well as the specialized Kaya Kalpa spiritual treatments.

Light Miller has written "Ayurvedic Remedies for the Whole Family," and co-authored, "Ayurveda and Aromatherapy," both published by Lotus Press, and has self-published an "Ayurveda Correspondence Course." Light's current book in progress is, "Honoring the Feminine Within All Life." Light travels extensively and can be emailed at Earthess@aol.com. Call this number if you are interested in more information on classes, customized product design, customized recipes for special events, or treatments.

....

Bryan Miller is a Chiropractic and Ayurvedic Practitioner. He loves cooking and helps to organize Light's Vata nature when they are in the kitchen together. They take turns cooking and creating nutritious menus for their clients and you will see a few of Bryan's delicious recipes in this cookbook.

Bryan is also an instructor for Everglades University, teaching classes in alternative medicine. He is co-creator of the Ayurveda Health Program at the Florida College of Integrative Health where he will teach a state approved degree program in Ayurveda as well as certification classes. Bryan co-founded a massage school, co-founded the essential oil company "EcoVeda," co-founded the Ayurvedic Center, and co-authored "Ayurveda & Aromatherapy" and a four volume Ayurvedic Correspondence Course.

Bryan practices an Ayurvedic lifestyle, teaches health and bodywork classes internationally, is a Pancha Karma Practitioner, and trained as a Kaya Kalpa (spiritual bodywork) practitioner, of which there are only a few in the world.

On a professional level, Bryan loves providing the services of Cross Fibre Massage, Shirodhara, and Tarpana (Ancient Forgiveness Ritual), as well as teaching. On a personal level, his great loves are surfing and gliding.

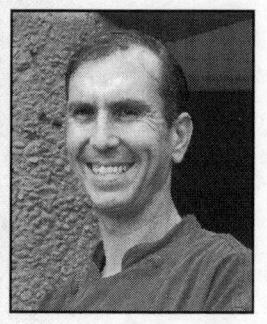

Chef Bodhie Miller has an extensive background in the design and creation of an ayurvedic diet. Being my son, he has been taught from a very early age how to incorporate an ayurvedic diet into a lifestyle. Chef Miller has taken the basic ayurvedic recipes and turned them into flavorful dishes. Chef Miller currently resides in Sarasota, Florida, with his wife and two children.

For the past 18 years he has gained the majority of his culinary skills apprenticing with Executive Chef's of local country clubs and 5 star restaurants.

Chef Miller opened up an ayurvedic restaurant inside the "Ayurvedic Center of Well Being" in Sarasota, Florida, where several of the dishes in this book were created

Chef Bodhie Miller has an extensive background in the design and creation of an ayurvedic diet. Being My son, he has been taught from a very early age how to incorporate an ayurvedic diet into a lifestyle. Chef Miller has taken the basic ayurvedic recipes and turned them into flavorful dishes. Chef Miller currently resides in Sarasota Fl. with his wife and 2 children where, for the past 18 years he has gained the majority of his culinary skills apprenticing Executive Chef's of local country clubs and 5 star restaurants.

Chef Miller opened up an ayurvedic restaurant inside the "Ayurvedic Center of Well Being" in Sarasota Fl. where many of the dishes in this book were created.

Raw Tips Provided by:

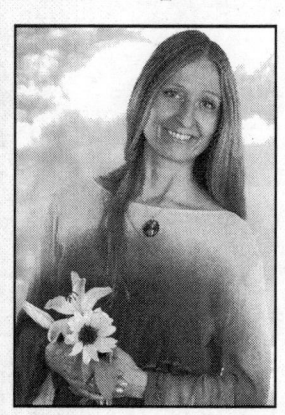

Brigitte Mars, a professional member of the American Herbalist Guild, is a nutritional consultant who has been working with Natural Medicine for over forty years. She teaches Herbal Medicine at Naropa University, Omega Institute, Hollyhock, Boulder College of Massage and Bauman Holistic College of Nutrition. She has a weekly local radio show called "Naturally" and a private practice.

Brigitte is the author of twelve books, including The Desktop Guide to Herbal Medicine, Beauty by Nature, Addiction Free Naturally, The Sexual Herbal, Healing Herbal Teas, and Rawsome!. Ms. Mars has been featured on NBC Dateline. www.brigittemars.com

Raw Food Recipes

Before you get started, there are a few basic points to consider:

- All ingredients should be raw, of course (raw carob powder, raw tahini, raw almond butter, unpasteurized miso, and so on).
- Use organic produce whenever possible.
- Wash all produce.
- Peel what needs to be peeled (bananas, avocados, waxed produce, jicama, papaya, and so forth); in all other cases (carrots, apples, unwaxed cucumbers), leave the peel on.
- Remove large hard seeds, such as those from from dates and prunes. Remove woody stems, such as those from figs and apples.
- When a recipe calls for soaking nuts, seeds, or dried fruits, soak them in twice as much water as their volume. Large nuts are generally soaked 8 to 12 hours. Small nuts and seeds are generally soaked 4 to 6 hours. Dried fruit should be soaked until it is tender. Rinse nuts, seeds, and dried fruits after soaking, and allow to drain well before using in a recipe.
- Use pure water in all your recipes.
- It's fine to substitute! Try using almonds for walnuts, raisins for dates, lemon juice for lime juice, and so forth.
- If what you are processing in the food processor needs more water, add some.
- Feel free to omit any seasonings, including salt, that you do not care for.
- Many raw soups can also be used as salad dressings.
- Be joyous in your food preparation. Pray, sing, chant, and smile.
- It takes only a moment to decorate. Love, good cheer, and humor conveyed through beautiful food will inspire others to try it and like it!
- Use your imagination!

Measurement Chart

Cup	Fluid Ounces	Tablespoons	Teaspoons	Milliliter
1/16 C	.5 oz	1 Tbsp	3 tsp	15 ml
1/8 C	1 oz	2 Tbsp	6 tsp	30 ml
1/4 C	2 oz	4 Tbsp	12 tsp	59 ml
1/3 C	3 oz	5 Tbsp	16 tsp	79 ml
1/2 C	4 oz	8 Tbsp	24 tsp	118 ml
2/3 C	5 oz	11 Tbsp	32 tsp	158 ml
3/4 C	6 oz	12 Tbsp	36 tsp	177 ml
1 C	8 oz	16 Tbsp	48 tsp	237 ml

Index

BEANS

Adzuki	253, 254
Bean Sprouts	3, 20, 249
Black-Eyed Peas	255, 256
Chickpeas	257
Fava	261, 262
Kidney Beans	263
Lentils	252, 266
Lima Beans	268, 269
Mung Beans	270
Peanuts	272, 273, 403
Soybeans	274
Split Peas	278
Tofu	273, 276, 277

BREAKFAST

Amaranth a la Saffron	287
Apple Juice	133
Beet juice	133, 134
Buttermilk Pancakes	432
Carrot juice	133, 147, 153, 160
Celery-Carrot Juice	153
Citrus Delight	114
Coconut Amaranth	287
Cottage Cheese Supreme	436
Eggs of the Sea	440
Fruit Lassi	449
Green Shake	244
Khichari	270, 271
Longevity Shake	244, 430
Miso Nourishing Soup	347
Oatmeal a la Bryan	299
Pancakes a la Bryan	311
Peach Porridge	96
Smoothie	45, 79
Spicy Yogurt	106

CASSEROLES

Bitter Melon Casserole	136
Breadfruit Casserole	47
Plantain Casserole	41

CHUTNEYS

Cilantro Mint Chutney	363
Date Chutney	60
Ginger Mint Chutney	372
Mango Chutney	83
Papaya Chutney	91

DAIRY

Cheese Blintzes	434
Cottage Cheese Supreme	436
Cream Cheese Celery	438
Curried Cream Cheese & Herbs	438
Eggs of the Sea	440
Ghee - Preparation	441
Goat Cheese Quesadilla	443
Goat Cheese & Spinach	443
Paneer	212, 430
Spinach Mozzarella Sauce	434

DAIRY PRODUCTS

Butter	209, 268, 431, 466
Buttermilk	428, 431, 432
Cheese	210, 382, 433, 434, 435, 436, 437, 438, 442, 443
Cottage	427, 435, 436, 465
Cream	72, 81, 125, 162, 180, 341, 408, 437, 438, 444, 445, 446, 447
Eggs	439, 440
Ghee	68, 441
Goat's Milk	443
Ice Cream	72, 81, 444, 445
Kefir	446
Paneer	212, 430

Ayurvedic Curative Cuisine for Everyone

Sour Cream 446, 447	Tapioca Pudding 220
Yogurt 106, 112, 394, 448, 449	Vanilla Flan 440

Desserts

Blackberry Corn Muffins 43	
Blackberry Pie 43	
Carrot Halvah 147	
Cherimoya Custard 52	
Cherry Pie 54	
Chocolate Banana Cream Topping 341	
Chocolate Chip Cookies 341	
Coconut Custard 411	
Fig Pudding 62	
Guava Amaranth Pudding 68	
Healthy Jello 232	
Ice Cream & Cinnamon 445	
Joy Balls 421	
Kiwi Gel 70	
Kumquat Ice Cream 72	
Lemon Ice 75	
Lemon Three Layer Cake 75	
Lychee Ice Cream 81	
Nectarine Pudding 87	
Oatmeal Cookies 298	
Orange Kiwi Delight 89	
Peach Pie 96	
Persimmon Ginger Crisps 100	
Persimmon Pudding 100	
Pineapple Pie 102	
Plum Pudding #1 104	
Plum Pudding #2 104	
Raspberry Cobbler 106	
Rice Pudding #1 304	
Rice Pudding #2 304	
Sapote Pudding 108	
Sooji Halva 310	
Spelt Berry Muffins 308	
Strawberry Parfait 110	
Strawberry Topping 110	

Dressings

Avocado Dressing 37
Buttermilk Salad Dressing 432
Cashew Salad Dressing 408
Dill Almond Dressing 367
Green Tara Mint Dressing 384
Hazelnut Dressing 413
Infused Juniper Berry Vinegar 376
Infused Parsley Oil or Vinaigrette 390
Kumquat Dressing 72
Marjoram Dressing 382
Mayonnaise - Eggless 344, 345, 374
Parsley Tomato Dressing 390
Pecan Salad Dressing 415
Pumpkin Seed Salad Dressing 419
Sesame Dressing 421
Sour Cream Dressing 447
Sour Cream Pineapple Dressing 447
Sunflower Seed Dressing 423
Tamarind Yogurt Dressing 112

Drinks

Almond Nut Milk 406
Apple Ginger Juice 32
Apple Juice 133
Beet juice 133, 134
Blueberry Divine 45
Blueberry Smoothie 45
Carob Tonic 50
Carrot Juice 133, 147, 153, 160
Celery Juice 152, 153, 176, 438
Coquito 411
Date Coconut Malt 60
Draksha Digestive Herbal Wine 64
Fig Shake 62
Fresh Currant Juice 58

Grape Liver Flush	64
Green Shake	244
Kiwi Shake	70
Lassi & Mango	83
Lemon Ginger Blast	74
Longevity Shake	244, 430
Loquat Apple Smoothie	79
Mint Limeade	77
Mint-Raspberry Lemonade	384
Nutmeg-Almond Drink	387
Nut or Seed Milk	405
Orange-Almond Drink	89
Papaya Shake	92
Passion Fruit Coconut Drink	94
Passion Lemon Drink	94
Saffron Drink	394
Watermelon Juice	85

ENTRÉE OR VEGETABLE SIDE DISH

Baked Celery	153
Baked Leeks	379
Baked Parsnips with Carrots	200
Baked Spaghetti Squash	216
Bamboo Shoots & Tomatoes	127
Beet Greens	134
Beet Medley	133
Beets in Lemon	134
Beets in Lime	134
Broccoli Subzi	137, 138, 300, 378
Brussels Sprouts	139, 140, 141
Brussels Sprouts Endive	141
Celeriac Root & Greens	151
Chana Marsala	258
Chard Veggie Combo	155
Cilantro Quesadillas	363
Curried Potato Patties with Carrots	206
Curry Sabudana (Tapioca)	221
Eggplant & Almond Sauté	170
Eggplant Bhurta	171
Eggplant Subzi	169
Eggplant Supreme	170
Elizabeth's Green Beans	129
Fava Stew	262
German Potato Salad	206
Green Bean Salad	130
Greens a la Coconut	194
Hiziki Bok Choy Combo	238
Jicama Fries	178
Jicama Stir Fry	178
Kale a la Cream	180
Kale Ambrosia	180
Kohlrabi Mint Delight	182
Lamb's Lettuce Scramble	184
Lemon Kale	74
Lotus Root Stir Fry	189
Marinated Artichokes	121
Marinated Fresh Artichokes	121
Mashed Celeriac Root	151
Mashed Parsnips	200
Mashed Taro	223
Mushroom Tambay	191
Nettles & Potatoes	386
Nutty Lettuce Wraps	186
Okra Coconut Tomato Curry	196
Okra Delight	196
Peanuts, Greens, Tofu	273
Peas & Potatoes	203
Pecan Balls	415
Pine Nut Eggplant Bites	417
Polenta	162
Potatoes & Kale	205
Potato Spinach Fennel Curry	205
Pumpkin Seed Squares	419
Punjab-Style String Beans and Kale	131
Rainbow Chard Pepper Combo	155
Raita	166
Roasted yams	227, 423

Ayurvedic Curative Cuisine for Everyone

Rosemary Potatoes 392
Rose Mushrooms 192
Rutabaga Steamed & Mashed 208
Saag Paneer 212
Sauerkraut 145, 376
Shiitake and Spinach 191
Snow Peas & Watercress 203
Spinach and Goat Cheese 210
Steamed Artichokes 121
Steamed Sunchokes & Carrots 176
Stir Fry Arugula 123
Stuffed Acorn Squash 215
Stuffed Chayotes 157
Stuffed Collard Greens 160
Stuffed Cucumber Boats 166
Stuffed Endive 173
Sunchoke Stir Fry 486
Sunchokes, Tomatoes & Celery Combo 176
Sweet Potato Lasagna 218
Sweet Potato Subzi 218
Sweet Rutabaga with Chard 208
Tomato Mushroom Skewers 117
Turnip Combo 225
Vegetarian Cabbage Rolls 145
Veggie Combo 155, 369
Wilted Spinach With Nuts 210
Yucca Patties 227
Zucchini Ratatouille 214

Entrees

Almond Croquettes 406
Baked Salmon 333
Baked Tofu 277
Beef Stew 320
Bodhie's Beef Scallopini with
Maderia Wine Demi-Glace 320
Bodhie's Prosciutto-wrapped
Apricot-stuffed Pork Tenderloin 324
Bodhie's Tuscan Lamb 322

Lamb Marsala 322
Lemon Curry Chicken 314
Mint Cilantro Pork Chops 324
Pasta Primavera 306
Rabbit ala Fricassee 325
Shrimp Salad & Peppers 335
Turkey Wraps 316
Veal Parmesan 326

Fish

Fish 3, 329, 330, 331, 332, 333
Salmon 333
Shellfish 334

Fruits

Apple Fritters 33
Apples 3, 25, 28, 29, 30, 243, 340, 342, 475
Apple Sauce 33
Apricot Delight 35
Apricots 34
Avocado 36, 37, 38, 462
Avocado a la Mexicana 37
Baked Papaya with Syrup 92
Banana 39, 40, 341
Blackberry 42, 43
Blueberries 44
Breadfruit 46, 47
Carob 49, 50
Cherimoya 51, 52
Cherries 53
Cranberries 55, 413
Currant 57, 58
Date 59, 60
Fig Pudding 62
Grape 63, 64
Grapefruit 65, 66
Guava 67, 68
Healthy Guacamole 38
Kiwi 69, 70, 89

Kumquat	71, 72
Lemon	24, 73, 74, 75, 94, 134, 314
Lime	24, 76, 77, 134
Loquat	78, 79
Lychee	80, 81
Mango	82, 83
Melon	84, 85, 135, 136
Nectarines	86
Orange	25, 88, 89
Papaya	90, 91, 92
Passion Fruit	93, 94
Peach	95, 96
Pear	97, 98
Persimmon	99, 100
Pineapple	101, 102, 213, 447
Plantains a la Coconut	41
Plum	78, 103, 104
Raspberry	105, 106, 384
Sapote	107, 108
Spicy Yogurt Raspberries	106
Strawberry	109, 110
Stuffed Apples	31, 32
Stuffed Grapefruit	65, 66
Stuffed Tomatoes	115, 116, 127, 176, 187
Tamarind	111, 112, 160
Tangerine	113, 114
Tomato	115, 116, 117, 196, 390, 392

GRAINS

Amaranth	68, 286, 287
Amaranth a la Saffron	287
Amaranth & Coconut	287
Baked Thyme Rice	398
Barley	288, 289, 470
Buckwheat	290, 291
Buckwheat Seaweed	291
Bulgur	292
Chayote & Rice	157
Corn	43, 161, 162, 293, 294, 454, 464
Couscous	306
Dill Millet	367
Ginger Rice Balls	372
Lotus Saffron Rice	189
Macaroni a la Seaweed	308
Marjoram Rice or Quinoa	382
Millet	295, 296, 367
Oatmeal a la Bryan	298
Oats	297
Pancakes a la Bryan	310
Peach Porridge	96
Polenta	162
Quinoa	299, 300, 382
Quinoa Pasta & Broccoli & Seaweed	300
Quinoa & Saffron	300
Rice	157, 189, 269, 301, 302, 303, 304, 311, 358, 372, 382, 398, 400, 444
Rice and Capers	358
Rice and Saffron	302
Rice Biriyani	303
Semolina	305
Spelt	307
Tabouli	292
Wheat	305, 309
Wild Rice	311
Yellow Rice and Turmeric	400

HERBS & SPICES

Ajwan	353
Allspice	353
Anise	354
Asafoetida	355
Basil	260, 355
Bay Leaf	356
Black Pepper	356
Borage	357
Capers	357, 358
Caraway Seeds	359
Cardamom	359

Ayurvedic Curative Cuisine for Everyone

Cayenne 360
Cilantro 324, 362, 363
Cinnamon 364, 445
Cloves 365
Dill 149, 240, 366, 367
Fennel 66, 149, 205, 368, 369
Fenugreek 370
Ginger 32, 74, 100, 242, 371, 372, 405
Horseradish 373, 374
Juniper Berries 375, 376
Leeks 377, 378
Lemongrass 379, 380
Marjoram 381, 382
Mustard Seed 385
Nettles 385, 386
Nutmeg 387
Onions 388
Parsley 389, 390
Poppy Seeds 391
Rosemary 391, 392
Saffron 189, 287, 300, 302, 303, 393, 394
Savory 395, 396
Tarragon 395, 396
Thyme 397, 398
Turmeric 399, 400

IMMUNE SYSTEM

Green Immune Soup 473
Immune Broth for Pitta & Kapha 471
Immune Broth for Vata 472

LEGUMES

Adzuki Moon Cakes 254
Black Eyed Peas & Collard Greens 256
Falafel 259
Khichari 270, 271
Kidney Bean Stew 264
Lentil Patties 267
Lima Bean Patties 269

Lima Beans and Rice 269
Sprouted Lentil Sauté 252

LOAFS

Banana Bread 40
Cashew Nut Loaf 409
Cauliflower Loaf 149
Cranberry Bread 56
Fava Loaf 262
Millet Loaf 296
Tropical 40, 46, 48, 49, 51, 65, 69, 71, 76, 78, 88, 90, 93, 101, 107, 109, 111, 113, 156, 177, 219
Turkey Loaf 316
Walnut Loaf 425

MEAT

Lamb 183, 184, 321, 322
Pork 323, 324
Rabbit 325
Veal 326

MISCELLANEOUS

Baking Powder 337
Bragg's Liquid Aminos 37, 38, 41, 47, 72, 74, 102, 114, 116, 117, 121, 123, 125, 130, 136, 140, 141, 145, 149, 151, 153, 155, 160, 162, 166, 167, 170, 173, 175, 176, 180, 182, 184, 186, 187, 191, 192, 196, 200, 202, 203, 205, 208, 211, 216, 218, 221, 223, 227, 254, 258, 259, 260, 262, 264, 265, 267, 273, 277, 279, 281, 282, 291, 296, 300, 314, 316, 328, 338, 367, 378, 382, 386, 392, 398, 413, 415, 417, 419, 423, 425, 434
Breadcrumbs 339
Chocolate 340, 341
Currant Energy Bars 58
Graham Cracker Crust 54
Guar Gum 342
Hazelnut Stuffing 413
Homemade Yogurt 449
Kuzu/Kudzu 343
Loquat Cough Syrup 79

Mayonnaise.................................. 344, 345, 374	Turkey.. 315, 316, 448
Miso 289, 346, 347	**SALADS**
Salt 121, 130, 149, 166, 167, 184, 187, 196, 205, 208, 221, 223, 225, 348, 386, 398, 415	Arame Salad... 234
	Arugula Salad.. 123
Soy Sauce 349	Asparagus Salad.. 125
Tamari 349, 382	Cherimoya Fruit Salad 52
Vinegar 350, 376, 390	Curry Chicken Salad 314
NUTS & SEEDS	Dulse Salad 236
Almonds.. 405	Eastern Salad 167
Cashews 407	Grape and Apple Salad..............................64
Coconut 41, 60, 94, 194, 196, 221, 280, 287, 350, 380, 404, 410, 411, 464	Green Bean Salad 130
	Green Papaya Salad....................................91
Hazelnuts & Filberts 12	Grilled Romaine Salad............................. 187
Nut or Seed Milk 405	Kidney Bean Salad.................................... 265
Pecans 414	Kohlrabi Salad... 182
Pine Nuts 416	Kombu Dill Salad 240
Pumpkin Seed................................... 418, 419	Melon Salad 85
Roasted Nut Seeds 423	Nectarine Salad...87
Sesame Seeds.. 420	Olive Salad 198
Sunflower Seeds... 422	Pineapple Salad... 102
Walnuts 424	Selene's Grapefruit and Fennel Salad........ 66
OILS	Shrimp Salad... 335
Avocado Oil 462	Strawberry Salad 110
Canola Oil... 463	Tangerine Salad.. 114
Castor Oil 463	Wakame Salad... 246
Coconut Oil 464	Watercress Salad 164
Corn Oil.. 464	**SAUCES, DIPS, SPREADS**
Flaxseed Oil 465	Artichoke Dip 121
Lard... 465	Basil Hummus 260
Margarine... 466	Bodhie's Demi-Glace................................ 328
Mustard Oil 466	Brussels Sprout Sauce.............................. 141
Olive Oil.. 467	Carob Sauce or Topping 50
Sesame Oil 468	Carrot Sauce 147
Soy... 349, 469	Cashew Cream 408
Sunflower Oil 469	Cherimoya Sauce 52
POULTRY	Cranberry Sauce 56
Chicken... 313, 314	Currant Sauce...58

Ayurvedic Curative Cuisine for Everyone

Guava Ghee	68
Guava Paste	68
Horseradish Sauce	374
Horseradish Vegan Mayonnaise	374
Hot Mole Sauce	487
Lamb's Lettuce Sauce	184
Loquat Preserves	79
Lychee Ambrosia for the Gods	81
Marjoram Cheese Dip	382
Mint Sauce	384
Miso-Tahini Sauce	347
Nori Ginger Sauce	242
Olive Pâté	198
Peanut Sauce	273
Pear Sauce	98
Pico de Gallo	361
Plum Sauce	104
Rosemary Tomato Sauce	392
Saffron Yogurt Sauce	394
Savory Sauce	396
Sour Cream Dressing	447
Spinach Mozzarella Sauce	434
Spinach Sauce #1	211
Spinach Sauce #2	211
Spinach Sauce #3	211
Tamarind Sauce	112
Tapioca Sauce	221
Taro Sauce	223
Tarragon Sauce	396
Thyme Sauce	398
Turmeric Sauce	400

Seaweeds

Agar Agar	231
Arame	229, 233, 234
Dulse	229, 235, 236
Hiziki	229, 237, 238
Kombu	149, 229, 239, 240
Nori	229, 241, 242
Wakame	229, 245, 246

Soups

Brussels Sprouts Soup	140
Burdock Soup	143
Cauliflower - Dill - Fennel Soup	149
Cold Avocado Soup	38
Corn Tortilla Soup	294
Cream of Asparagus Soup	125
Cream of Corn Soup	162
Creamy Soybean Soup	275
Dhal with Coconut	280
Fennel Soup	149, 369
Fish Caldo	333
Green Immune Soup	473
Immune Broth for Pitta & Kapha	471
Immune Broth for Vata	472
Indian Dahl Soup	282
Kombu Soup	240
Lemongrass Coconut Soup	380
Miso Barley Soup	289
Miso Nourishing Soup	347
Nettle Soup	386
Potato Leek Soup	378
Pumpkin Soup	216
Seaweed Soup	230
Split Pea Soup	279
Summer Tomato Soup	117
Sunchoke Soup	175
Tapioca Soup	220
Tomato Delight Soup	116
Turnip Soup	225
Watercress Soup	164

Sweeteners

Agave Sugar	452
Brown Sugar	453
Corn Syrup	454
Fruit Sugar	454

Honey 49, 455
Jaggery 456
Lactose 427, 456, 457
Maltose/Malt Syrup 457
Maple Sugar 458
Molasses 458
Rock Candy 459
Stevia 252, 459
Sugar Cane 453
White Sugar 460

VEGETABLES
Artichoke 120, 121, 174, 175
Arugula 122, 123, 141
Asparagus 124, 125
Bamboo Shoots 126, 127
Beans 25, 128, 129, 131, 247, 248, 250, 253, 257, 261, 263, 268, 269, 270
Beets 132, 134
Bitter Melon 135, 136
Broccoli 137, 138, 300, 378
Brussels Sprouts 139, 140, 141
Burdock 142, 143
Cabbage 144, 145
Carrots 146, 176, 200, 206
Cauliflower 138, 148, 149, 378
Celeriac 150, 151
Celery 152
Chard 154, 155, 208
Chayote 156, 157
Chicory 158
Collards 159
Corn 43, 161, 162, 293, 294, 454, 464
Cress 163
Cucumber 165, 166
Eggplant 168, 169, 170, 171, 417
Endive 141, 158, 172, 173
Jerusalem Artichoke 174
Jicama 177, 178

Kale 74, 131, 179, 180, 205
Kohlrabi 181, 182
Lamb"s Lettuce 183
Lettuce 183, 184, 185, 186, 235
Lotus Roots 188
Mushroom 117, 190, 191
Mustard Greens 193
Okra 195, 196
Olive 197, 198, 467
Parsnip 199
Peas 201, 202, 203, 255, 256, 272, 278
Polenta 162
Potato 204, 205, 206, 217, 218, 226, 378
Rutabaga 207, 208
Spinach 160, 191, 205, 209, 210, 211, 434, 443
Squash 168, 213, 215, 216
Sweet Potato 217, 218, 226
Tapioca 219, 220, 221
Taro Root 222
Turnip 224, 225
Yam 217, 226

Food Enzymes for Health & Longevity
3rd Edition –Revised and Enlarged
by Dr.Edward Howell

This new, enlarged edition of the classic book contains over 400 references to scientific literature that contributed to the formulation of Dr. Howell's revolutionary "food enzyme concept". The second incorporated an interview of the author by Victoras Kulvinskas.

There is also an extensive new foreword by Viktoras Kulvinskas that has been added to this revised 3rd edition, as well as a new research appendix at the end. The Foreword adds a very substantial body of recent and updated research to support the food enzyme concept of Dr.Howell and underline the importance of food enzymes.

Dr.Edward Howell, a pioneer researcher in food enzymes and human nutrition, was born in Chicago. After obtaining a limited medical license from the state of Illinois, he spent six years on the professional staff of the Lindlahr Sanitarium, a well known 'nature cure' hospital predominantly utilizing nutrition and physical therapies. In 1930, he established his own facility for the treatment and research of chronic ailments through nutrition and physical modalities. He is also the author of treatise, Enzyme Nutrition, published in 1985.

ISBN : 978-81-9326-43-3-1, Edition : PB, Pages : 250

Place order at : moonlightbooks2016@gmail.com/ info@moonlightbooks.in